RESEARCH LITERACY

RESEARCH LITERACY

A Primer for Understanding and Using Research

JEFFREY S. BEAUDRY
LYNNE MILLER

THE GUILFORD PRESS
New York   London

Library of Congress Cataloging-in-Publication Data

Names: Beaudry, Jeffrey S. | Miller, Lynne, 1945–
Title: Research literacy : a primer for understanding and using research / by
   Jeffrey S. Beaudry and Lynne Miller.
Description: New York : Guilford Press, 2016.
Identifiers: LCCN 2015033613| ISBN 9781462524624 (paper)
   | ISBN 9781462524631 (cloth)
Subjects: LCSH: Research—Methodology. | Qualitative research. | Decision
   making.
Classification: LCC Q180.55.M4 B385 2016 | DDC 001.4/2—dc23
LC record available at *http://lccn.loc.gov/2015033613*

To our grandchildren,
Callie Leikam and Jackson and Anna Clark

Preface

"Research says. . . ." Every one of us who works in schools, social services, or health care has heard these words from someone in authority who wants to implement a new approach, program, or organizational arrangement. Because we are called upon daily to make informed decisions about our work, we need to act as responsible and "research-literate" consumers. This requires having the skills and knowledge to make thoughtful judgments about the possibilities and limitations of available research, about whether and how to apply findings to particular contexts, and about how to communicate findings to multiple audiences. This textbook engages readers in close readings of high-quality research articles that represent diverse traditions, designs, and procedures. It emphasizes applications to practice and decision making, and it leads readers through a step-by-step process that culminates in a full-length methodological review essay on a topic of a reader's choosing. Although the examples used in this volume are specific to education, the methods described here apply to other fields as well. The ultimate goal of this text is to help readers lay the foundation for becoming informed, critical, and literate consumers of research who can advocate convincingly for evidence-based practice and who stand on solid ground when they question mandates and directives beginning with the statement "Research says. . . ."

ORGANIZATION OF THE VOLUME

This book is divided into seven parts and provides an integrated and thematic approach to research literacy. It is replete with examples of both iconic and current studies, and it provides criteria for evaluating the different approaches it covers. Part I introduces the concepts of *research literacy* and *information literacy* and is meant to serve as a starting point for novice readers of research. Part II focuses on qualitative research. It includes three chapters with topics ranging from the underlying assumptions of the qualitative paradigm and its approach to data collection and analysis, to discussions of the specific designs of ethnography, case studies, phenomenological studies, narrative studies, and two types of text analysis (qualitative document analysis and critical discourse analysis). Parts III, IV, and V focus on quantitative research; they include seven chapters that describe premises and concepts basic to the quantitative paradigm, explain the process of quantitative reasoning and its use of descriptive and inferential statistics, and describe various experimental and nonexperimental designs.

We realize that this order of presentation is at odds with that of most research textbooks, which begin with quantitative research. We have chosen to introduce qualitative research first in order to ensure that it not be given short shrift and hurriedly introduced at the end of a course, as is often the case. We have also found that students are less intimidated by qualitative work than by other types of research, and that it provides a gentler introduction to the research landscape. Having said this, the order in which qualitative and quantitative research are presented in this volume may be easily be reversed when these parts of the book are taught.

Part VI describes research that mixes methods and creates new ones; these are approaches that challenge the traditional dichotomy between qualitative and quantitative research and/or address more diverse audiences. This part includes three chapters on academic mixed methods research, program and teacher evaluation, and practitioner research. This part of the book is best presented after students have encountered and come to terms with the premises and methods of more orthodox research approaches.

Part VII concerns research syntheses or reviews; it consists of two chapters that introduce various forms of professional reviews and provide guidelines for writing a student review essay. The second of these chapters, Chapter Seventeen, provides step-by-step procedures and exemplars for writing a student review essay that describes and evaluates the methodologies employed in six articles on a topic of one's choosing.

PEDAGOGICAL FEATURES

Based on sound pedagogical principles, this volume builds on prior knowledge and balances academic rigor with accessibility for diverse learners. It provides concise and readable definitions of key terms and concepts, as well as checklists for understanding, and it introduces new ideas and skills as necessary to support learning. It activates learning through advanced organizers; it helps build mental maps of research concepts by way of visual images, concept maps, graphs, and charts; it supports academic writing with written guides, templates, rubrics, and exemplars; and it shows how to use technology to access information and resources. At the end of each chapter, summaries and lists of relevant terms and concepts are provided, as well as activities designed to consolidate, extend, and apply learning. Examples of responses to these activities are included in an Appendix at the end of the book. Our reflections on research methods and meanings add further insights into the conduct of research.

ACKNOWLEDGMENTS

We extend thanks to several members of the editorial staff at The Guilford Press: C. Deborah Laughton, Publisher, Research Methods and Statistics; Martin Coleman, Associate Managing Editor; Marie Sprayberry, Copyeditor; Louise Farkas, Senior Production Editor; and Katherine Sommer, Editorial Assistant. We also thank our reviewers, who offered thoughtful and critical feedback on our drafts, and Joshua

Leikam, who produced the illustrations for the part openings. A special thank-you is in order to the hundreds of graduate students at the University of Southern Maine who used and commented on our materials as we developed them over the course of 10 years, and to our former Dean, BettyLou Whitford, who first suggested that we convert our teaching materials into a textbook.

On a personal note, we want to thank our spouses, Judy Beaudry and Larry Simon, for their patience and support. Jeff extends a special thank-you to his mother, Jeanne Beaudry, who continues to provide love, guidance, and inspiration to all who know her. We wish our readers success in their educational and professional endeavors.

Brief Contents

Extended Contents

III. Quantitative Research: The Basics

6. Introduction to Quantitative Research

7. Descriptive Statistics and Data Displays

PART I

Introduction to Research and Information Literacy

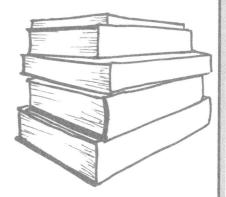

" Research is formalized curiosity. It is poking and prying with a purpose. "

—Zora Neale Hurston

Part I defines *research* and introduces the concepts of *research literacy* and *information literacy*, which are foundational to understanding how to read and critique research.

CHAPTER ONE

Introduction to Research Literacy

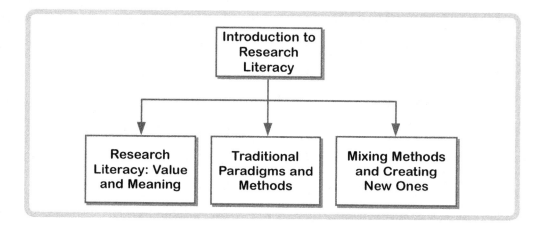

T his chapter introduces the idea of *research literacy*, explains its value and its meaning, and provides a brief overview of the methods of research that appear in education.

CHAPTER OBJECTIVES

✓ Understand research literacy, its value, and its meaning.

✓ Understand the qualitative and quantitative paradigms and methods, and their shared and distinctive characteristics.

✓ Understand what is meant by *primary, empirical, peer-reviewed* research and its key elements.

✓ Understand American Psychological Association (APA) formatting for citations and references.

✓ Understand the new and evolving approaches that mix research methods and create new ones.

RESEARCH LITERACY: VALUE AND MEANING   MAP 1.1

The word *research* has its roots in the French word *rechercher*, which means "to search for" or "to go about seeking." Educational researchers go about seeking the answers to questions that concern teaching, learning, and educational practice. In so doing, they use a variety of methods and tools. For educational practitioners, these methods and tools may seem a bit intimidating. That's why research literacy is important.

> *Research literacy* is the ability to locate, understand, discuss, and evaluate different types of research; to communicate accurately about them; and to use findings for academic and professional purposes.

In effect, research literacy is not just one literacy; it is a combination of literacies that, taken together, empower educators to access, understand, and apply "what the research says" to both their academic and professional work.

- *Information/technological literacy* is the ability to use resources such as electronic media and databases to locate and retrieve research articles; this requires knowing how to access resources that are useful in both academic research and evidence-based practice.

- *Verbal literacy* is the ability to understand, discuss, and critique written texts and to communicate about them both in writing and orally; this requires a working knowledge of the vocabulary and conventions of writing and citing research.

- *Numeracy* is the ability to understand and apply mathematical calculations and symbols; this requires an understanding of statistics and statistical reasoning, and of how these are best applied to research and practice.

- *Visual literacy* is the ability to understand how to "read" and construct non-verbal texts; this requires a familiarity with how research findings are represented

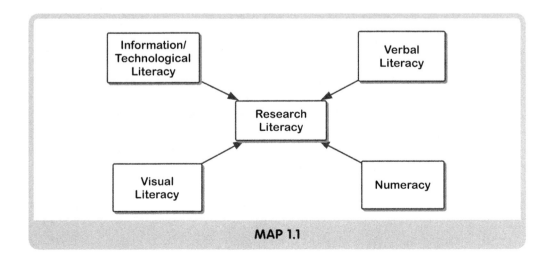

MAP 1.1

in tables, charts, and other displays of data, and how to use concept maps, graphic organizers, and images to unpack complex ideas and procedures.

TRADITIONAL PARADIGMS AND METHODS: QUALITATIVE AND QUANTITATIVE RESEARCH

MAP 1.2

Researchers use methodological approaches that represent particular ways of thinking. At the root of each approach are philosophical assumptions about what is knowable and how it can be known. Thomas Kuhn (1962) coined the term *paradigm* to describe "an integrated cluster of substantive concepts, variables and problems attached with corresponding methodological approaches and tools" (p. 32). In social science research, there traditionally have been two competing paradigms: *qualitative* and *quantitative*. At the root of the differences between the two paradigms are philosophical assumptions about what is knowable, who creates knowledge, and for whom the knowledge is intended and used.

The two traditions privilege *empirical* and *primary* research. This means that the authors of the study are the people who actually conduct the research, collect observable information (*data*), and analyze results. "Think pieces" (reflective and theoretical essays) and secondhand, filtered accounts of what "research says" are not included in primary, empirical research.

Qualitative and quantitative researchers publish their studies in peer-reviewed journals that are directed to an audience of fellow researchers and other interested parties who read those journals. *Peer-reviewed research journals* publish studies that have been vetted by other researchers, who assess the studies' quality and make

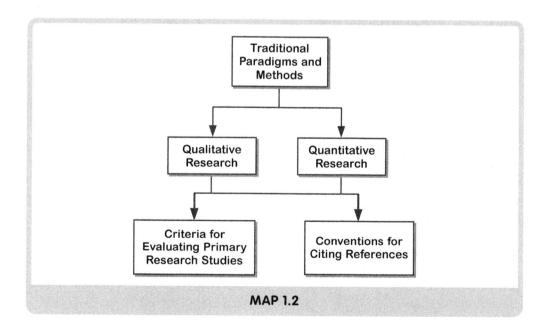

MAP 1.2

recommendations for or against publication or offer suggestions for revision. Primary, empirical, peer-reviewed articles include the following key elements:

- *A review of relevant and recent research.* This review may frame a topic or methodology, or it may illuminate findings. Its location varies in accordance with conventions of the research method.

- *A statement of the research purpose and the design.* The purpose may be presented as a statement, a research question, or a hypothesis that makes a prediction of outcomes. The particular design within each tradition will be clearly identified.

- *A description of sampling.* The sample is described in terms of the number of participants, the way they were selected, the role(s) they played in the study, and their characteristics.

- *A description of data collection methods.* The methods for collecting empirical evidence is explained in terms of what evidence was collected, how it was collected, and under what conditions.

- *Data analysis/results.* The approaches, tools, and procedures that were applied to make sense of the data and communicate findings are described in detail. This description may include charts, tables, and diagrams.

- *Conclusion and discussion.* Here the researchers discuss the results and their implications for further research and practice, and may also include an acknowledgment of any limitations of the study.

Qualitative Methods

The qualitative paradigm is rooted in the philosophy of *naturalism*, which assumes that people are best studied in their natural settings, and rejects the idea that individuals and human societies can be understood as a single, objective reality. Rather, it is based on the assumption that reality is best understood by uncovering how people make meaning of their particular situations. The qualitative paradigm of social research is the paradigm of *antipositivism* or *postpositivism*. It seeks to uncover subjective realities holistically. It emphasizes researcher engagement; it describes phenomena from the point of view of those who live and experience them; and it depends on interpretive processes for analysis.

Because qualitative researchers want to know how a particular group of people makes sense of phenomena or events within a particular context, they engage with the actors and make themselves visible and known to them in both data collection and analysis.

Qualitative researchers use conventions, approaches, tools, and procedures that are unique to the method.

The research review serves to enhance or elaborate findings and makes comparisons to prior studies; it is embedded in sections of the article or appears at or near the end of the study.

The most frequently occurring qualitative methods or designs in educational research include the following:

• *Ethnography* describes a culture or group and is the original qualitative design. Ethnographic case studies apply ethnographic methods of data collection and analysis to specific, bounded contexts, such as an event, program, or activity.

• *Phenomenological studies* (also known as *interview studies*) focus on individuals and how they understand and make sense of an experience or phenomenon.

• *Narratives* also focus on individuals and how they make meaning and bring order and coherence to their life stories.

• *Qualitative document analyses* describe and interpret existing written documents that are produced by actors without being solicited by researchers.

• *Critical discourse analyses* use critical theory to interpret texts and talk, with the goal of uncovering power relationships that reproduce those existing in society.

Sampling is *purposeful* and identifies participants, called *actors*, based on a researcher's subjective judgments about who can provide the richest information. Samples tend to be small in number. Because samples are purposeful, they are not meant to represent anyone beyond the boundaries of the study. The researcher does not generalize the findings to other samples or settings; rather, the researcher invites readers to decide whether the findings resonate with their own experience and contexts.

Data collection and analysis depend on the researcher as "the key instrument." This means that the researcher interacts personally with actors, conducts and records observations and interviews with them, and collects relevant documents. Data analysis is an inductive, iterative process in which the researcher develops and applies a coding strategy in order to organize data and develop themes and understandings, using words, metaphors, and images. Interpretation is an essential element in data analysis and involves the application of a particular interpretive lens that the researcher makes transparent to readers. Results are presented in an extended essay that includes detailed descriptions and verbatim accounts.

Quantitative Methods

The Greek letter Σ, *sigma*, is the symbol for *sum of.* This signifies a reliance on quantifiable data—that is, the use of mathematical calculations to reach results. Research in the quantitative tradition is a well-planned itinerary that gets a researcher from point A to point B with no diversions along the way. The quantitative paradigm is rooted in the philosophical school known as *positivism,* which is based on the assumption that human beings and human societies are subject to laws that are similar to the laws of nature, and which accepts as knowledge only those ideas that are empirically verifiable and grounded in sensory experience. Positivism views reality as being objective and the duty of a scientist as uncovering reality through data and facts. The quantitative paradigm of social research is the paradigm of positivism. It seeks to describe and explain objective reality bit by bit. It emphasizes the researcher's distance from subjects, quantifies and measures phenomena, and depends on statistical procedures for analysis.

Because quantitative researchers want to know how phenomena can be described or explained objectively, they maintain a distance from their subjects and seek to be invisible in data collection and analysis. Similar to qualitative researchers, they use conventions, approaches, tools, and procedures that are unique to the method.

The research review makes a case for doing the research. In general, the research review examines prior research in order to establish a theoretical foundation and to generate a hypothesis that the study will confirm or disconfirm.

The quantitative methods or designs that appear most frequently in educational research include the following:

- *Test and survey reports* summarize information about subjects.

- *Experiments* investigate cause and effect by introducing an intervention and analyzing outcomes that result from the intervention.

- *Nonexperimental group comparisons* investigate differences that exist between membership groups.

- *Correlations research* investigates the direction and strength of relationships and makes predictions about how one part of a relationship will influence outcomes on another.

Sampling may be *random* or *nonrandom*. Randomization is preferred since it makes it more likely that findings can be generalized to other subjects and settings.

Data collection and analysis depend on objective measurement and mathematical calculations. Unlike qualitative researchers, quantitative researchers keep a distance from the people they are studying in order to maintain objectivity. The results of data analysis are reported statistically; verbally in texts; and visually in tables, charts, graphs, and maps.

Criteria for Evaluating Studies

Although qualitative and quantitative methods have different specific criteria for judging the quality of a study, the following general questions are useful in guiding an evaluation of either type.

- What is the purpose of the study? Is the purpose clearly stated? Is this a researchable topic? Are research questions or problems of practice posed? Are hypotheses stated? Are the purpose, method, and design aligned?

- Is there a research review? If yes: Does the author review relevant, prior research? If so, for what purpose? To what extent does the research review fulfill its purpose? Given the design, is the review appropriately placed? How does the author contextualize the study?

- Does the author provide sufficient information about how many participants are in the sample and how they were selected and a description of their relevant characteristics? Are the sample size and the sampling strategy appropriate to the purpose and design?

- Does the author provide a detailed description of how data were collected and under what conditions? Are the data collection tools and procedures appropriate for the purpose?

- Does the author clearly describe the approach to data analysis? To what extent are conclusions or interpretations justified by the purpose and the conduct of the research? Does the author avoid overconcluding?

- Are results and their value clearly communicated and in line with the purpose?

Conventions for Citing References   MAP 1.3

Although professional researchers can choose from among several styles for citing and preparing full references of sources, most scholars in the social sciences and education use the format of the American Psychological Association (APA), and most university programs in education require it of students. Other formats, such as those of the Modern Language Association (MLA) and *The Chicago Manual of Style*, are more common in the humanities. Most empirical educational research uses APA style for both in-text citations and full references at the end of each article or chapter.

In-text citations occur within the body of an article or chapter and indicate the original source of an idea or a quote.

The *list of references* is located at the end of an article or chapter under a separate heading ("References").

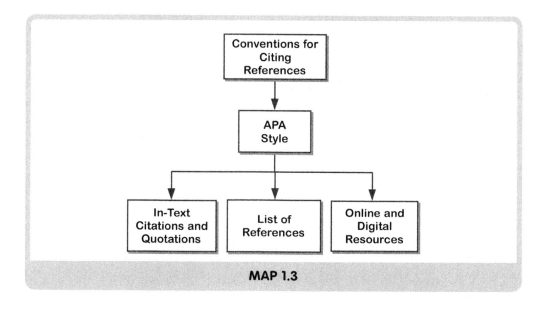

MAP 1.3

The most complete guide to APA style is the *Publication Manual of the American Psychological Association*, currently in its sixth edition (APA, 2010), which can be ordered through the APA website (*www.apastyle.org/index.aspx*). Intended primarily for scholars and researchers, this publication includes chapters on research ethics, the structure of scholarly and research papers, guidelines for writing clearly, the correct use of mechanics and style, the use of graphics, and correct formats for citations and references. It also provides examples of citations and end-of-chapter references. There are several websites that are more appropriate for a general population of users. Among them are the following:

APA Style Essentials
   www.vanguard.edu/psychology/faculty/douglas-degelman/apa-style
Purdue Online Writing Lab
   https://owl.english.purdue.edu/owl/resource/560/05
Son of Citation Machine
   www.citationmachine.net

Library databases, which are discussed in the next chapter, also provide citations in the correct format.

MIXING METHODS AND CREATING NEW ONES   MAP 1.4

Map 1.4 captures the essence of relatively recent research approaches that cross the traditional divide between the qualitative and quantitative paradigms by mixing methods and creating new ones. The philosophy that undergirds these methods is *pragmatism*, which is a quintessentially American philosophy and was advocated by William James, Charles S. Peirce, and John Dewey. The basic premise of pragmatism is that the value of an inquiry can best be judged by its practical consequences. Research that combines methods and invents new ones is pragmatic research, which is, in effect, a new paradigm. This book highlights three such methods: *mixed methods research*, *program and teacher evaluation*, and *practitioner research*.

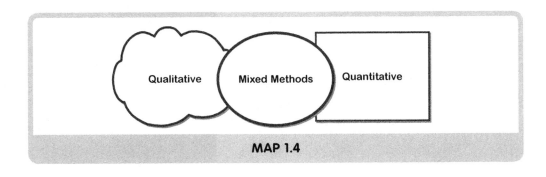

MAP 1.4

Mixed Methods Research

Of the three approaches discussed here, mixed methods research is most similar to traditional approaches: It is a form of primary and empirical investigation that is peer reviewed and appears in established research journals. It is different in that it combines traditional qualitative and quantitative methods in a single study, in order to respond to broad-based questions that are not adequately addressed by either type of method by itself. The research review is usually presented at the beginning of the study and generates research questions rather than a hypothesis. The qualitative and quantitative strands are treated separately in discussion of sampling, data collection, and initial analysis; they may be balanced or unequally weighted. In a concluding section, the data analyses are combined in a final interpretive discussion.

Program and Teacher Evaluation

Like mixed methods research, program evaluation mixes qualitative and quantitative methods, but does so for a different purpose and for a different audience. Its purpose is to investigate the progress or merits of a program, curriculum, teacher effectiveness, or policy for an audience of decision makers, stakeholders, and policy makers, and to make formative and summative judgments. Program evaluations are both primary and empirical, but may not be peer reviewed; they are most commonly published in reports that carry recommendations for future action. As is the case with mixed methods research, program evaluation may equally balance qualitative and quantitative methods, or they may weight one more heavily than the other. Program evaluation reports usually omit a research review and instead include a commentary about the program under study and for whom and what purpose the evaluation is being conducted. Data collection and analysis proceed along traditional lines and are combined in a final conclusion that provides suggestions for improvement of a program or makes a judgment about its effectiveness.

Educator effectiveness is a good example of a policy that requires this type of evaluation. When individual teachers rather than programs are being evaluated, however, the evaluation is usually referred to as *teacher evaluation*. It goes back to the 1980s, as teacher evaluation has been at the center of policy making for school improvement since 2011 (Darling-Hammond, 2013; Popham, 2013). Each individual state in the United States has its own unique policy regarding teacher evaluation, all of which focus on the connection between teachers' classroom practices and student growth. There are dual purposes for teacher evaluation programs: formative for improvement, and summative for decisions to retain teachers or let them go.

Practitioner Research

Practitioner research is a more radical departure from the assumptions and practices of the traditional paradigms than are mixed methods research and program/teacher evaluation. It takes issue with the notion that research is best conducted by professionals whose primary purpose is to describe or explain educational practice. It privileges educators as both the research audience and as the authors who examine, reflect on, and seek to improve practice and to contribute to the practice of others. Practitioner research employs an amalgam of methods for data collection and analysis, including qualitative, quantitative, and inventive approaches. While practitioner research relies heavily on qualitative methods, it also employs quantitative methods of data collection and analysis in establishing the need for the research and in documenting results. There are no agreed-upon structures or formats for practitioner research, and presentations vary quite a bit. There is a focus on commentary and reflection throughout the process.

Table 1.1 summarizes these three approaches.

CHAPTER SUMMARY   MAP 1.5

✓ *Research literacy* is the ability to locate, understand, discuss, and evaluate high-quality research; to communicate accurately about it; and to use the findings for academic and professional purposes.

✓ Research literacy combines information/technological literacy, verbal literacy, numeracy, and visual literacy.

✓ Qualitative and quantitative methods represent the traditional paradigms of research. Quantitative research is based on positivism; qualitative research is based on postpositivism.

✓ Qualitative research is descriptive and interpretive; it seeks to describe and interpret a particular setting or phenomenon from the subjective perspective of the people who live in a setting,

TABLE 1.1. Mixing Methods and Creating New Ones			
	Mixed methods research	Program and teacher evaluation	Practitioner research
Purpose	To investigate broad-based questions that are not adequately addressed singly by qualitative or quantitative methods	To render judgments about the progress or outcomes of a policy, curriculum, or program, or the performance of teachers	To illuminate, inform, and improve practice
Audience	Fellow researchers and other readers of research journals	Decision makers, stakeholders, and policy makers	The author and other education practitioners
Authors	Research professionals	Evaluation professionals	Practitioners
Methods	A mix of traditional qualitative and quantitative methods of data collection and analysis	A mix of traditional qualitative and quantitative methods of data collection and analysis	Adaptation of traditional qualitative and quantitative methods of data collection and analysis, and invention of new ones
Results	Published in established, refereed journals	Presented as a summary of findings and recommendations	Presented as commentary and reflection in a variety of formats

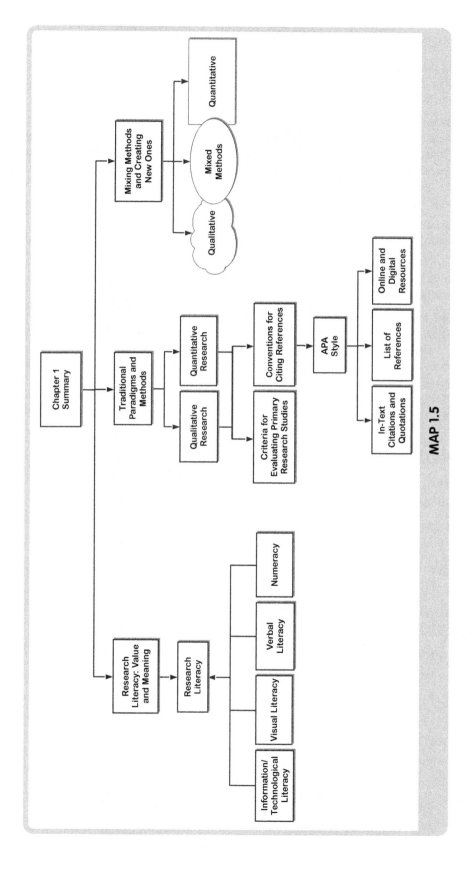

MAP 1.5

and it uses words and images to communicate findings. Qualitative methods or designs include ethnographies and ethnographic case studies, phenomenological interviews, narratives, and text analyses (qualitative document and critical discourse analyses).

✓ Quantitative research is descriptive and explanatory; it seeks to describe and explain phenomena that are quantified as variables from an objective perspective; and it uses numbers, statistics, charts, and tables to communicate findings. Descriptive designs, like test and survey reports, use descriptive statistics to investigate the state of variables at a given time; causal, comparative, and predictive designs use inferential statistics to investigate relationships between and among variables in experiments and nonexperiments.

✓ Quantitative and qualitative articles are primary and empirical, and they appear in peer-reviewed journals. Articles include a research review; descriptions of purpose and design, sampling, data collection, and data analysis/results; and a conclusion/discussion.

✓ Most social sciences and education researchers use the format of the American Psychological Association (APA), and most university programs in education require it of students.

✓ A third paradigm of research, based on pragmatism, has recently emerged for responding to questions that require flexible and adaptive approaches. This paradigm mixes qualitative and quantitative methods and creates new ones. Mixed methods research combines traditional methods to answer questions that one method alone cannot answer; program evaluation and teacher evaluation combine traditional qualitative and quantitative methods to investigate the progress or worth of an innovation or the performance of individual teachers; and practitioner research combines traditional and newly created methods to answer problems of practice.

KEY TERMS AND CONCEPTS

antipositivism

correlations research

data analysis

data collection

educator effectiveness

empirical research

ethnography/case studies

experiments

information/technological literacy

mixed methods research

narratives

nonexperimental group comparisons

numeracy

peer-reviewed research

phenomenological interview studies

positivism

postpositivism

practitioner research

primary research

program evaluation

purpose statement

qualitative research

quantitative research

research literacy

research review

results and conclusion

sampling

teacher evaluation

test and survey reports

text analysis

verbal literacy

visual literacy

REVIEW, CONSOLIDATION, AND EXTENSION OF KNOWLEDGE

Below are abstracts of articles on bullying. Read each abstract, and then answer the questions that appear below.

1. **Penning, S. L., Bhagwanjee, A., & Govender, K. (2010). Bullying boys: The traumatic effects of bullying in male adolescent learners.** *Journal of Child and Adolescent Mental Health, 22*(2), 131–143.

ABSTRACT

Objective: This study investigated the nature and extent of the relationship between bullying and trauma among male adolescent learners. Trauma was operationalised through the multiple constructs of posttraumatic stress, anxiety, depression, dissociation and anger.

Method: In this quantitative study, two objective measures were administered (viz. the Olweus Bullying/Victimisation Scale and the Trauma Symptom Checklist for children) to a sample of male adolescent learners between the ages of 12 and 17, from a South African male-only high school ($n = 486$).

Results and Discussion: Statistical analysis (correlational analysis and MANOVA) produced evidence to suggest that there was a statistically significant relationship between bullying and trauma, and this was strongest for the victim role. The relationship between bullying and trauma was dependent on the frequency of bullying; as the frequency of being bullied increased, so too did the mean scores of all the five trauma subscales. In general, the findings indicated that learners presented with elevated levels of internalising trauma outcomes. Depression demonstrated the highest correlation with the victim role, followed by posttraumatic stress. In addition, 22.4% of learners could be clinically and sub-clinically diagnosed with posttraumatic stress and 21.0% with dissociation. Overall, the findings corroborate the argument that repetitive stressful events (such as bullying) are related to symptom-clusters of ongoing trauma.

QUESTIONS

1. What was the purpose of the study?
2. How would you categorize the research method?
3. What was the sample? Size (n) =
4. Describe any other information about the sample.
5. What were the methods (tests or measures) used in data collection?
6. What (statistical) methods were used for data analysis?
7. What were the results?

2. **Cranham, J., & Carroll, A. (2003). Dynamics within the bully/victim paradigm: A qualitative analysis. *Educational Psychology in Practice, 19*(2), 113–133.**

ABSTRACT

The present research examined whether high school students ethically justify bullying behaviour within a school context. Ten students, purposefully selected because of their specific roles within the bully/victim paradigm, participated in semi-structured interviews. Data analysis using the constant comparative method associated with grounded theory revealed complex social structures that existed within the purposefully selected sample. These structures are dynamic and demand compliance by students. The consequences for dissent are social isolation and exclusion. A student's categorization within the bully/victim paradigm may be determined by their ability to comply with the requirements of the complex constructs in the school social environment.

QUESTIONS

1. What was the purpose of the study?
2. How would you categorize the research method?
3. What was the sample? Size (n) =
4. Describe any other information about the sample.
5. What were the methods used in data collection?
6. What method was used for data analysis?
7. What were the results?

3. **Peters, R. D., Bradshaw, A. J., Petrunka, K., Nelson, G., Herry, Y., Craig, W. M., . . . Rossiter, M. D. (2010). The Better Beginnings, Better Futures Project: Findings from grade 3 to grade 9. *Monographs of the Society for Research in Child Development, 75*(3), 1–174.**

ABSTRACT

Although comprehensive and ecological approaches to early childhood prevention are commonly advocated, there are few examples of long-term follow-up of such programs. In this monograph, we investigate the medium- and long-term effects of an ecological, community-based prevention project for primary school children and families living in three economically disadvantaged neighborhoods in Ontario, Canada. The Better Beginnings, Better Futures (BBBF) project is one of the most ambitious Canadian research projects on the long-term impacts of early childhood prevention programming to date. Bronfenbrenner's ecological model of human development informed program planning, implementation, and evaluation. Using a quasi-experimental design, the BBBF longitudinal research study involved 601 children and their families who participated in BBBF programs when children were between 4 and 8 years old and 358 children and their families from sociodemographically matched comparison communities. We collected extensive child, parent, family, and community outcome data when children were in Grade 3 (age 8–9), Grade 6 (age 11–12), and Grade 9 (age 14–15). The BBBF mandate was to develop programs that would positively impact all areas of [a] child's development; our findings reflect this ecological approach. We found marked positive effects in social and school functioning domains in Grades 6 and 9 and evidence of fewer emotional and behavioral problems in school across the three grades. Parents from BBBF sites reported greater feelings of social support and more positive ratings of marital satisfaction and general family functioning, especially at the Grade 9 follow-up. Positive neighborhood-level effects were also evident. Economic analyses at Grade 9 showed BBBF participation was associated with government savings of $912 per child. These findings provide evidence that an affordable, ecological, community-based prevention program can promote long-term development of children living in disadvantaged neighborhoods and produce monetary benefits to government as soon as 7 years after program completion.

QUESTIONS

1. What was the purpose of the study?
2. How would you categorize the research method?
3. What was the sample? Size (n) =
4. Describe any other information about the sample.
5. What were the methods used in data collection?
6. What method was used for data analysis?
7. What were the results?

4. **Guerra, N. G., Williams, K. R., & Sadek, S. (2011). Understanding bullying and victimization during childhood and adolescence: A mixed methods study. *Child Development, 82*(1), 295–310.**

ABSTRACT

In the present study, quantitative and qualitative data are presented to examine individual and contextual predictors of bullying and victimization and how they vary by age and gender. Two waves of survey data were collected from 2,678 elementary, middle, and high school youth attending 59 schools. In addition, 14 focus groups were conducted with 115 youth who did not participate in the survey. Changes in both bullying and victimization were predicted across gender and age by low self-esteem and negative school climate, with normative beliefs supporting bullying predicting increases in bullying only. Focus group comments provided insights into the dynamics of bullying, highlighting its connection to emergent sexuality and social identity during adolescence. Findings are discussed in terms of their implications for preventive antibullying interventions in schools.

QUESTIONS

1. What was the purpose of the study?
2. How would you categorize the research method?
3. What was the sample? Size (*n*) =
4. Describe any other information about the sample.
5. What were the methods used in data collection?
6. What method was used for data analysis?
7. What were the results?

5. DiBasilio, A. (2008). *Reducing bullying in middle school students through the use of student-leaders.* **Retrieved from ERIC database. (ED501251)**

ABSTRACT

The purpose of this action research project report was to reduce bullying in middle school students through the use of student-leaders. Twenty-eight 8th graders, two counselors, and 24 teachers participated for a total of 54 participants. The study was conducted between September 11, 2007, and December 20, 2007. This project focused on four types of bullying: physical, verbal, social, and electronic. The three tools that the teacher-researcher used to document evidence of the problem were a counselor survey, a teacher survey, and a student survey. The data gathered on the student survey allowed the students to identify ways in which they had viewed and/or experienced the roles of victim, bully, and bystander. Seventy-one percent of the student-leaders reported being victims of verbal bullying at least once last spring. Twenty-six percent of students reported observing social and verbal bullying a minimum of every week. The data gathered from the teacher and counselor surveys allowed the teachers and counselors to identify ways they had viewed bullying or when it had been brought to their attention. The teacher survey showed that 67% (*n* = 16) of teachers believed that bullying was an average problem last spring (2007). Both counselors believed that bullying was at least an average problem last spring. Student-leaders were enlisted and trained to go into classrooms to share information about bullying. The teacher-researcher included in this program direct instruction on bullying prevention, team-building activities, and group discussions. These interventions were intended to reduce the amount of bullying school-wide. The students were also taught leadership and pro-social skills that prepared them to go into classes to share what they had learned and pass along the skills necessary to reduce bullying. The post survey results showed some positive changes. Overall, more teachers considered bullying either not a problem or a small problem in the past month as compared to last spring, where 67% (*n* = 16) saw it as an average problem. Students widened their definition of bullying throughout the intervention, and the amount of social and verbal bullying they participated in decreased. There was an 11% increase in student-leaders helping the victim if they were bullied. According to the counselor post survey, based on the students they worked with, bullying improved slightly. The teacher-researcher believes that this intervention needed more time than one semester to make more of an impact. . . .

QUESTIONS

1. What was the purpose of the study?
2. How would you categorize the research method?
3. What was the sample? Size $(n) =$
4. Describe any other information about the sample.
5. What were the methods used in data collection?
6. What method was used for data analysis?
7. What were the results?

CHAPTER TWO

Information Literacy
Accessing and Searching Digital Resources

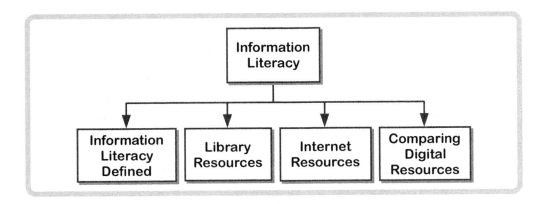

This chapter focuses on *information literacy*, which is the ability to "locate, analyze, evaluate, and use information resources to support research and learning" in "a variety of digital age media and formats" (International Society for Technology in Education, 2008). It also introduces the digital resources that store and make it possible to retrieve vast amounts of research. These digital resources are available in libraries and on the World Wide Web, and can be used to locate and access primary, empirical, peer-reviewed research articles and research reviews. They can be used to inform both practice and academic work. They provide practitioners with information about innovative programs and methods, and they offer students a place to start in developing academic papers.

CHAPTER OBJECTIVES

✓ Understand the concept of information literacy in the digital age.

✓ Understand digital library resources (professional commercial databases, online journals, and interlibrary loan) and their uses.

✓ Understand how to combine keywords in a three-keyword search to retrieve primary research articles from professional commercial databases.

✓ Understand web-based resources (search engines, directories, and user-created content) and their uses.

✓ Understand the types of user-created content: blogs, wikis, and video-sharing sites.

✓ Understand the difference between library and web-based resources for retrieving primary, empirical, peer-reviewed journal articles.

LIBRARY RESOURCES

MAP 2.1

Along with the digital age have come major shifts in libraries and the role of librarians. The library is no longer a place filled with rooms of shelved books and journals, and librarians are no longer custodians of and guides to print resources. Instead, contemporary librarians are information specialists who organize and provide access to both print and digital resources. Each library has its own procedural mechanisms, visual interfaces, and technological tools for searching and retrieving articles and papers. For educational research consumers, the most important of these resources are professional databases, online journals, and interlibrary loans. These are accessed through *portals,* which appear on library websites and provide entryways to the library's databases. Portals vary considerably in their appearance and may be updated as often as once or twice a year.

Professional Commercial Databases

Professional commercial databases are general collections of articles of all types (primary research, research reviews, program descriptions, personal narratives, book reviews, etc.) gathered into a single resource.

There are numerous professional databases that provide access to primary, empirical, peer-reviewed journal articles in education. The most frequently used in education are presented in Table 2.1. One of the benefits of a database search is that it provides information for both in-text citations and entries in the References list in various formats (APA, *The Chicago Manual of Style*, MLA, etc.).

Searching Databases

There are two ways to search a database: by the name of the database or by the topic of interest. In searching by database name, the first step is to select the database that promises to be most productive for a particular search. The next step is to go to "ALL Databases." A screen may look like this or similar to it:

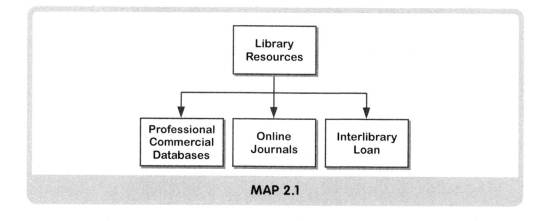

MAP 2.1

TABLE 2.1. Professional Databases Frequently Used in Education

Database	Description
Academic Search Complete	Comprehensive, scholarly, interdisciplinary database; over 13,800 indexed/abstracted and 9,000 full-text journals included; major collection in education (K–12, higher education, adult education); published by EBSCO Host.
JSTOR Arts and Sciences VI Collection	Covers disciplines across the social sciences, with clusters focused in economics, education, linguistics, political science, and area studies. Often these are interdisciplinary titles, which broaden the scope of coverage for the social sciences and expand the range of international scholarship.
Education Full Text	Provides full copies in electronic files (usually .pdf), ready to download.
PsycINFO	Devoted to peer-reviewed literature in the behavioral sciences and mental health; nearly 4 million records; published by the American Psychological Association (APA) general collection for psychology, counseling, special education.
PsycARTICLES	A database of full-text articles from (at this writing) 110 psychology journals published by the APA, the APA Educational Publishing Foundation, the Canadian Psychological Association, and Hogrefe & Huber. The database includes all material from the print journals, with the exception of ads and editorial board lists. The database is updated daily. Coverage from 1985.
Education Resources Information Clearinghouse (ERIC)	One of the largest databases, with journal articles, books, research syntheses, conference papers, technical reports, policy papers, and other education-related materials; a service provided by the U.S. government.

ALL Databases
A B C D E F G H I J L M N O P R S T U V W X Y Z

A simple click on the first letter of the name of the selected database provides a list of all databases with names beginning with that letter. A click on the name of the desired database provides a brief description of the database; this is often followed by a requirement to enter a user name and ID that a library or institution provides to users. The next step is the actual search, which requires the use of keywords and Boolean operators.

Keywords (also called *tags* or *meta tags)* are phrases that identify the topic of the search.

Boolean operators are words used to make the keywords search more precise.
The three Boolean operators are AND, OR, and NOT.

AND narrows the search by retrieving only those documents that contain both of the words specified.

OR broadens the search by retrieving any of the words that are included.

NOT narrows the search further by excluding unwanted words or terms.

A good way to search is to begin with one keyword and then progress to a three-keyword search. The first keyword command focuses on the topic of interest. It begins with typing in one or more keywords in the spaces provided—for example,

Inclusive education

This yields approximately 2,238 *records* or documents, far too many to review in a reasonable time. The second keyword command may be used to indicate the level of education of particular interest—for example,

inclusive education AND *secondary*

This reduces the number of records to 336, which is still unwieldy. The third keyword may be used to indicate the method of research of interest—for example,

inclusive education AND *secondary* AND *qualitative*

This yields only 26 records. Using this three-keyword search allows a user to create a customized folder that can be labeled "Inclusive education, secondary, qualitative," with 26 articles to review and evaluate to see which articles meet the criteria for primary, empirical, peer-reviewed research.

The other strategy for searching is to search by subject matter. This casts a wider net than searching by name of database; it also has a greater chance of leading to non-peer-reviewed secondary articles. This type of search begins by finding the prompt that says, "Select a subject to begin." This will produce an exhaustive subject menu, which includes the topic *education*. A click on that button yields an array of databases and their descriptors, by several databases that provide primary, empirical, peer-reviewed articles.

Online Journals

Online journals are either digital versions of print journals or journals that are published exclusively online.

Almost all professional organizations have at least one journal that is available online (see Table 2.2 for a selection); membership in an organization often includes access to its electronic publications. In addition, there are journals dedicated to either qualitative or quantitative research methods (see Table 2.3 for a sampling).

Searching Online Journals

Though each library has unique procedures for searching online journals, most use portals that follow a format similar to the one from the University of Southern Maine Libraries, shown in Figure 2.1. There are two effective ways to access journals through this online journal portal: by title or International Standard Serial Number (ISSN) and by subject.

Browsing by title or ISSN usually begins with a pull-down menu that provides several options, such as these:

| "Title begins with" | "Title equals" |
| "Title contains all words" | "ISSN equals" |

TABLE 2.2. Selected Journals by Professional Organizations and Associations

Journal title	Professional organization
Reading Research Quarterly	International Literacy Association
Exceptional Children	Council on Exceptional Children
Journal for Research in Mathematics Education	National Council of Teachers of Mathematics
Journal of Research of Science Teaching	National Science Teachers Association
Anthropology and Education Quarterly	Council on Education and Anthropology
Educational Administration Quarterly	University Council for Education Administration
Canadian Journal of Education	Canadian Society for the Study of Education
American Educational Research Journal and *Educational Researcher*	American Educational Research Association
British Educational Research Journal	British Educational Research Association

TABLE 2.3. Selected Qualitative and Quantitative Journals

Qualitative journals

Anthropology and Education Quarterly
International Journal of Qualitative Studies in Education
Journal of Contemporary Ethnography
Qualitative Sociology
Qualitative Sociology Review
Qualitative Inquiry
Qualitative Studies in Education

Quantitative journals

American Educational Research Journal
Journal of Educational Measurement
Journal of Experimental Education
Psychological Review
Journal of Educational Psychology
Journal of Sport and Exercise Psychology
British Journal of Educational Psychology

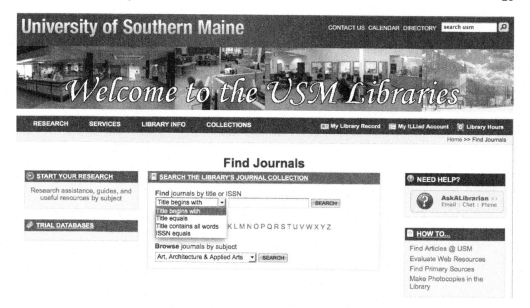

FIGURE 2.1. USM Libraries: Portal for e-journal searching. Copyright by the University of Southern Maine. Reprinted by permission.

A good place to begin is with "Title contains all words." Let's assume that you are searching for journals that are specific to early childhood special education and beginning the search with the words *special education*. This search will yield 17 *records* or entries. It is important to add keywords when a search yields too many or not enough records. In this example, by adding the words *early childhood*, you can retrieve more specific records:

> *International Journal of Early Childhood Special Education* (1308-5581) from 2009 to present in Directory of Open Access Journals Topics in early childhood special education (0271-1214)
> from 03/01/1990 to 03/31/2008 in Academic Search Complete
> from 03/01/1990 to 03/31/2008 in Health Source: Consumer Edition
> from 03/01/1990 to 03/31/2008 in Health Source: Nursing/Academic Edition
> from 03/01/1990 to 03/31/2008 in MasterFILE Premier
> from 04/01/1996 to 09/30/2007 in Education Full Text
> from 01/01/1999 to present in SAGE Premier 2010

Browsing by subject also usually begins with a pull-down menu. In the University of Southern Maine portal, the menu lists subjects from Art and Architecture to Social Science. Here are some examples:

Book Studies & Arts (53)	College & School Publications (45)
Education—General (368)	Education, Special Topics (244)
Educational Institutions (12)	History of Education (80)

Education does not appear on the list; it is a subheading under Social Science. By clicking on Social Science and then clicking on Education, you can retrieve a list of topics and the number of journals dealing with each.

Interlibrary Loan

Sometimes a library will not have the desired research article or book. In these cases, there is interlibrary loan.

> *Interlibrary loan* is "the process by which a library requests material from, or supplies material to, another library. The purpose of interlibrary loan as defined by this code is to obtain, upon request of a library user, material not available in the user's local library" (American Library Association, 2013).
>
> Most libraries belong to a consortium or alliance that shares databases and resources. These groups may be regional, statewide, national, or international; their members may include university and state library systems, or they may be limited to specific users or disciplines. For example, the New York State Library's interlibrary loan program serves government agencies as well as the general public through local libraries, whereas the Harvard Law Library limits its interlibrary loan services to faculty, students, and staff at Harvard University. In both cases, negotiations are completed through libraries and not individuals. Each library provides explicit steps for electronically accessing its interlibrary loan site.

INTERNET RESOURCES   MAP 2.2

So far we have focused on searches for expert content—that is, content in peer-reviewed journals and academic professional databases. These sources are vetted for content accuracy and research integrity; to borrow a term from the arts, they are "selectively curated." The Internet has introduced new sources of information and has shifted our mental model of what counts as knowledge. Search engines, directories, and user-created content sites are now reference points for accessing knowledge and information. The serious warning here is that users of these resources have to follow principles of good judgment.

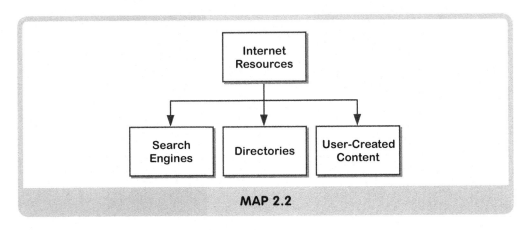

MAP 2.2

Search Engines

Search engines (like Google, Bing, and Yahoo! Search) are tools that can be used by anyone who has access to the Internet to retrieve resources about a specific topic.

Since its debut in 1998, Google has dominated the market by offering an increasingly wide array of content and by providing multiple levels for searching, including Google Scholar and other advanced searching functions. For example, we may do a Google search for *middle school technology* in two ways: by using the standard Google search engine and by using the Google Scholar search engine.

In the standard Google search, immediately after you enter the phrase *middle school technology*, the screen fills with a list of references from the Web. This includes titles, authors, and URLs that you can explore in your search. At the top of the page are several other buttons. A click on Images provides access to free photos and graphic art that may be used to communicate ideas visually and to add to written texts. A click on Maps provides information and directions to nearby locations where the topic is in use. A click on More adds links to Videos, Books, Flights, and Apps.

To access Google Scholar, you can type the keywords *Google Scholar* into the browser. The purpose of Google Scholar is to index "articles, theses, books, abstracts and court opinions, from academic publishers, professional societies, online repositories, universities and other websites." Google Scholar provides tools to refine searches, using keywords and search limiters. An advantage of Google Scholar is that it yields no commercial ads or invitations as results. A disadvantage is that it may connect to publications that require membership in professional organizations or registration as a library user.

In addition, Google Scholar permits users to see all the citations of each article by using the link "Cited by . . ." at the bottom of each resource listing. The cross-links in citations provide a valuable way to broaden a search through the network of scholars in a profession.

Advanced Scholar Search provides several tools for refinement. To do an advanced search on Google Scholar, use the pull-down arrow at the top of the search bar. That will show the advanced search options. This allows you to search by words and phrases, author, journal, or a range of dates. As in the standard Google search, a user may select Images, Maps, and Videos.

Directories

Directories are organized lists of links to organizations, activities, events, publications, addresses, and media that are assembled and edited by professional groups, commercial organizations, and self-organized Internet organizations.

The Library of Congress has a very large collection of directories, which are organized into what it calls *Alcoves*. For instance, as shown below, Alcove 9: An Annotated List of Reference Websites has a section dedicated to general education (Library of Congress, 2011; *www.loc.gov/rr/main/alcove9/education/general.html*).

Alcove 9: An Annotated List of Reference Websites

Education: General Educational Resources and Directories

U.S. Department of Education

The home page for the Department of Education has many links and directories for finding current educational policy, education topics in the news, priorities of the President and the Secretary of Education, national educational efforts, speeches, a calendar of events, and other timely information. This site also includes a page of the most requested items on such topics as financial aid, educational statistics, and educational grants.

National Library of Education

The National Library of Education, the research arm of the U.S. Department of Education, has approximately 100,000 items in its collections which must be accessed in person.

Education World

Sponsored by several corporate sponsors, this website offers a database indexing over 100,000 websites with a K–12 focus. The site includes lesson plans, directories of schools and colleges, news stories, professional development, and many additional sources of information.

Librarians' Index to the Internet: Education

"The Librarians' Index to the Internet is a searchable, annotated subject directory of more than 7,000 Internet resources selected and evaluated by librarians for their usefulness to users of public libraries."

The Digital Librarian on Education

This site includes hundreds of links for local and national organizations, as well as home pages from many teachers, schools, and school districts. This is "a librarian's choice of the best of the Web."

Yahoo! Education Index

Broad categories of this well-known search engine lead to thousands of educational sites. K–12 links are particularly extensive, but all included sites seem well-chosen and up-to-date.

DMOZ (*www.dmoz.org*), formerly known as the Open Directory Project, calls itself "the republic of the Web" and is perhaps the most comprehensive and accessible directory on the Internet. The About page of its website explains:

> DMOZ follows in the footsteps of some of the most important editor/contributor projects of the 20th century. Just as the Oxford English Dictionary became the definitive word on words through the efforts of volunteers, DMOZ follows in its footsteps to become the definitive catalog of the Web.
>
> DMOZ was founded in the spirit of the Open Source movement, and is the only major directory that is 100% free. There is not, nor will there ever be, a cost to submit a site to the directory, and/or to use the directory's data. DMOZ data is made available for free to anyone who agrees to comply with our free use license. ("About DMOZ," 2014)

TABLE 2.4. Categories of DMOZ	
Search DMOZ	
Arts	Recreation
Business	Reference
Computers	Regional
Games	Science
Health	Shopping
Home	Society
Kids and Teens	Sports
News	World

DMOZ uses a hierarchy of categories and subcategories. The 16 major categories are represented in Table 2.4. A search through the Open Directory is a series of selections from lists. A user starts with one of the major categories and then types in a subtopic, which then links to a list of more subtopics. The results continue; lists in categories are generated until the user reaches the final subcategory for the specific topic of interest.

The Participative Web: User-Created Content

User-created content (UCC) is "(i) content made publicly available over the Internet, (ii) which reflects a 'certain amount of creative effort', and (iii) which is 'created outside of professional routines and practices'" (Wunsch-Vincent & Vickery, 2006).

CC allows anyone with Internet access to create a repository of writing, images, or video that others can comment on and edit. It relies on "the collective intelligence of all users" to create knowledge, to disseminate information, and to exchange ideas. User-created content sites are omnipresent on the Web. Provided that their information is accurate, UCC sites like blogs, wikis, and media-sharing sites (see Table 2.5) can be of assistance to both educational researchers and research consumers.

COMPARING DIGITAL RESOURCES   MAP 2.3

Both libraries and the free commercial internet provide access to a wealth of digital resources on a variety of topics and in a variety of formats. Although library searches ensure access to high-quality research, they are not the only way to access these texts. When vetted properly, the free commercial Internet can provide a useful starting place for searches that complement the resources offered by libraries. Table 2.6 presents a comparison of library resources and free commercial resources.

TABLE 2.5. User-Created Content (UCC) Types and Sample Sites

Type	Sample sites
Blog: A website where a person writes regularly about recent events or topics that interest him or her, usually with photos and links to other websites that he or she finds interesting.	InformED: Research and journalism on educational trends (*http://educationpolicy.air.org/blog/2013/09/building-on-a-strong-foundation-edsectorair.html*) Qualitative Inquiry: Teaching and mentoring qualitative research (*http://qualitativeinquiry.com*)
Wiki: A website or database that allows users to add and edit content.	Wikipedia: Free online encyclopedia (*https://en.wikipedia.org/wiki/Main_Page*) Mind Mapping in Education: Mind-mapping software (*www.mindmapping.com/mind-mapping-in-education.php*)
Media-sharing site: A website that allows users to download videos and other media.	YouTube: Video sharing (*www.youtube.com*)

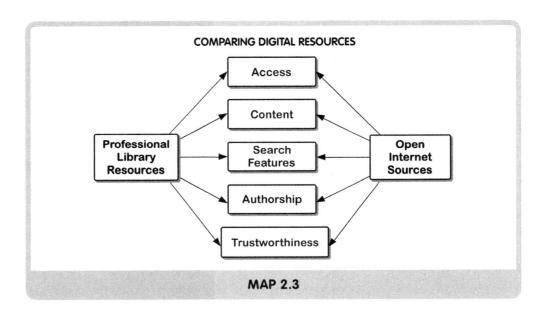

MAP 2.3

TABLE 2.6. Comparing Library and Internet Resources

Feature	Library resources	Free commercial resources
Access	Provide limited access to subscribers through institutions, particularly libraries.	Provide free and wide access to individual Internet users.
Content	Include wide range of "selectively curated" resources; inclusive depository for primary, empirical, peer-reviewed research articles.	Include wide range of all kinds of resources; limited depository for primary, empirical, peer-reviewed research articles.
Search features	Provide numerous filters. Provide citations in APA format.	Provide limited filters. Do not provide citations in APA format.
Authorship	Are confined to expert authors.	Include nonexpert users and expert authors.
Trustworthiness	Ensure high levels of trustworthiness.	Highly variable; may be "just good enough."

CHAPTER SUMMARY

MAP 2.4

✓ *Information literacy* is the ability to "locate, analyze, evaluate, and use information resources to support research and learning" in "a variety of digital age media and formats" (International Society for Technology in Education, 2008). Digital tools use computer technologies that support the storage and retrieval of vast amounts of research and are located in libraries and on the World Wide Web.

✓ Digital library resources include professional commercial databases, online journals, and interlibrary loan.

✓ Digital library resources are available to qualified users on library sites.

✓ Database searches involve the use of keywords and Boolean operators.

✓ The three-keyword search is an effective strategy for retrieving primary research articles from professional commercial databases.

✓ Web resources include search engines, directories, and user-created content (UCC).

✓ Web resources are usually free and available to a variety of users.

✓ UCC includes blogs, wikis, and media-sharing sites.

✓ Library and Web searches provide different, and often complementary, strategies for retrieving primary, empirical, peer-reviewed journal articles.

KEY TERMS AND CONCEPTS

Advanced Google Scholar Search

Blogs

Boolean operators

Directory

Google Scholar search

Information literacy

Interlibrary loan

Keywords

Media-sharing sites

Meta tags

Online journals

Participative Web

Portal

Professional commercial databases

Search engines

Selectively curated

Standard Google search

User-created content (UCC)

Wikis

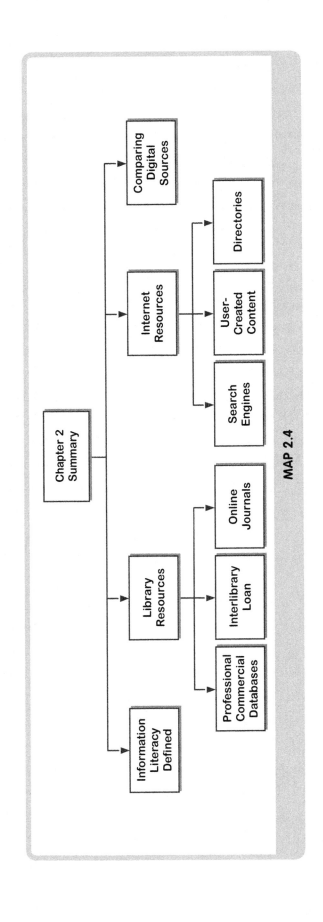

MAP 2.4

REVIEW, CONSOLIDATION, AND EXTENSION OF KNOWLEDGE

1. What do you consider the most relevant and highest-quality database for your area of research? Why?

2. Select a topic of interest to you and follow these steps:

   a. Go to a library website where you are or can be a licensed user, and use a three-keyword search to find one qualitative, one quantitative, and one integrative primary, empirical, peer-reviewed article. Then enter the bibliographic information in APA format. (You may want to use *citationmachine.net.*)

   b. Go to your library's database and find the interlibrary loan portal. Read the procedures for completing an interlibrary loan request, and complete a request for an article on your topic of interest.

   c. Go to the Library of Congress Alcove 9 section on general education (*www.loc.gov/rr/main/alcove9/education/general.html*), and search one of the websites listed for references related to your topic of interest.

   d. Go to DMOZ (*www.dmoz.org*) and find a resource that applies to your topic of interest.

   e. Search for (i) a blog, (ii) a wiki, and (iii) a YouTube video that relate to your topic of interest, and enter their URLs below.

      Blog URL:

      Wiki URL:

      YouTube URL:

3. Rate the resources you found in exercise 2, from highest to lowest, in terms of their usefulness to you as a research consumer.

PART II
Qualitative Research

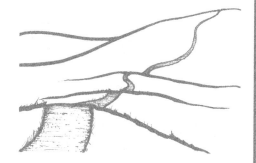

"Discoveries are often made by not following instructions, by going off the main road, by trying the untried."

—FRANK TYGER

Part II goes into more depth about qualitative research, "a form of social inquiry that focuses on the way people interpret and make sense of their experiences and the world in which they live" (Holloway, 1997, p. 2). It provides a broad overview of the method and describes the various designs and approaches.

The image of a long and winding road in the picture above is meant to capture the idea that qualitative research is a journey over unexplored territory that encounters many twists and turns along the way. It takes uncharted routes to explore settings, events, and phenomena; it seeks to uncover subjective realities holistically. It emphasizes researcher engagement; it describes phenomena from the point of view of those who live and experience them; and it depends on interpretive processes for analysis.

CHAPTER THREE

Qualitative Research

Introduction and Overview

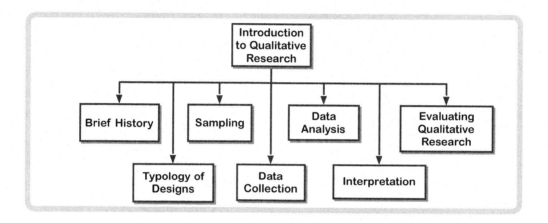

This chapter introduces the core concepts and practices of qualitative research.

CHAPTER OBJECTIVES

✓ Understand the historical background of qualitative research in social science and education.

✓ Understand the key characteristics of qualitative research.

✓ Understand the major research designs and their purposes.

✓ Understand qualitative sampling strategies: purposive and theoretical.

✓ Understand how qualitative researchers collect and record data.

✓ Understand the three sources for data collection: observations; interviews; and documents and discourses.

✓ Understand the constant comparative method of data analysis and its global usage in qualitative inquiry.

✓ Understand commonly used interpretive approaches in qualitative work.

✓ Understand criteria for evaluating the quality of qualitative studies.

A BRIEF HISTORY OF QUALITATIVE RESEARCH

Qualitative research has a long history, reaching back to the late 19th and early 20th centuries, when cultural anthropologists spent prolonged periods of time observing and recording the behaviors and social patterns of distant—and what were then termed "primitive"—cultures. Malinowski's study of the Trobriand Islanders (1922) and Mead's *Coming of Age in Samoa* (1928) are iconic texts in early ethnography. American sociologists brought anthropological techniques closer to home in their studies of small-town and urban cultures. In their ethnography titled *Middletown*, Lynd and Lynd (1929) noted that they "approached an American community as an anthropologist does a primitive tribe" (p. iv). Whyte (1955) left his office at Harvard daily to observe and record Italian American culture on the street corners of Boston's North End.

Willard Waller and Margaret Mead were among the first social scientists to apply qualitative methods to the study of schools and schooling. Waller's landmark study, *The Sociology of Teaching* (1932), developed a detailed description of how teachers experienced the school culture. Mead's *An Anthropologist Looks at the Teacher's Role* (1942) described the different types of interactions that occurred between teachers and students in various locales. After World War II, however, qualitative research became marginalized when the quantitative paradigm, with its roots in positivism, offered the promise of rigor, precision, and scientific proof to the study of social life. This approach dominated the research landscape during the Cold War era of the 1950s and 1960s; input–output studies proliferated in education.

By the late 1960s and early 1970s, many researchers became disillusioned with quantitative research and its ability to deliver on its promise. Social scientists like Bruyn (1966), Glaser and Strauss (1967), and others looked to philosophies other than positivism to ground their study of social life, ushering in a renaissance of interest in the qualitative paradigm. This generated an intense methodological debate between qualitative and quantitative researchers that did not subside until later in the 1970s. During this time a large number of educational researchers, seeking to capture the nuances of educational practice, moved away from input–output studies toward qualitative methods of inquiry. Chief among them were Ray Rist (1970) and Harry Wolcott (1973), who published landmark studies of the experiences of children and adults in schools that were emulated by other researchers.

In the 1980s, another strand developed within the qualitative paradigm—one that questioned the paradigm itself and viewed a researcher's perspective as offering just one among many possible representations of a social situation. This challenge to the researcher's representation of social reality highlighted the power relations between the researcher and the researched, and thus had political implications. It led to the development of such methods of social critique as feminism, postcolonialism, and race theory, which have gained traction and continue to be significant. In addition, a currently emerging movement further distances qualitative research not only from the positivist foundations of the quantitative paradigm, but from its own roots: It uses poetry and drama to represent and communicate findings.

This brief history does not assume a linear progression of qualitative approaches. In fact, what it is meant to demonstrate is the diversity, flexibility, and inventiveness of qualitative methods as ways to understand and value the social world as humans experience it. What remain constant across the diverse approaches to qualitative research are these distinguishing characteristics:

- The research focuses on people in their natural settings.
- Designs are varied, flexible, and adaptive.
- Samples are small, either purposeful or theoretical, and sensitive to setting and purpose.
- Data collection is limited to observations, interviews, available documents/ artifacts, and discourse.
- The researcher is the key instrument for data collection and is engaged with and visible to actors.
- Data analysis is inductive and iterative.
- Interpretive methods range from emic to etic.
- Words and images are the means of communication.

This last point is very important. The story goes that Albert Einstein had this quotation on his bulletin board: "Not everything that can be counted counts, and not everything that counts can be counted." Qualitative researchers work from the assumption that "what counts" is best described in words and visual images rather than by numbers and calculations. Qualitative researchers use words to develop detailed descriptions of cases, to communicate with actors and with readers, to reproduce direct quotes, to describe the meanings actors ascribe to their social situations, to develop codes and analytic frameworks, and to capture the essence of an understanding or interpretation through metaphor. And they often translate words into images and visual representations like drawings, photographs, concept maps, diagrams, word trees, and "word clouds" (by using programs like Wordle), to further develop understandings.

TYPOLOGY OF DESIGNS   MAP 3.1

Developing a typology of qualitative designs is no simple matter. In fact, some researchers have identified as many as 39 designs! Although such minute distinctions make sense to academics, they do little to serve practitioners who are the consumers of educational research. To simplify matters, we have settled on five designs: ethnography, case study, phenomenological study, narrative study, and text analysis (which includes qualitative document analysis and critical discourse analysis). Our typology is based on two criteria: the specific purpose of each design, and its method of data

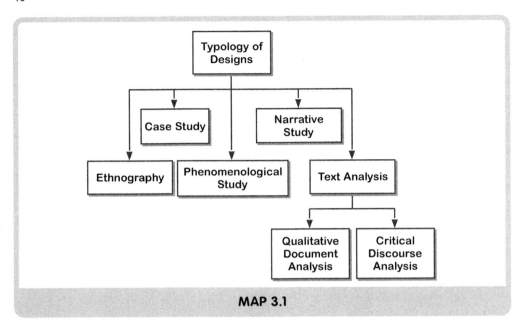

MAP 3.1

collection. These designs are represented in Table 3.1 and are discussed more fully in Chapters Four and Five.

Qualitative designs are always open to modification as new understandings develop or new discoveries emerge. A qualitative researcher "follows the bread-crumb trail" much as Hansel and Gretel do in finding their way through the forest, looking for clues about where to go next in hopes of reaching a final destination. This is an apt metaphor for qualitative work: Researchers follow clues to find their way through an unfamiliar culture or subculture; to understand a particular event or phenomenon; or to gain insights into how people think, feel, and behave.

TABLE 3.1. Qualitative Designs

Design	Purpose	Data
Ethnography	To describe and interpret a culture or group	Observations, interviews, texts
Case study	To describe and interpret a particular event, program, or activity	Observations, interviews, texts
Phenomenological study	To describe and interpret phenomena from the actors' points of view	Interviews
Narrative study	To bring order and coherence to a life story or collection of stories	Life story interviews
Text analysis: Qualitative document analysis	To describe and interpret official and personal written documents	Print and electronic documents produced and used by actors
Text analysis: Critical discourse analysis	To describe and interpret written texts and speech from a critical theory perspective	Texts and talk

SAMPLING

MAP 3.2

The selection of a sample in terms of setting and actors is arguably the most important decision that qualitative researchers make, and it requires a strategic and thoughtful approach. In selecting samples, qualitative researchers look for settings and actors that will provide illumination and insight into the culture, phenomenon, or event under study. They seek to study people, termed *actors*, in ways that are as natural as possible. In most instances, this requires researchers to collect data from *natural settings*, the environments where people live and work. In this way, the researcher is in a position to the grasp the nuances of a particular context and to develop a holistic understanding of a culture, a phenomenon, or an event. The focus on lived experience in natural settings distinguishes qualitative from quantitative research. Qualitative researchers look for *information-rich* samples that fit their particular interests, and usually depend on small samples that are either *purposeful* or *theoretical*.

Purposeful Sampling

Purposeful sampling refers to the deliberate process of selecting an appropriate setting and people for inquiry.

There are various approaches to purposeful sampling. A researcher may choose samples that are (1) *typical samples*, composed of average settings or actors; (2) *extreme or deviant samples*, composed of extreme or marginal settings or actors; (3) *maximum variation samples*, composed of a heterogeneous mix of settings or actors; (4) *homogeneous samples*, composed of settings or actors who share a narrow range of characteristics; (5) *critical samples*, composed of settings or actors who provide a rich example of the phenomenon under study; or (6) *snowball samples*, composed of settings or actors who are nominated by other settings or actors to be part of a sample.

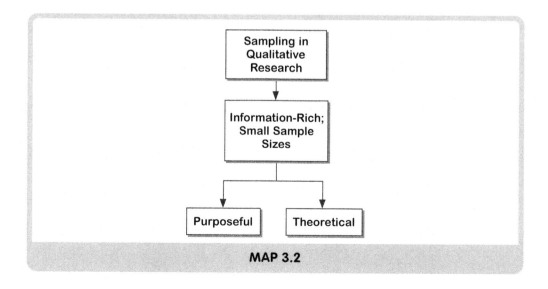

MAP 3.2

Theoretical Sampling

> *Theoretical sampling* seeks out settings, actors, or texts that the researcher views as being able to make a contribution to the process of data collection and analysis.

Theoretical sampling may involve returning to previous samples or accessing new ones. There are two types of theoretical samples that access new settings and actors. These are (1) *confirming samples*, composed of settings and actors who strengthen emerging themes, patterns, and interpretations and (2) *negative case samples*, composed of settings and actors who counter emerging themes, patterns, and interpretations. Theoretical sampling continues until *saturation* is reached—the point at which a researcher decides that no further inquiry is necessary to establish a concept.

DATA COLLECTION   MAP 3.3

In qualitative research, all data are mediated through a researcher. Researchers have three kinds of data available: *observations*; *interviews*; and *documents* and *discourses*. In order to capture these data, the researchers have to come into close contact with the settings and actors they are studying and serve as the key instrument for data collection. Qualitative researchers continue to collect data until *data saturation* has been reached.

> *Data saturation* is the endpoint in data collection; it occurs when the researcher determines that information has become repetitive and that no new insights or ideas are being revealed.

Observations

Observation is basic to all qualitative research. It is the defining characteristic of classical anthropological fieldwork and remains central to contemporary qualitative practice. It provides researchers with direct access to social phenomena as they occur in real-world situations. Qualitative observation depends on the researchers' ability to capture and record everything they see and hear—the details of settings and

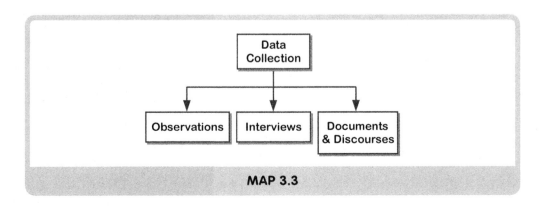

MAP 3.3

existing texts and of behaviors and conversations. An observer may engage with actors in a variety of ways.

In *covert observation,* an observer does not reveal him- or herself to actors. If a researcher has a natural role in the setting and is known to actors, but hides the research intentions from the group, this is called *full participation.* Another form of covert observation has been informally referred to as "under-the-bed" or " behind-the-mirror" observation. Its formal name is *complete observation,* and as the name indicates, it involves observers who hide not only their intentions, but also their physical selves from those being observed.

In *overt observation,* a researcher fully discloses the research and its purpose to actors. A researcher who has a natural role in the group is termed a *participant-as-observer.* A researcher who does not have a natural role in the group, but participates in it and its activities in order to collect data, is termed an *observer-as-participant.* As Adler and Adler (1994, p. 380) explain, "this peripheral membership role enables the researcher to observe and interact closely enough with members to establish an insider's identity without participating in those activities constituting the core of group membership."

Interviews

Interviews uncover how people feel, think, and make sense of their lives, a social situation, or a specific event or phenomenon; they allow researchers to gain access to insights and information that might not otherwise be available. Qualitative interviews are always open ended. This sets them apart from the closed-response questionnaires and surveys that are used in quantitative research. Interviews allow the actors to present interpretations of events as they, and not their interviewers, see them. A good qualitative interview is one in which an actor does most of the talking; an interviewer says little, listens actively, and interjects only to paraphrase, summarize, or prompt the actor for further elaboration or explanation. Interviews may be conducted with individuals or with groups of individuals. Group interviews are called *focus groups.*

In recording interviews, researchers may choose to use an audio recorder for later transcription; they may opt to take copious notes during the interviews; or they may prefer to make brief notations during the interviews, and to fill in more information and reconstruct direct quotes soon after the interviews are completed.

There are numerous ways to conduct an interview. Generally, there are four types of qualitative interviews: (1) an *unstructured interview,* which is like a conversation in that it proceeds as a natural dialogue between a researcher and actor; (2) a *semistructured interview,* which is more focused and has a specific set of topics or questions to be covered, but in which the researcher proceeds in no particular order and thus allows the actor a great deal of leeway in responding; (3) a *structured* or *standardized interview,* which is the most focused type of interview and in which the same questions are asked of all actors in the same order; and (4) a *life story interview,* in which people are simply asked to tell their life stories in their own words and in a free-flowing narrative style, without too many questions from the interviewer.

Within an interview, a researcher may ask different types of questions. James P. Spradley (1979), a noted anthropologist and a pioneer in applying anthropological methods to education, divided interview questions into three types: (1) *descriptive questions*, which ask for concrete accounts of events that stay clear of abstractions or emotions; (2) *structural questions*, which ask for explanations that place the descriptive events in context; and (3) *contrast questions*, which ask for analyses of similarities and differences.

Michael Patton (1990) has offered another typology of questions: (1) *behavior* or *experience questions*, which ask about actions and behaviors that an actor observes or has observed; (2) *opinion* or *value questions*, which ask about understandings; (3) *feeling questions*, which ask about an actor's emotional responses; (4) *knowledge questions*, which ask about factual information that the actor knows; (5) *sensory questions*, which ask about physical reactions; and (6) *background/demographic questions*, which ask about the characteristics of the people being interviewed.

Documents

Documents are verbal and visual texts that are produced by actors and provide information about a culture or group. They are the least obtrusive data sources in qualitative researchers' repertoire. A document may be a written or electronic document created and used by actors. There are two major kinds of documents: *official* and *personal*.

Official documents provide information about how a culture or group is formally organized, about its demographics and characteristics, and about the formal relationship of the group to the community and to larger entities. These may include policy manuals, curriculum guides, administrative letters, memos, textbooks, attendance reports, student records, flow charts, transcripts, minutes from meetings, mission statements, and course syllabi. *Personal documents* provide insights into what matters and is valued by actors, which may not be revealed in observations or interviews or official texts. They may include diaries and journals, letters, personal lists, and other private documents.

Discourses

Discourses are written or spoken units of language that are carefully scrutinized for "all the linguistic devices employed by the persons who produced the discourse, taking into account the social and ideological setting of the discourse" (Wilson, 1993). Scholars make the distinction between discourses and conversations, discourses being the written words and conversations being the spoken words that are being analyzed. For our purposes, we consider both types of data as discourses. Unlike the traditional qualitative analyses of documents and interviews, which seek to uncover the meanings that actors ascribe to their communications, the analysis of discourses looks at the context of language and how it shapes and is shaped by the context in which it occurs.

DATA ANALYSIS

MAP 3.4

Data analysis in qualitative research depends on procedures for organizing and reducing data and for summarizing results. As in data collection, analysis flows through a researcher—making the researcher the instrument for both data collection and data analysis.

Data Reduction

The goal of data analysis is to reduce the data into manageable units, so that the researcher can make sense of it and provide a cohesive summary and interpretation of findings. Qualitative data analysis is a rigorous and complex process that requires a considerable investment of time and persistence, and that entails several approaches. For instance, some researchers identify patterns and themes in the data through a process of reading and rereading all field notes and making comments in the margins or underlining important sections before proceeding to categorize and code the data. The process is recursive and iterative; that is, the researchers revisit the raw data until they settle on themes and patterns that capture the way people live and make meaning of their experiences. Most qualitative researchers use *codes*, or labels that assign meaning to chunks of data so that the data can be sorted into categories for analysis, to organize their data. There are two ways in which researchers approach coding: They may use *generative codes* or *a priori codes*.

    Generative codes are developed directly from the data during and/or after data collection. The *constant comparative method* of coding is the most frequently used strategy for generative coding; it is considered the default method of coding in much of

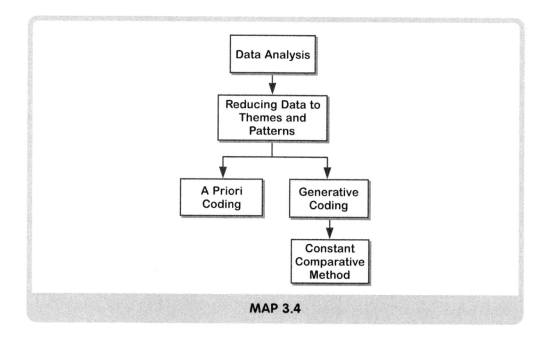

MAP 3.4

qualitative research. The method involves "(a) comparing different people (such as their views), situations, actions, accounts and experiences, (b) comparing data from the same individuals with themselves at different points in time, (c) comparing incident with incident, (d) comparing data with category, and (e) comparing a category with other categories" (Charmaz, 2000, p. 515). Analysis of data begins early in the research and begins a process of theory development that involves the interplay of three vital elements: coding, memo writing, and theoretical sampling. Coding organizes data in three stages. The first step is *open coding,* which involves coding line by line in order to generate initial concepts about what is occurring in the setting and what people are doing. The second step is *axial coding* (also called *action coding*), which involves making comparisons within and across the data and linking concepts to each other. The final step is *selective coding,* which identifies "core categories" that are central to the theory being generated.

A priori codes are developed before data collection begins. They are derived from a comprehensive review of theory and prior research, which provides useful perspectives for understanding the topic of inquiry. In education, a priori codes are commonly developed from work in psychology (e.g., motivation, cognitive development, self-esteem) and in sociology (e.g., hierarchies, identity, socialization).

Computer-Assisted Qualitative Data Analysis Software

Computer-assisted qualitative data analysis software (CAQDAS) provides tools that assist researchers in organizing and analyzing data. This is a relatively new method for coding and analyzing data; it did not take hold in qualitative research until the 1990s. The most frequently used CAQDAS programs in qualitative research are NVivo, ATLAS.ti, and Ethnograph.

Among the advantages of CAQDAS are the following: freedom from clerical tasks; efficiency and flexibility in dealing with large datasets; the ability to generate visual images and graphics that allow for arranging and rearranging coding categories; and support for collaborative work (Rademaker, Grace, & Curda, 2012; St John & Johnson, 2000). However, there are also several disadvantages: the time and energy required to master the software; the distancing of researchers from their data; and mistaken assumptions about what the software can do. The software does not develop codes; the researcher does the initial coding of data. The software does not do the analytical thinking; the researcher continues to be in charge of the analysis and interpretation of the data (Gibbs, Lewins, & Silver, 2005).

INTERPRETATION   MAP 3.5

Central to qualitative research is the idea of *interpretation*—the stance the researcher takes in collecting data and in making meaning from them. Also known as *verstehen* from the German, interpretation is a complex and multilayered concept that distinguishes between *emic* and *etic* perspectives.

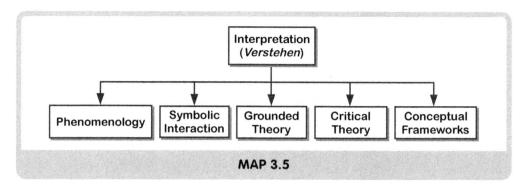

MAP 3.5

Emic refers to the "insider" perspectives and interpretations of actors: it acknowledges the multiple and often diverse perspectives of reality that different actors may hold.

Etic refers to the "outsider" perspectives and interpretations of the researcher; it makes sense of reality from an external, social-scientific viewpoint.

It is helpful to view these two perspectives as "markers along a continuum of styles or different levels" (Fetterman, 1989, p. 3). Next, we briefly describe five approaches to interpretation that frequently appear in qualitative studies in education, and we place them along the continuum from emic to etic as represented in Figure 3.1.

Phenomenology

Closest to the emic perspective is the *phenomenological* approach. In brief, phenomenology seeks to understand the essence of a phenomenon from the point of view of the actors, and it depends on in-depth interviews and personal writing and reflections of the actors. Phenomenology is associated with the early 20th-century philosopher Edmund Husserl, who wanted to understand *phenomena* as the ways that things appear in people's experience and the meanings that people attribute to those experiences. The philosophy of phenomenology assumes that reality is not objective and is subjectively experienced by individual actors. It "assumes the relativism of multiple social realities, recognizes the mutual creation of knowledge by the viewer and the viewed, and aims toward interpretative understandings of subjects' meanings" (Charmaz, 2000, p. 510).

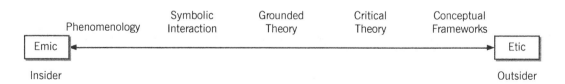

FIGURE 3.1. The emic–etic continuum.

Symbolic Interaction

The *symbolic interaction* approach is next along the emic–etic continuum; it assumes a process of negotiation among actors, leading to shared meanings that are socially rather than individually constructed. The ideas behind symbolic interaction first appeared in the writings of John Dewey in the early 20th century at the University of Chicago, and were elaborated by George Herbert Mead in 1934 and by later sociologists in the 1950s and 1960s. As defined by Herbert Blumer (1969), the symbolic interaction approach is based on three premises:

> (1) Human beings act toward things on the basis of the meanings things have for them. (2) The meaning of such things is derived from, or arises out of, the social interactions that one has with one's fellows. (3) These meanings are handled in, and modified through, an interpretative process that is used by the person in dealing with the things he encounters. (pp. 2–3)

Symbolic interaction assumes that meanings are not inherent, that they are shaped through interaction with others, and that people develop perceptions of themselves based on how others see them. Symbolic interaction requires researchers to enter into the worlds of the people they are observing, and to dig deep to come to an understanding of the meanings actors attach to their actions as well as the consequences of those actions. Blumer (1969) explained:

> The metaphor that I like is that of lifting the veils that obscure or hide what is going on. The task of scientific study is to lift the veils that cover the areas of group life that one proposes to study. The veils are not lifted by substituting, in whatever degree, pre-formed images for firsthand knowledge. The veils are lifted by getting close to the area and by digging into it through careful study. (p. 39)

One of the major concepts of symbolic interaction is *labeling*; this is a social process by which the actors in the setting assign identifying labels (e.g., "class clown" or "computer nerd") to other actors, who take on behaviors that reinforce the expectations the labels connote.

Grounded Theory

Grounded theory is derived from symbolic interaction, but goes one step further and seeks to generate and verify a theory that emerges from the data. Though its ultimate aim is to develop explanatory theories that represent etic understandings, its analysis depends on emic understandings as a starting point. The grounded theory approach goes one step further than symbolic interaction: It uses the descriptive data and social constructions to generate a theory that explains behaviors and perceptions.

Grounded theory was introduced by Barney Glaser and Anselm Strauss in 1967 in their book *The Discovery of Grounded Theory*. The idea that qualitative research could lead to the generation of theory was considered revolutionary at that time; it moved qualitative research beyond description toward explanation. Grounded theory elaborated symbolic interaction by introducing the constant comparative method for generating codes and theories, discussed earlier. It also advocated for the use of *negative case sampling,* in which researchers use theoretical sampling to identify actors or settings that disconfirm the researchers' emerging analysis or hypotheses.

Critical Theory

The *critical theory* (also known as *activist/emancipatory*) approach also seeks explanation, but it does so by applying theories of social critique with the aim of uncovering the unarticulated "meanings that sustain powerlessness and that people's conscious models exist to perpetuate, as much as to explain, social phenomena" (Anderson, 1989, p. 253). Critical approaches fall further along the emic–etic continuum, relying more heavily on an etic perspective. While these approaches acknowledge the emic understandings of actors, their ultimate aim is to arrive at etic understandings that explain how the underlying realities of power and social control distort understandings and keep actors oppressed and marginalized.

Critical theory was originally developed by the Frankfurt school of philosophers in Germany to explain how ideology contributes to the oppression and marginalization of people and groups. It is used here as an umbrella term for theories of social critique that explain how power relationships, privilege, and social control shape social situations. The goal of these theories is to lay bare to actors and readers how dominant ideologies and interests distort perceptions of reality. Their ultimate goal is to help actors emancipate themselves from oppression and marginality. As Thomas (1993) explained,

> The roots of critical thought spread from a long tradition of intellectual rebellion in which rigorous examination of ideas and discourse constituted political challenge. Social critique by nature is radical. It implies an evaluative judgment of meaning and method in research, policy, and human activity. The act of critique implies that by thinking about and acting upon the world, we are able to change both our subjective interpretations and objective conditions. (p. 81)

This approach usually employs one, or a combination, of four social theories: (1) *Marxism and neo-Marxism* use social class, ideology, and false consciousness as organizing concepts to explain understanding how social forces oppress groups of people; (2) *feminism* uses gender as its organizing concept to explain how patriarchal institutions and values undermine and oppress women; (3) *queer theory* uses sexuality as its organizing concept to explain how the idea of "otherness" undermines and oppresses people who are different from the norm; and (4) *critical race theory* uses race as its organizing concept to explain how the idea of "whiteness" that dominates society undermines and oppresses people of color.

Conceptual Frameworks

Although inductive data analysis has long been foundational to the qualitative method, some researchers have adopted *conceptual frameworks* as an interpretive lens. This is a more deductive stance that depends on a priori categories derived from a review of the literature, rather than on generative coding, to interpret findings. It begins with preestablished codes and considers emic understandings secondarily as they add to or refine etic understandings. The use of conceptual frameworks to organize and interpret qualitative data has gained traction in qualitative work. Frameworks are not "steel girders"; they are "like the scaffolding of wooden planks . . . that facilitate more comprehensive ways to investigate a research problem" (Eisenhart, 1991, pp. 210–211). In the course of conducting the research, a researcher reworks and refines the framework, taking into account the actions, behaviors, and perspectives of actors.

EVALUATING QUALITATIVE RESEARCH   MAP 3.6

The question of how to evaluate the quality and integrity of qualitative work is answered in terms of *trustworthiness* and *transferability*.

Trustworthiness

Trustworthiness is synonymous with *verisimilitude*; it refers to the authenticity and credibility of the data and the dependability of the analysis and interpretation of the data. The use of the term *trustworthiness* in this context was coined by Lincoln and Guba (1985), who offered this explanation:

> The basic issue in relation to trustworthiness is simple: How can an inquirer persuade his or her audiences that the findings of a particular inquiry for the subjects (respondents) with which and the context in which the inquiry was carried out are worth paying attention to? What arguments can be mounted, what criteria invoked, what question asked, that would be persuasive on this issue? (p. 290)

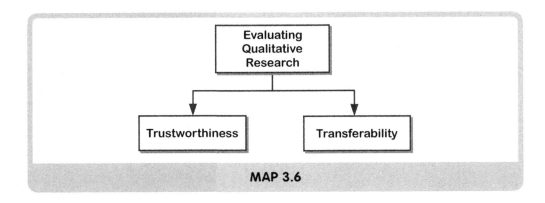

MAP 3.6

In general, an article that is strong in trustworthiness has these qualities:

• *A research stance* that is fully described. This refers to the position the researcher takes in regard to actors, context, and content and to the process of research itself. In describing the research stance, a researcher should provide a rationale for choices about content and design, and should make explicit the theoretical approaches and interpretive assumptions that are used.

• *Thick descriptions* of the study's context and of the actors' actions, thoughts, words, and feelings. In developing thick descriptions, researchers not only fully describe context and actors; they present the actual language of the actors, including dialect and idiosyncratic usage, as well as the personal meanings that the actors ascribe to their own words and actions and those of others.

• *Sampling* that demonstrates a strategic and thoughtful process for selecting the context and the actors for the inquiry, and that makes a case for using a purposeful or theoretical sample.

• *Triangulation* of data, which combines multiple sources of information or different investigators. Triangulation may involve making comparisons among actors, among multiple researchers, or among data collection methods. The term is borrowed from the U.S. Army's method of ensuring the accuracy of radio transmissions during World Wars I and II, where in order for information to be considered sound, the same signal had to be received from two different locations. In qualitative research, triangulation performs the same function: It provides assurances that the researcher has checked on more than one "signal."

• *Checks for accuracy*, which verify the authenticity of the data through member checks and/or peer reviews/audits. *Member checks* ask actors for feedback on the accuracy of the data and for elaboration on data the research has recorded. *Peer reviews/ audits* draw on researchers from outside the study to lend a neutral perspective on the research and review processes for data collection and analysis.

• *Transformation of data into themes*, which involves a process of data analysis that reduces data into categories. A researcher may use generative or a priori codes, or may provide a detailed description of how themes were generated without referring to coding. The researcher may mention a specific software program to assist in the process.

• *Engagement*, which provides sufficient time for the researcher to develop trust and collect sufficient data to achieve data reduction.

• *Reflection*, which may involve the use of tools and processes that enable the researcher to examine his or her role as a researcher and the ongoing progress of the inquiry. Tools may include (1) *reflexive journals*, or private diaries in which a researcher makes continuing entries about decisions concerning data collection and analysis, and reflects on any personal values, interests, and biases; (2) *bracketing*, or the placement of [brackets] around any phrases in research notes that may suggest personal values, interests, and biases, and that may also suggest further avenues to pursue in data collection; and (3) *memos*, or written reflective notes in which the researcher records insights about what he or she is learning during data collection. All of these tools enable a researcher to "catch your thoughts, capture the comparisons and connections you make, and crystallize questions and directions you want to pursue" (Charmaz, 2006, p. 72).

Transferability

Transferability refers to readers' personal assessment of the application of findings beyond the boundaries of the study and to their own situation. In qualitative research, it is the readers' responsibility to make connections, and it is the researchers' responsibility to provide sufficient information for the readers to make those connections. Transferability depends on the degree to which the readers resonate with the study—its purpose, sample, descriptions, data analyses, and interpretations. Thick description and careful sampling are particularly important in making judgments about transferability. Again, while it is the researchers' responsibility to provide sufficient information for the readers to make judgments about trustworthiness, it is left to readers to make subjective judgments about transferability and the degree to which the content, actors, contexts, and findings resonate with their personal concerns and interests.

The rubric in Figure 3.2 describes the qualities to consider in evaluating the trustworthiness and transferability of qualitative research.

CHAPTER SUMMARY   MAP 3.7

✓ Qualitative research studies social phenomena and events, human relationships and experiences, and the meanings that people ascribe to them.

✓ Qualitative research has a rich history, dating back to early 20th-century ethnography.

✓ Samples are small, purposeful, or theoretical, and sensitive to setting and purpose.

✓ Types of qualitative designs include ethnography, case study, phenomenological study, narrative inquiry, and two types of text analysis (qualitative document analysis and critical discourse analysis).

✓ Data collection is limited to observations, interviews, and documents/discourses.

✓ The researcher is the key instrument for data collection and analysis.

✓ Data analysis often uses generative or a priori codes.

✓ Interpretation (*verstehen*) makes meaning from the data analysis and is based on phenomenology, symbolic interaction, grounded theory, critical theory, or conceptual frameworks.

✓ Data are presented and analyzed in words and images.

✓ Results are case specific and cannot be generalized to other settings or actors.

✓ The quality indicators of qualitative research come under the umbrella of trustworthiness and transferability.

	Strong	Moderate	Weak
Trustworthiness: The verisimilitude of findings, credibility of data, and dependability of analysis and interpretation.			
	Strong	**Moderate**	**Weak**
Research stance	Full description of researcher's relation to the research project, rationale for exploring the issue, and interpretive lens.	Some detail provided for relation to project and rationale.	Scant or no discussion of relation to project and rationale.
Thick description	Detailed descriptions of context and actors' actions, thoughts; verbatim language from interviews and documents.	Adequate descriptions provided; some detail lacking.	Limited descriptions; no direct quotes.
Sampling	Detailed description of selection of context and actors; rationale for selecting; detailed description of key actors.	Information provided, but lacking in detail.	Scant information provided.
Triangulation	Explicit reference to triangulation and to multiple data sources used in the study.	Reference to multiple data sources used; triangulation implied.	Scant or no evidence of multiple data sources or of how these were triangulated.
Checks for accuracy	Detailed description of checks for accuracy (member checks or peer reviews/audits).	Description of checks for accuracy; some details lacking.	No explicit checks for accuracy.
Transforming data into themes	Detailed description of data reduction or coding strategy and of who was involved.	Mention of data reduction, but details lacking.	Scant or no indication of data reduction/coding.
Reflection	Detailed description of reflective tools and processes.	Mention of reflective tools or processes, but lacking in detail.	No mention of reflective tools or processes.
Engagement	Detailed description of time spent in the context and with actors (sufficient time to gain trust and to gather information until data saturation was reached).	Description of time spent in the context and with actors (sufficient time to gain trust and to gather information, but details lacking to judge data saturation).	Inadequate description of time with the context and actors (insufficient time to gain trust, gather information, or reach data saturation).
Transferability: The reader's ability to resonate with findings and connect them to other contexts and actors.			
	Strong	**Moderate**	**Weak**
Thick description	Detailed description of context and actors' actions, thoughts; verbatim language from interviews and documents.	Adequate descriptions provided; some detail lacking.	Limited descriptions; no direct quotes.
Sampling	Detailed description of selection of context and actors, as well as rationale for selecting; detailed description of key actors.	Information provided, but lacking in detail.	Scant information provided.

FIGURE 3.2. A rubric for the evaluative criteria of trustworthiness and transferability.

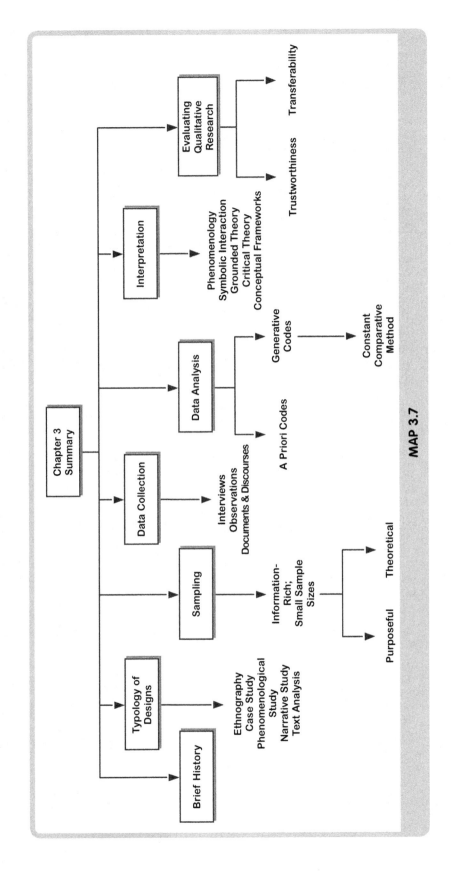

MAP 3.7

KEY TERMS AND CONCEPTS

a priori code

axial code

CAQDAS

case study

complete observer

constant comparative method

covert observation

critical race theory

critical theory

discourses

emic and etic perspectives

ethnography

feminism

full participant

generative code

grounded theory

life story interview

Marxism/neo-Marxism

narrative inquiry

observation

observer-as-participant

official documents

open code

overt observation

participant-as-observer

Patton and Spradley questions

personal documents

phenomenological study

phenomenology

purposive sampling

qualitative research

queer theory

selective code

semistructured interview

standardized interview

structured interview

symbolic interaction

text analysis

theoretical sampling

transferability

trustworthiness

verstehen

REVIEW, CONSOLIDATION, AND EXTENSION OF KNOWLEDGE

1. Using the list of key terms and concepts on page 55, place a check next to each term/concept you are clear about, and place an X next to each one that is still fuzzy in your mind. Then go back into the chapter, review the terms that are fuzzy, and develop a personal glossary.

2. Using an electronic database, search for a qualitative article, read the abstract, and answer the following questions:

   a. What does the abstract tell you about the methodology of the study?

   b. What does it tell you about the design?

   c. What does it tell you about the findings?

3. Indicate the appropriate study design for each research purpose from these choices:

   a. ethnography

   b. case study

   c. phenomenological study

   d. text analysis

   e. narrative study

   ____ This study investigates the way special education teachers in an urban school district think about their working relationship with regular education teachers in the building.

   ____ This study seeks to understand the culture of special education, from the inside out, within a middle-sized suburban school district.

   ____ This study investigates how the decision was made to refuse playground privileges to a child with Asperger's syndrome in a rural elementary school.

   ____ This study aims to understand how one veteran special education teacher has made sense of and given order to her professional and personal life over the past two decades.

   ____ This study investigates how definitions of qualifying disabilities differ in documents in a K–12 district and a local university.

CHAPTER FOUR

Ethnography

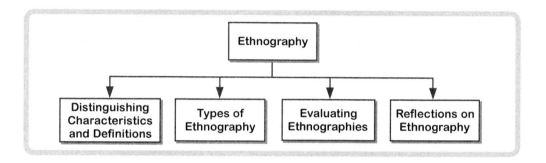

This chapter describes ethnography. It is the original form of qualitative inquiry and is rooted in early 20th-century cultural anthropology, which aimed to describe "native" or "exotic" cultures to a Western audience. From these early beginnings, ethnographic research has evolved and changed to meet new demands.

CHAPTER OBJECTIVES

✓ Understand that ethnography is the original qualitative design.
✓ Understand the major concepts and terms associated with ethnography.
✓ Understand fieldwork/participant observation and field notes as signature ethnographic practices.
✓ Understand that participant observation interweaves data from observations, interviews, and texts to produce a convincing narrative.
✓ Understand the types of ethnographies and their relation to interpretive frameworks.
✓ Understand how to evaluate ethnographies for trustworthiness.
✓ Understand the contribution of ethnographic research to education.

DISTINGUISHING CHARACTERISTICS AND DEFINITIONS   MAP 4.1

Ethnography: Describing and Interpreting Culture

Ethnography describes and interprets a culture or a cultural group.

The term *ethnography* is derived from the Greek, meaning "writing of culture." Traditionally, culture was defined as a people's "way of life," consisting of social structures and patterns of behavior that are passed down from generation to generation. A more contemporary account defines culture as "webs of significance that actors spin for themselves" (Geertz, 1973, p. 5). Both definitions provide a view of culture as a complex organism with intricately connected patterns of interactions among actions, relationships, and meanings.

Ethnographic researchers engage personally with *actors* (the research participants) over a prolonged period of time in order to develop understandings about their social situation from the actors' own perspectives. Depending on themselves as the instruments for data collection, the researchers observe and record people and events, interview actors, and collect documents in an ongoing way. They engage in an iterative process of analysis and use a variety of lenses to interpret findings. The signature practices of the ethnographer are *participant observation* and the recording of *field notes*.

Participant Observation

Participant observation is the method of data collection that occurs during fieldwork and involves the researcher's participation in the setting and the systematic collection of data through observations, interviews, and texts.

One of the most cogent explanations of participant observation and fieldwork appeared in a classic book by the anthropologist Hortense Powdermaker (1966), entitled *Stranger and Friend*:

Fieldwork and participant observation require both involvement and detachment. Taken together, they are both an art and a science. Involvement is necessary to understand the

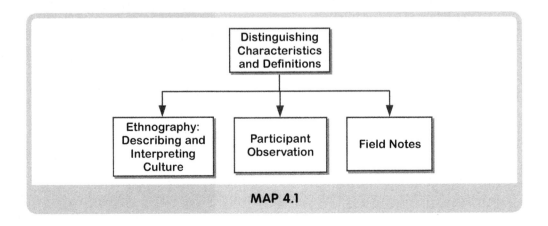

MAP 4.1

psychological realities of a culture, that is, its meanings for the indigenous member. Detachment is necessary to construct the abstract reality: a network of social relations, including the rules and how they function—not necessarily real to the people studied. (p. 9)

The term *participant observation* may be misleading. It is a broad term that depends on the interweaving of three sources of data (observations, interviews, and documents/discourses) into a holistic narrative. As a participant observer, a researcher tries to collect data in an organic way and may focus on various combinations of the following: (1) actors—their physical appearance and dress, their use of language, their body language and nonverbal cues (called *kinesics*), the individual actions they perform, and the group activities in which they engage; (2) informal and formal events that occur; (3) the physical environment and physical objects that are present and the ways in which they use space (called *proxemics*); (4) the dialogues and informal conversations that take place; (5) the goals that actors are trying to accomplish; and/or (6) the feelings and emotions that are felt and expressed (Spradley, 1980, p. 78; Bogdan & Biklen, 1982, pp. 85–86).

As a participant observer, a researcher may simply observe and record occurrences and events without systematic planning, may choose to focus on critical incidents that have special meaning and importance, or may schedule interviews and observations with the actors. Some observers prefer simply to listen and look, and to record their observations later in a field journal. Others prefer to take notes, to jot down ideas, or to use audio or video technology to record events as they occur. Interviews are informal, resembling natural conversations at first, and going deeper as the situation warrants and as the researcher begins to embed questions into the conversation. Official and personal documents that are readily available in a setting offer another perspective on what a group values and uses; they can also provide an opening for conversation and also corroborate other sources of data. Generally, researchers conducting full-fledged ethnographies depend on unobtrusive measures like unannounced observations and informal conversations, while case study researchers generally schedule observations and use a variety of interview formats and semistructured interviews.

Chapter Three makes a distinction between *covert* and *overt* observations and their various research stances. The same distinction holds for the broader concept of participant observation. In terms of ethics, an overt approach is the better choice: It is based on an honest relationship between researcher and actors; it allows a researcher to collect and record data openly; and it minimizes the risk of the researcher's "going native" and becoming so immersed in the participant role as to lose objectivity. An overt participant observation stance involves the researcher as either a *participant-as-observer* or an *observer-as-participant*, depending on whether the researcher plays a natural role in the setting. However, overt observation is not without its disadvantages and can lead to an *observer effect*. Although covert participant observation avoids the risk of observer effect and allows the researcher to study groups and situations that might otherwise be inaccessible, its disadvantages outweigh its advantages. It runs the risk of leaving actors with whom a trusting relationship has been built feeling upended by the researcher's precipitous and unexplained exit, or resentful of having been studied without their full knowledge and consent. Most contemporary ethnographies and all ethnographic case studies use overt participant observation.

Although the unit of analysis differs in ethnographies and ethnographic case studies (the former focusing on a culture, group, or setting, and the latter on an event or program), in both cases researchers rely heavily on individuals as *key informants*. Such informants are "a few individuals selected on the basis of criteria such as knowledge, compatibility, age, experience, or reputation who provide information about their culture" (Definitions of anthropological terms, 2013). Although a researcher may have an initial idea about whom to select as key informants, that often changes once the researcher is in the field. Key informants may be the people with the most knowledge about a setting, or those who are of the highest or lowest status, or leaders or followers, or the most communicative, or members of different role groups or social formations who can articulate a point of view that is not usually heard. In the final analysis, selecting key informants relies on the judgment of the researcher.

Field Notes

Field notes are "the written account of what the researcher hears, sees, experiences, and thinks in the course of collecting and reflecting on the data of a qualitative study" (Bogdan & Biklen, 1982, p. 74).

Field notes are descriptive, interpretive, and reflective. Clifford Geertz (1973) coined the term *thick description* to capture the interaction of description and interpretation in field notes, and he distinguished this from *thin description*, which only records facts and observations.

Descriptive field notes describe in detail settings, actors, events, and activities, and reproduce the actual language, dialect, and idiosyncratic usage of the actors.

Reflective field notes describe the researcher's view of the process and progress of the inquiry, and contribute to interpretation.

In descriptive field notes, the emphasis is on concreteness; good descriptions do not use evaluative or abstract language. For example, instead of reporting, "Jane looked happy," an ethnographer would write, "Jane's lips were parted in a smile; her eyes were crinkled; and her head was tilted to one side." In describing a setting, the ethnographer would note every detail of the physical space and might make drawings and diagrams of the placement of desks or books and other visual representations.

In reflective field notes, "the more subjective side of the researcher's journey is recorded. The emphasis is on speculation, feelings, problems, ideas, hunches, and impressions. Also included is material in which the researcher lays out plans for future research as well as clarifies and corrects misunderstandings in the field notes" (Bogdan & Biklen, 1982, p. 86). Ethnographic researchers intersperse reflective commentary throughout their field notes; they separate such comments from descriptions by the bracketed notation *[oc]* (for *observer comment*), as a way to protect against their imposing their own experience and meanings upon a situation, and as a guide to what data may need confirmation through triangulation and member checks.

TYPES OF ETHNOGRAPHY

MAP 4.2

Realist Ethnography

The focus of ethnography has been and continues to be on describing and interpreting culture. However, contemporary ethnography is not the *realist* ethnography of the early 20th century, which emerged just as cultural anthropology was becoming established as a discipline. Realist ethnography is representative of "a mode of writing in which the author enters a culture or group and seeks to represent the reality of a whole world or form of life" (Marcus & Cushman, 1982, p. 29). It rests on the premise that researchers can leave personal experiences and biases at the door, and can develop a neutral, objective, and true-to-life description of how actors view and make sense of their world.

Realist ethnographers viewed culture from what is called a *functionalist* perspective, which sees each human society as an organic whole consisting of related parts, each with a specific purpose. The purposes may be as diverse as meeting the differing psychological needs of individuals or meeting the needs of the society as a whole to sustain itself. In any case, the focus is more on social structures and less on individual actors, who usually remain nameless. Later in the 20th century, various intellectual and social influences challenged this idea of ethnography, and ethnographers' methods moved away from "taxonomic descriptions of behavior and social structure toward thick descriptions and interpretations of symbol and meaning" (Anderson, 1989, p. 249). Contemporary approaches use the interpretive lenses that have been described in Chapter Three along the emic–etic continuum (see Figure 3.1). The

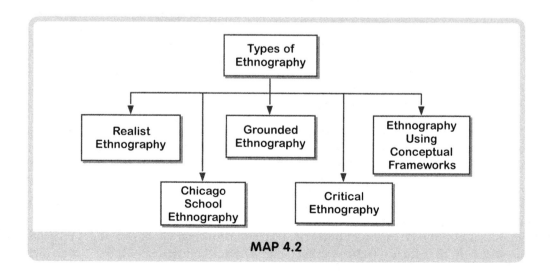

MAP 4.2

following approaches and interpretive lenses are discussed below, and an example of each approach is provided.

> Chicago school ethnography: Symbolic interaction
>
> Grounded ethnography: Grounded theory
>
> Critical ethnography: Critical theories
>
> Ethnography using conceptual frameworks

Chicago School Ethnography

The term *Chicago school ethnography* identifies ethnographies that use symbolic interaction as their interpretive lens. As noted in Chapter Three, symbolic interaction was first developed by members of the sociology department at the University of Chicago in the 1930s, who wanted to uncover the negotiated meanings of actors within a setting, and to understand the process by which a group or subculture ascribed behavioral expectations or labels to actors and how those actors assumed the behaviors of their assigned labels. Phil Cusick (1983) described the role of Chicago school ethnographers as "to unravel and explain the complexity of the events so that others who share similar circumstances may find ways to express and understand their world" (p. 143).

Example of Chicago School Ethnography

Rist, R. (1970). Student social class and teacher expectations: The self-fulfilling prophecy in ghetto education. *Harvard Educational Review, 40*(3), 411–451.

Rist spent 3 years as a participant observer in a school where all of the students and teachers were African American, and he followed one group of students as they progressed from kindergarten through second grade. Rist undertook this study as a graduate student under the direction of Jules Henry. He wrote 30 years later:

> From the beginning Jules Henry directed the study according to an intensive field-based and observational/ethnographic methodology. The expectation was there would be up [to] fifteen hours of fieldwork. . . . We were to prepare elaborate and detailed field notes on each site visit and then subsequently code according to a coding scheme that the team developed. (Rist, 2000, p. 135)

After just 8 days observing the kindergarten class, Rist observed that the teacher had assigned students to one of three tables. In an early interview, the teacher explained to Rist that she had placed at Table 1 those students whom she labeled were "fast learners," that students at Table 2 were those she labeled "average learners," and that students at Table 3 were those she described as having "no idea what was going on in the classroom." Noting that no formal assessment had taken place, Rist looked for clues that might provide insight into the teacher's thinking. He observed the physical presentation of students at the various tables and noted differences in skin coloring,

conditions of hygiene and clothing, interactions with the teacher, and uses of language at the three tables. He also examined official school documents that reported
family income, enrollment in welfare programs, parental employment status, level of
parental education, and the number of children in each family. When he compared
these data with the table assignments, he uncovered a pattern of placement that coin-
cided with the social and economic status of the children. In a later interview with
the teacher, Rist discovered that she had been raised in a middle-class, two-parent
family similar to those of the children at Table 1. This led Rist to view the teacher's
labeling of students as a search for "an ideal type" that reflected her own life experience and biases.

As the year progressed, Rist observed the following teacher behaviors: (1) She
moved the blackboard in front of Table 1, making it most difficult for students at
Table 3 to see the material; (2) she positioned herself close to Table 1 students and at
a distance from those at Tables 2 and 3; and (3) she directed her instruction to those
closest to her, and responded more frequently to raised hands from Table 1 students.
He also made note of student behaviors at the end of the school year, including the
following: (1) The students at Tables 2 and 3 made fewer attempts to gain the teacher's attention; (2) Table 1 students made frequent derisive remarks to those at Tables 2
and 3, while no student at those tables made such remarks to Table 1 students; (3) the
students at Tables 2 and 3 turned on each other with name calling and threats; and
(4) some students at Tables 2 and 3 withdrew physically from instructional activities,
while others began to teach each other. Summarizing his observations in the kindergarten classroom, Rist (1970) wrote:

> Lack of communication with the teacher, lack of involvement in the class activities and
> infrequent instruction all characterized the situation of the children at Tables 2 and 3. Dur-
> ing one observational period of an hour in May, not a single act of communication was
> directed towards any child at Table 2 or 3 by the teacher except for twice commanding "sit
> down." (p. 425)

Rist followed the students into second grade, where he observed repetitions of
the behaviors and interactions that he had observed in kindergarten. He consulted
official school documents that reported student test scores at the end of second
grade, and noted that they corresponded to the original placement of students at
Tables 1, 2, and 3 during the first 8 days of kindergarten. His visits to the class
in second grade confirmed his earlier observations. He ended his study with the
proposition that the labels and expectations the kindergarten teacher had imposed
on the children by the eighth day of kindergarten foreshadowed their later achievement and school success.

Grounded Ethnography

As the name implies, *grounded ethnography* uses grounded theory for data analysis and
interpretation. Grounded theory, as described in Chapter Three, expands on symbolic interaction in that researchers generate and validate a theory from their data.

In this approach, data collection and analysis go hand in hand, and researchers use the constant comparative method, theoretical sampling, and negative case sampling.

Example of Grounded Ethnography

Harry, B., Sturges, K. M., & Klingner, J. K. (2005). Mapping the process: An exemplar of process and challenge in grounded theory analysis: *Educational Researcher, 34*(2), 3–13.

This article reported on a grounded ethnography study of placements in special education. The ethnography lasted 3 years and involved three phases. In Phase 1, the researchers collected data that helped them select a purposeful sample of schools, where they audiotaped 71 interviews with school staff. They asked: "What do you think explains overrepresentation?" In Phase 2, the researchers assumed the roles of observer-as-participant. In this phase, they (1) observed all of the K–3 classrooms in the 12 schools, (2) observed a theoretical sample of two teachers and their classrooms 8–12 times each, and (3) completed "exit interviews" for a theoretical sample of 24 teachers. In Phase 3, the researchers selected a theoretical sample of 12 students for in-depth case studies. A detailed description of one of the cases is provided in this article.

Analysis involved open and axial coding. The researchers made clear that as they moved to axial codes, they were identifying categories or properties that "are being identified through the interpretive lens of the researcher, who is already beginning to abstract meaning from the data" (p. 5); this is always the case in grounded theory. Analysis proceeded through five levels toward the development of an explanatory theory:

Level 1: Open coding based on original interviews

Level 2: Categories developed from the codes

Level 3: Themes developed from the categories

Level 4: Testing the themes for explanations

Level 5: Interrelating the explanations

The researchers found three interrelated explanations: family stereotyping, internal deficits, and inequitable opportunity to learn. They made use of other researchers to review their data collection and analysis procedures, and they developed visual maps to represent the five levels of analysis and the three interrelated themes. In conclusion, they noted:

> Our interrelation of the explanations showed that no single explanation could stand alone. None could be supported or refuted without reference to another explanation with which it interacted. For research concerned with the nuances of human behavior, we consider this a realistic finding, one that underscores the difficulty of measuring complex social processes. (p. 10)

Critical Ethnography

Critical ethnography has been characterized as "conventional ethnography with a political purpose" (Thomas, 1993, p. 4). Applying a wide range of critical theories, it challenges the assumptions of realist ethnography in terms of the idea of culture and representation, and it questions the ideas of culture and of a researcher's authorial authority. Critical ethnography critiques the idea of culture on the grounds that "It freezes stereotypes; creates 'others'; enforces an artificial coherence within a group; dismisses within-group variations; ignores how external power relations, for example, in capitalism, affect culture; ignores how internal power relations oppress some members of a cultural group" (Eisenhart, 2001, p. 2). It challenges the authorial authority of the researcher as the sole agent of representation, beneath the "holistic analysis of structure and processes of culture" (McQueen & Knussen, 2002, p. 22), and it probes the external social, economic, and political forces that mediate meanings and that keep the oppressed in a continued state of oppression. In effect, critical ethnography rejects the view that ethnographers can be value-neutral in their interpretations and acknowledges a researcher as being very much a part of the power structure that is being critiqued. Critical ethnographers directly address how their own experiences, cultural backgrounds, and intentions influence the stories they tell. "This is a process . . . a process of self reference" (Davies, 1999, p. 4). In effect, reflexivity is critical reflection.

Although there is no agreed-upon way to conduct a critical ethnography, it is fair to say that a researcher first logs and codes data in ways similar to the Chicago school and grounded ethnography approaches, and then engages in a process of collaborative critique with the actors. This involves making connections to other settings and experiences, and seeking further understanding through the lens of critical theories. It is a collaborative and democratic process that has "the researcher attaining an insider's view of the cultural group and group members attaining an insider's view of research culture" (Carspecken, 1996, p. 207). It has as its ultimate goal an activist stance that leads to emancipation from oppression.

Example of Critical Ethnography

Motha, S. (2006). Racializing ESOL teacher identities in U.S. K–12 public schools. *TESOL Quarterly, 40*(3), 495–518.

Motha's study applied feminist and critical race theory to an ethnography of four novice teachers of English for speakers of other languages (ESOL); three of the teachers were European American, and one was Korean American. The author made explicit that she was assuming a critical approach and described the ethnography as "a year-long critical feminist ethnography . . . that examined the implications of teachers' privileged status as native speakers of standard English, a raced category, within an institutional culture that underscored the supremacy of both Whiteness and native speaker status" (p. 495). She further acknowledged how her past experiences with the four actors, whom she taught and supervised during their preparation program, created a "power imbalance" that—despite her best efforts—could not be completely eliminated (p. 501).

Motha collected data from observations of the four teachers in their classrooms and conducted interviews with them, as well as with students, administrators, and other faculty members. She also examined texts in the form of official school documents, examples of student work, email exchanges, and audiotaped phone conversations. In the final two stages of her research, she used transcripts of the conversations, or discourses that occurred during afternoon teas that she held with the four teachers. During these teas the teachers and the researcher reflected on their own racial and gendered identities, the impact of these identities on their students, and the ways in which school policies had gender and racial undertones. The teas also served as a setting where the teachers could support each other in developing teaching strategies that challenged the oppressive elements of school practices.

Motha began her analysis by using a constant comparative approach to coding the data from the afternoon teas, where she and the teachers had collaboratively constructed a "critical, racialized" analysis of school practices. She employed the constant comparative method of analysis to code and analyze the data. The major themes that emerged had to do with how the teachers negotiated their own racial identities and how language was being "racialized" within classrooms and the larger school community. Central to this last point was the development of a critique of Standard English and its seemingly value neutrality. The researcher concluded:

> Standard English often serves as a code for White English, with its ostensible neutrality suppressing the racialized nature of language discrimination. The tacit assumption that Standard English is racially neutral is related to the social, and particularly discursive, construction of White as neutral. . . . The inseparability of Whiteness from Standard English both reflects and reinforces White privilege. (p. 515)

Ethnography Using Conceptual Frameworks

Unlike the other ethnographic approaches, the fourth type of ethnography uses categories and concepts that are derived from a comprehensive literature review as initial codes. While this form of ethnography starts with a deductive theory, it also generates from the data secondary codes that describe unanticipated findings.

Example of a Conceptual Frameworks Ethnography

Hull, G. A., & Zacher, J. (2007). Enacting identities: An ethnography of a job training program. *Identity: An International Journal of Theory and Research, 71*(1), 71–102.

The authors used the general concept of *identity development* as the framework for their ethnography of an adult job training program. Having reviewed research that considered the complicated relationship between identity development and job-related skills development, they identified three concepts that elaborated on the original framework for their study. These were the psychological concepts of *enacted identities*, *mediational means*, and *performative moments*, and they were used to guide the coding and analysis of the data.

The two researchers took jobs as teachers of writing in the program and functioned as participants-as-observers for 18 months. They collected data from multiple sources and in multiple forms. They also took detailed field notes of their observations in class and during extracurricular activities; videotaped and audiotaped community events; taped and transcribed oral history interviews with the director and three students; conducted phone interviews with two students who had dropped out; and maintained contact with the director and several students for 2 years after the initial fieldwork. They also collected written student journals and scripts, flyers, newspaper articles about the program, and class handouts.

Data analysis proceeded in three stages. In the first stage, the researchers looked for patterns in their field notes, interviews, and texts; checked with the director and students on the accuracy of the data and themes; and divided the data into seven large units of analysis. In the second stage, the researchers revised the categories, eliminating some and combining others. In the third stage, they "reread and reorganized our categories, juxtaposing them to the sociocultural literature on identity formation" (p. 87). They reorganized the data under the original conceptual framework, added the category *reorientations of self* (p. 87), and described how the four concepts interacted with each other.

EVALUATING ETHNOGRAPHIES

MAP 4.3

In evaluating an ethnography, the reader should use the rubric provided in Chapter Three (see Figure 3.2). The guiding question for trustworthiness is this: Does the ethnography present a detailed portrait of the culture or group under study? The reader should pay particular attention to the stance of researchers and their theoretical and ideological commitments, the duration of their presence in the field, and the use of thick descriptions and triangulation.

Rist's (1970) ethnography of teacher expectations and student achievement in an urban elementary school provides a detailed portrait of three elementary classrooms.

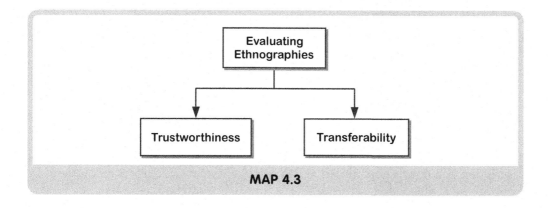

MAP 4.3

However, due to some omissions in the final text, the study earns only a moderate rating for trustworthiness. In regard to his research stance, the author describes how he chose the context for the study, but he does not describe the choices he made about the research process itself or his interpretive lens. Given his use of labeling theory, one can infer that he used a symbolic interaction approach, but this was not made explicit. Having spent 3 years in the field, Rist provides strong evidence of prolonged engagement as an observer-as-participant. There is ample thick description of student behaviors and physical characteristics and of teacher behaviors and movements around the room, as well as the use of direct teacher quotes and of official documents on file at the school. There is evidence that the author triangulated these data in the process of data collection. In addition, the researcher was in the field for a prolonged period of engagement. Absent, however, is any mention of checks for accuracy or reflection. More important, there is no mention of the process of analysis by which the author transformed data into themes. The study would be likely to resonate with a reader with an interest in the topic or experience with a similar circumstance, due to its use of thick description and the theoretical sampling.

Harry et al.'s (2005) grounded ethnography of special education placement provides a detailed portrait of the process of placements and is strong in trustworthiness. The authors have made their research stance clear by announcing their interpretive stance at the outset. In a grounded ethnography, we would expect authors to place less emphasis on thick description of actors and context, and more on how data are transformed into themes. However, this is not the case here, as the authors include a detailed account of a case study and its central actor. The prolonged engagement in the field, collaboration among the authors, and peer reviews by other researchers are indications of trustworthiness. The same is true for the use of member checks and triangulation during the ongoing processes of data collection and analysis, and for the reflective interaction among the researchers. The detailed descriptions of how data are transformed into themes and how theories are constructed are especially robust. Due to its thick description and thoughtful sampling, the study would be likely to resonate with a reader with an interest in the equity of special education or with direct experience with placement procedures.

Motha's (2006) critical feminist ethnography provides a detailed description of the experience of novice teachers in the school under study and is strong in trustworthiness. Its clear statement of research and its ongoing reflexivity are the hallmarks of critical ethnography. The author's use of first-person pronouns to describe her own life circumstances and those of the teachers she was studying, as well as her embedded reflections about method, relationships, and concern with power, are further evidence of critical stance and reflexivity. In addition, she was engaged in the setting for a prolonged period of time and provides thick description, replete with verbatim transcriptions of conversations, detailed observations, and descriptions of texts that triangulate data. In collaboratively constructing coding categories and interpretation, Motha maintained ongoing checks on the accuracy of data and the transformation of data into themes through the constant comparative method. The use of thick description and purposeful sampling makes it likely that a reader with an interest in feminist and racial analyses of schooling would find this study transferable.

Hull and Zacher's (2007) conceptual frameworks ethnography of a job training program also provides a detailed portrait of the setting and culture under study and demonstrates strong trustworthiness. The authors are explicit in describing their choice of their research position as participating teachers and observing researchers in the program under study, and are also clear about the use of conceptual frameworks as lenses for analysis and interpretation. They provide a detailed description of how they transformed data into themes and how they juxtaposed the conceptual frameworks with the data. They provide thick descriptions of the setting and the actors, reproducing actual language and describing a wide variety of events in detail. Triangulation is evident in the authors' use and cross-referencing of multiple data sources; there is also evidence of member checks with two key actors. Checks for accuracy were achieved through member checks with two key actors and through the ongoing interaction and reflection of the two researchers. Thick description and purposive sampling make it likely that a reader with an interest in the psychology of identity formation or experience in a similar setting would resonate with the study and find the findings transferable to another context.

REFLECTIONS ON ETHNOGRAPHY

As this chapter has demonstrated, ethnographic designs continue to evolve to meet new demands and interests. Their contribution to research in education cannot be overstated, as Harry Wolcott (1987) exhorted:

> Let educators of other persuasions do the counting and measuring they do so well. Ethnographers have their commitment and their unique contribution to make within the educational community. That commitment is not to technique per se. . . . the contribution is in helping educators better understand both the little traditions of schools and the bigger traditions of the larger society. (p. 50)

Ethnographic research helps educators see the familiar in unfamiliar ways: It illuminates practices; uncovers taken-for-granted assumptions; and provides insights about the multiple perspectives that various actors bring to the experience of a particular class, classroom, or school experience.

CHAPTER SUMMARY   MAP 4.4

✓ Ethnography is the original qualitative research design, and it describes and interprets a culture or a cultural group.

✓ The key practices of ethnography are participant observation and field notes.

✓ Field notes include thick descriptions, which are both descriptive and reflective/interpretive.

✓ The first ethnographies were realist ethnographies.

✓ Contemporary ethnographies and their interpretive lenses include the Chicago school ethnography (symbolic interaction), grounded ethnography (grounded theory), critical ethnography (critical theories), and ethnography using conceptual frameworks.

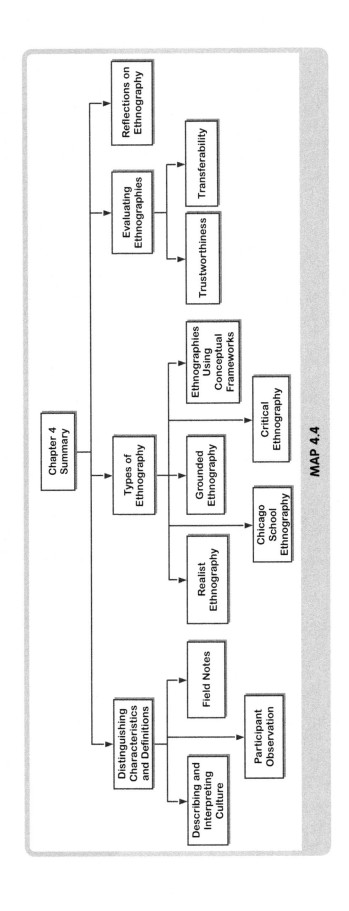

MAP 4.4

✓ Ethnography should be evaluated for trustworthiness and transferability, as described in Chapter Three. Trustworthiness includes evidence of research stance, thick description, sampling, triangulation, checks for accuracy, transforming data into themes, reflection, and prolonged engagement. Transferability is a matter of subjective judgment on a reader's part, but this judgment is based on thick description and sampling.

KEY TERMS AND CONCEPTS

actors/informants

Carspecken steps of critical method

Chicago school

critical ethnography

descriptive field notes

ethnography

field notes

grounded ethnography

grounded theory

labeling

reflective field notes

reflexivity

symbolic interaction

theoretical sampling

thick description

REVIEW, CONSOLIDATION, AND EXTENSION OF KNOWLEDGE

1. Using the list of key terms and concepts above, place a check next to each term/concept you are clear about, and place an X next to each one that is still fuzzy in your mind. Then go back into the chapter, review the terms that are fuzzy, and develop a personal glossary.

2. Using an electronic database, search for an ethnography on a topic of interest. Follow the Guide to Reading below as you work through the article. Then, using the Guide as a template, write a critique (about 750 words long) of the ethnography you have selected.

Guide to Reading

Research Review: What is the purpose of the review? Where is it located in the article? What research does the author choose to review? Is it relevant? Is it recent?

Purpose and Design: What is the purpose of the ethnography? Are research questions posed? If so, what are they? What type of ethnography is it? Is the type of ethnography appropriate for the purpose?

Sampling: What sampling strategy was used to select the culture, group, or setting? How were key actors selected? How many were selected? What were the characteristics of these key actors?

Data Collection: What was the researcher's role in the setting, and what was the researcher's relationship with the actors? What kinds of data were collected—interviews, observations, documents? How and where were data collected and recorded, and over what period of time?

Data Analysis, Interpretation, and Conclusions: How were the data transformed into themes and patterns? Was coding used? If so, was it identified and explained clearly? Did the researcher use any metaphors? Visual representations? How was analysis checked? What interpretive lens or theoretical perspective does the author apply to findings? What are the conclusions? Has the author overconcluded?

Evaluation: Rate the following as strong, moderate, or weak

Overall quality of the study: Strong, moderate, weak

Trustworthiness: Strong, moderate, weak

Transferability: Strong, moderate, weak

Sample Critique

Hull, G. A., & Zacher, J. (2007). Enacting identities: An ethnography of a job training program. *Identity: An International Journal of Theory and Research, 71*(1), 71–102.

Research Review

The research review is placed at the beginning of the article. Its purpose is to examine the theoretical and empirical literature concerning the sociological concepts of *enacted identity*, *performative moments*, and *mediational means* (p. 79) that the researchers used as the framework for the study. In addition, the review provided a context for the study by reviewing federal policy in regard to job training programs.

Purpose and Design

The purpose of the study was to explore how participants in a job training program experienced changes in their identity as the program progressed. Three research questions were raised:

(a) What kinds of identities did students enact, and how did these identities change in the course of the program? (b) What tensions or points of convergence were there between students' identities and the identities proffered by the program? and (c) How did those tensions or points of convergence play out in participants' identity work? (p. 80)

This is an example of a conceptual frameworks ethnography: The researchers used the concepts developed in the research review to frame the study. It qualifies as ethnography because the researchers participated in the setting over time and used multiple methods of data collection. This design allowed Hull and Zacher to gain access to the social world of the participants in a natural setting.

Sampling

The purposeful sampling involved the selection of the setting and the actors. The setting was a job training program that prepared adults for work in the computer and electronics industries and aimed to change their perceptions of themselves. The sample of actors consisted of nine students who completed a writing class in the program. Two of the students were identified as key informants. In addition, the director of the program was observed and interviewed.

Data Collection

The two researchers assumed roles as overt participants-as-observers by becoming writing instructors in the program:

> We came to City Jobs as researchers intending to study the workings of a promising vocational program. We soon realized, however, that were we to become party to the kinds of information that we sought we would need to find ways to take part legitimately in the day-to-day workings of the program. (p. 81)

Hull and Zacher spent 18 months collecting data in the form of observations, interviews, and documents. They took detailed field notes of their observations in class and during extracurricular activities; videotaped and audiotaped community events; taped and transcribed oral history interviews with the director and three students; conducted phone interviews with two students who had dropped out; and maintained contact with the director and several students for 2 years after the initial fieldwork. They also collected written student journals and scripts, flyers, newspaper articles about the program, and class handouts.

Data Analysis, Interpretation, and Conclusions

Data analysis proceeded in three stages. In the first stage, the researchers looked for patterns in their field notes, interviews, and artifacts; checked with the director and students on the accuracy of the data and themes; and divided the data into seven large units of analysis. They found, "These units of analysis in and of themselves were not sufficient to explain the intricate phenomenon of the identity work in which students engaged throughout the program; to further understand how it took place, we contrasted some of the larger units against each other" (p. 87). In the second stage, the researchers revised the categories, eliminating some and combining others. In the third stage, they "reread and reorganized our categories, juxtaposing them to the sociocultural literature on identity formation " (p. 87). They reorganized the data under the conceptual framework established in the research review (identity enactment, mediational means, and performative moments), and added the category *reorientations of self* (p. 87). The researchers described how these concepts interacted with each other.

Evaluation

This conceptual frameworks ethnography merits a rating of strong. First, it demonstrates strong trustworthiness. The authors are explicit in describing their choice of positionality as participating teachers and observing researchers in a job training program and are also clear about the use of conceptual frameworks as lenses for analysis and interpretation. They provide a detailed description of how they transformed data into themes and how they juxtaposed the conceptual frameworks with the data. They provide thick descriptions of the setting and the actors, reproducing actual language and describing a wide variety of events in detail. Triangulation is evident in the authors' use and cross-referencing of multiple data sources; there is also evidence of member checks with two key actors. Checks for accuracy were achieved through the member checks with two key actors and through the ongoing interaction and reflection of the two researchers. Thick description and purposive sampling make it likely that a reader with an interest in the psychology of identity formation or experience in a similar setting would resonate with the study and find the findings transferable to another context.

CHAPTER FIVE

Other Qualitative Designs

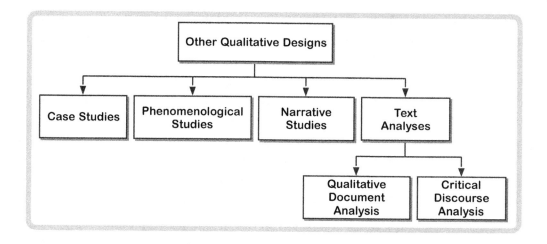

All qualitative research is rooted in ethnography. This chapter describes five qualitative designs that adapt ethnographic practices and interpretive lenses for purposes other than describing and interpreting a culture. These designs include case studies, phenomenological studies, narrative studies, and two types of text analysis (qualitative document analysis and critical discourse analysis).

CHAPTER OBJECTIVES

✓ Understand how case studies, phenomenological studies, narrative studies, and two types of text analysis (qualitative document analysis and critical discourse analysis) adapt the methods of ethnography for different purposes.

✓ Understand the bounded nature of case studies.

✓ Understand how case studies differ from ethnographies.

✓ Understand the types of case studies and methods of analysis and interpretation.

✓ Understand phenomenological studies and methods of data collection, analysis, and interpretation.

✓ Understand narrative studies; their nature and types; and methods of data collection, analysis, and interpretation.

✓ Understand the two types of text analysis, the various types of texts, and the ways in which texts are analyzed and interpreted.

CASE STUDIES   MAP 5.1

Definition and Characteristics

A *case study* describes and interprets a "phenomenon of some sort occurring in a bounded context" (Miles & Huberman, 1994, p. 25).

The case study researcher investigates a contemporary real-life event, program, or process. A *bounded context* is one that has a limited focus; it is "fenced in" so that it does not extend beyond the particular situation or program under study. Although ethnographic case studies use the same data sources and analytic procedures as ethnographies, they differ in important ways:

- Case studies provide an in-depth view of a particular program, event, or phenomenon, while ethnographies provide a description and interpretation of a group or culture.
- Data collection is more structured in case studies than in ethnographies, and a researcher relies more heavily on structured interviews with key actors.
- In case studies, quantitative data are often used to provide background information and to identify appropriate cases for a study.
- Case studies require less time in the field than do ethnographies.
- A case study researcher is engaged in the field for a less prolonged and continuous period of time.

Ethnographic case studies have become widely used in educational research because of their bounded nature, narrow focus, and workable time and resource demands. Robert Stake (1994, pp. 236–247) has developed a useful typology of case studies:

- *Intrinsic case studies* investigate a single case in order to develop insight because of an intrinsic interest of the researcher.

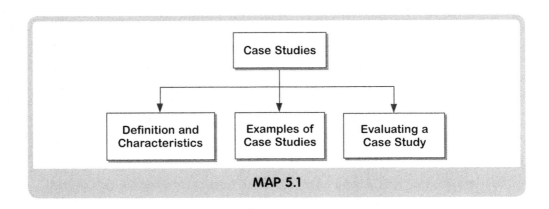

MAP 5.1

- *Instrumental case studies* investigate a single case in order to develop insights into a general issue, concept, or phenomenon that may be representative of other, similar cases.

- *Multiple/collective case studies* (also called *cross-case analyses*) investigate several cases in order to understand a common condition; these case studies are always instrumental and often lead to theorizing about the condition under study.

Three Examples of Case Studies

1. Intrinsic Case Study

Rhoads, R. A. (1995). Whales tales, dog piles, and beer goggles: An ethnographic case study of fraternity life. *Anthropology and Education Quarterly, 26*(3), 306–323.

Rhoads had a particular interest in the experiences of women in university cultures and conducted an intrinsic case study as a way to "highlight aspects of fraternity life that contribute to the ongoing marginalization, and in some cases the victimization of women" (p. 307). Over a period of 6 months, the researcher conducted 12 structured interviews with key actors, engaged in informal conversations, attended fraternity events as an observer-as-participant, and examined documents such as the fraternity handbook and minutes of meetings. Each person interviewed was provided a copy of the interview transcript for comment and clarification. The researcher used Patton's approach to inductive organization in analyzing the data. Using the feminist theory of patriarchy and the critical theories of power and culture, the researcher uncovered the following themes: (1) hostile representations of women, (2) viewing women as passive participants, and (3) a "machismo conception of manhood" (p. 316).

2. Instrumental Case Study

Duke, D., & Landahl, M. (2011). "Raising test scores was the easy part": A case study of the third year of school turnaround. *International Studies in Educational Administration, 39*(3), 91–114.

Duke and Landahl conducted an instrumental case study that was designed to answer a question of concern to educators: How can a school sustain academic gains that occur as a result of a reform initiative? To explore this issue, the researchers looked at an elementary school that had participated in a school turnaround project that had achieved gains in student achievement during the first 2 years of the project and was now in its third year of implementation. When achievement data showed a decline in gains during the third year, the researchers refocused their inquiry in order to gain an understanding of what undermined the school's goal of sustaining the academic gains that had been achieved. The second author was the principal of the school and the key informant. This perspective was triangulated with staff interviews, on-site observations, documents (e.g., minutes of grade-level meetings and school improvement plans), and collected reflections. Using open and axial coding, the researchers concluded that the goal of institutionalizing the reforms of Years 1 and 2 might have undermined the very goal of sustaining academic achievement in Year 3. They suggested the following: (1) An innovative team structure that had been implemented in Years 1 and 2 might have eroded individual teacher responsibility; (2) the focus on reading and math might have led to decreased attention to instruction in science and social studies; (3) the emphasis on the needs of low-achieving students might have overshadowed those of higher-achieving students; and (4) efforts to fully implement a new instructional approach might have taken attention away from focusing on student achievement.

3. Cross-Case Analysis

Hafeil, M., Stokrocki, M., & Zimmerman, E. (2005). Cross-site analysis of strategies used by three middle school art teachers to foster student learning. *Studies in Art Education, 46*(3), 242–254.

The three researchers conducted a cross-case analysis of the instructional practices of three middle school art teachers. They raised the following questions for research: (1) What were the similarities and differences among the teachers' philosophies at the three sites? (2) What art curriculum content and instructional strategies did the teachers use? (3) What instructional resources and new technologies were used to enhance the learning environment? (4) In what ways did the teachers assess their students' learning?

The researchers conducted observations and formal and informal interviews with students and teachers, collected lesson plans, audiotaped classes, and examined student work. They analyzed the data for each site separately, using for initial analysis the conceptual frameworks of teacher philosophies, curriculum emphasis, instructional strategies, and assessment practices. From these data, they generated themes and clustered data into units of meaning for each site. They then "conducted a cross-site analysis in which interrelated, conceptual themes were used to generate insights that illuminated and clarified instructional strategies and contexts in which student learning took place" (p. 243).

The researchers had assumed that they would find geographical differences in curriculum, instruction, and assessment, and were surprised that the cross-case analysis uncovered more similarities than differences. The fact that the three teachers all taught in middle schools serving white, middle-class students led the researchers to conclude, "The type and magnitude of the art curricula developed in the middle schools we studied can be attributed more to middle class contexts than to the impact of geographical location on how and what middle school students were taught" (p. 253).

Evaluating Case Studies

In evaluating a case study, readers should use the rubric provided in Chapter Three. The guiding question for judging the trustworthiness of a case study is this: Does the study answer the research question and capture the complexities of the case? In assessing research stance, the reader should consider whether the case and its boundaries are clearly defined. Below, the three case studies discussed in this section are evaluated.

In terms of trustworthiness, the authors of the three studies discussed above have succeeded in answering the research questions they posed and in capturing the complexity of the cases, each of which had clearly defined boundaries. All three studies are strong in trustworthiness. The authors provide thick descriptions of the context and actors; the reports include direct quotes throughout; and the researchers spent sufficient time in the field to reach data saturation. In the three studies, the researchers collected documents, conducted observations, and triangulated all data. In order to check the accuracy of data, Rhoads provided transcripts for review and comment to the actors, and Duke and Lindahl asked teachers for written reflections. The three researchers in the cross-case study provided checks on each other. The authors of the three studies also provide detailed descriptions of how they reduced data and developed themes. In terms of reflection, the Rhoads study and the Duke and Lindahl study are strong; the cross-case study is less so. In terms of transferability, the thick descriptions and appropriateness and richness of the samples in both cases allow the reader to make connections with other settings and to resonate with and learn from findings.

PHENOMENOLOGICAL STUDIES   MAP 5.2

Definition and Characteristics

Phenomenological studies investigate human experiences (referred to as *lived experiences*) and the meanings these experiences hold for actors.

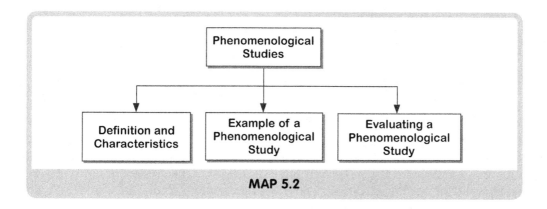

MAP 5.2

Phenomenological researchers search for the "essences" of a phenomenon from the perspective of those who experience it. The goal of the research, then, is to identify the "essence" of a shared experience from the vantage points of actors. This requires researchers to suspend their own prior beliefs, assumptions, and feelings about the phenomenon they are investigating.

Bracketing or *epoche* is the term that describes the process of separating a researcher's world view from that of an actor.

As Keen (1975) explained,

> We want not to see this event as an example of this or that theory that we have; we want to see it as a phenomenon in its own right, with its own meaning and structure. Anybody can hear words that were spoken; to listen for the meaning as they eventually emerged from the event as a whole is to have adopted an attitude of openness to the phenomenon in its inherent meaningfulness. (p. 38)

The major sources of data for phenomenological studies are open-ended interviews of a small number of actors. The interviews are audio- or video-recorded and transcribed for data analysis.

Phenomenological reduction (also known as *eidetic reduction*) is the process of data analysis in phenomenological research.

The process of phenomenological reduction includes (1) a reading of the interview transcriptions to get a sense of the whole; (2) a closer reading that considers the literal words of the actors and the descriptions they provide; (3) developing units of meanings and clustering them into themes that capture commonalities; and (4) identifying the "essence" of the experience or phenomenon through *reflection and synthesis*—the integration of descriptions to produce an understanding of the phenomenon and its meaning to the persons being interviewed.

Example of a Phenomenological Study

McClelland, J. (1995). Sending children to kindergarten: A phenomenological study of mothers' experiences. *Family Relations, 44*(2), 177–183.

The goal of this phenomenological interview study was to understand how mothers experienced the phenomenon of their children's starting kindergarten. More specifically, the researcher was interested in understanding how mothers who had had unsuccessful school careers themselves experienced a common phenomenon. The researcher was forthright in describing her own interest in the phenomenon as a mother, but noted, "When I have drawn on my own experiences, they are designated as such. I tried to maintain fidelity with the transcripts of interviews and used the words of the mothers where possible to express the essence of their experiences" (p. 178).

McClelland identified her sample through a local adult education program. The sample consisted of nine mothers in their 20s and 30s who were all enrolled in an adult education program; all but one had dropped out of junior or senior high school; most were receiving Aid to Families with Dependent Children (AFDC) payments and were unemployed. Each mother was described in detail and interviewed three or four times, either at the adult education center, in her home, or in a public space.

In order to gain an understanding of each mother's own school experience, McClelland began the initial interviews with this statement: "Tell me about going to school when you were a child." The interviews were unstructured and conversational, and shifted to discussions of the experiences the mothers were having with their children's schools and what it was like to send their children to kindergarten. Each conversation was tape-recorded and transcribed. After each interview, McClelland wrote a summary and checked to see whether she had captured the meanings the mothers intended. The author described the process of analysis and interpretation as follows:

> A holistic approach was used to uncover the themes as the conversations progressed, I read the transcripts over and over to grasp the threads of themes and returned to talk again with the mothers, asking them more questions to clarify and develop the themes. I reflected on what they had said and asked them what their experiences meant to them. I read both scholarly work and popular accounts of children disengaging from their parents at varying stages of development. Successive conversations with the mothers helped me to confirm and sharpen the themes after I wrote them in one- or two-page summaries. More extensive drafts of the themes were written, critiqued by other phenomenologists, and rewritten. (p. 179)

The four themes that the researcher identified were "change," "worry," "mixed feelings," and "letting go." Phenomenological, or eidetic, reduction led to an understanding of the "essence" of the experience as one that signaled a major change in the lives of the mothers.

Evaluating a Phenomenological Study

In evaluating a phenomenological study, the reader should again use the rubric provided in Chapter Three. The guiding question for evaluating trustworthiness is this: Does the study capture the "essence" of the experience? In assessing the research stance, a reader should pay particular attention to the use of bracketing; in assessing thick description, a reader should look for copious direct quotes; and in assessing data transformation, take into account the use of phenomenological reduction.

In terms of trustworthiness, the McClelland study is strong in capturing the essence of the experience of sending a child to kindergarten. The author has (1) clearly stated her research stance and made every effort to separate her own experience from that of the participants in her study (this demonstrates *epoche*); (2) provided in-depth descriptions of each of the nine mothers, replete with information about where they lived, their own school experiences, and their relationships and connections to others, as well as verbatim transcripts of the interviews; (3) cross-referenced and compared data from within and across interviews; (4) asked other phenomenological researchers to critique her work; (5) used a process of phenomenological reduction to arrive at themes; and (6) reflected on her method and her relationship to the topic throughout the study. In terms of transferability, a reader with an interest in the phenomenological method and/or in preparing a child for kindergarten would resonate with the findings, due to the thick description of data and portraits of the sample.

NARRATIVE STUDIES   MAP 5.3

Definition and Characteristics

> *Narrative studies* describe and give meaning to the lived experiences of individuals through a collaborative process of storytelling that brings order and coherence to the complexity of human lives.

While at first glance studies appear similar to phenomenological studies, they differ in an important way. Unlike phenomenological interviews, which focus on a clearly limited and defined phenomenon, narratives involve the inquirer and the narrator in a process of storytelling. Connelly and Clandinin (2006) have described the importance of storytelling in this way:

> People shape their daily lives by stories of who they and others are and as they interpret their past in terms of these stories. Story, in the current idiom, is a portal through which a person enters the world and by which their experience of the world is interpreted and made personally meaningful. Narrative inquiry, the study of experience as story, then, is first and foremost a way of thinking about experience. (p. 375)

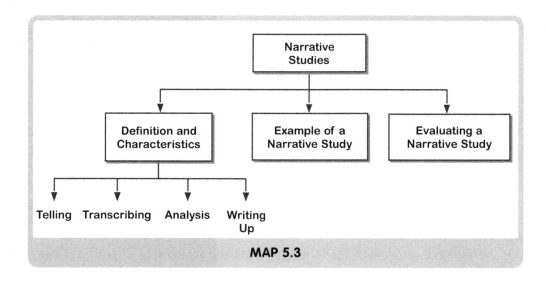

MAP 5.3

The purpose of narrative inquiry is to develop a coherent and well-ordered story that provides insight into the narrator's life experiences. This is done through telling and retelling a story in a dialogic process where the voice of the narrator is privileged and the voice of the researcher is secondary. This process, known as *storying and restorying*, is the central data collection method of narrative inquiry. It may involve several narrators in telling stories about a similar experience, or it may involve one narrator in telling a story of his or her life. Narrative inquiries usually proceed in three stages—*telling, transcribing*, and *analysis* (Reisman, 2002)—before the actual writing up begins.

Telling

There is no set way for telling to occur. In inquiries that collect stories from multiple narrators, the telling may take place in a one-on-one situation or in a group setting. In the one-on-one situation, the telling may begin with interview questions, with informal conversations, or with triggers such as photographs. In the group setting, two or more narrators meet and tell their stories at the same time. In inquires based on a single narrator, the telling involves the narrator in giving a uniquely ordered life history. Lieblich, Tuval-Mashiac, and Zilber (1998) recommended a process that begins by asking the narrator to write a chapter heading for each period of his or her life, and then to fill in each chapter by answering these questions: (1) "Tell me about a significant episode or a memory that you remember from this stage," (2) "What kind of a person were you during this stage?" (3) "Who were significant people for you during this stage, and why?" and (4) "What is your reason for choosing to terminate this stage when you did?" (p. 26).

Transcribing

Transcribing involves transforming the spoken and recorded words into print. This is a time-consuming process; transcribing a 1-hour narrative interview may take up to 6 hours. For this reason, many researchers depend on contracted transcribers, though there are also good reasons for the researchers to do their own transcriptions. In the process of listening to the recorded narratives, the researchers can gain a familiarity with the material and can make note of voice inflections, pauses, and other linguistic indicators. As in interviews, transcriptions serve as the texts for analysis.

Analysis

Analysis begins with a reading and rereading of the transcribed narratives. A researcher usually parses each narrative into segments, generates codes and themes for each segment, and then goes back to reading the whole transcript. These codes and themes are developed via general inductive or constant comparative methods. The researcher uses the words of the narrator to create a plotted story that has a beginning, middle, and end. This process of restorying allows the researcher to identify elements and themes that occur across the autobiographical or the collected narratives. In general, the researcher either conducts an inductive analysis of the narrative's content or engages in a *discourse analysis*, which looks at how language is used at the word, sentence, and text levels to describe, interpret, and explain transcribed data.

Writing Up

After completing the analysis, the researcher usually writes an initial *research text* and brings it back to the narrators for further inquiry. As Clandinin & Huber (2010) explain:

> Interim research texts are often partial texts that are not closed to allowing participants and researchers to further co-compose storied interpretations open to negotiation of a multiplicity of possible meanings. Bringing back interim research texts to further engage in negotiation with participants around unfolding threads of experience is central in composing research texts. The dialogue with participants around interim research texts can lead the inquirer back for more intensive work with the participant if further field texts are needed in order to compose a more complex account of the participants' experiences. (p. 439)

By *further field texts*, Clandinin and Huber mean observational notes, letters, documents, or other media that can add to the final research report or research text. The final written product is meant to be a finely crafted literary work that includes visual images, metaphors, and poetry to represent the complex and multilayered nature of the narrative.

Example of a Narrative Study

DeMilk, S. A. (2008). Experiencing attrition of special education teachers through narrative inquiry. *High School Journal, 92*(1), 22–32.

The author completed separate narratives with five special education teachers, with the aim of uncovering what drove them either to remain as teachers or to leave the field. Acknowledging her own interest in special education and a concern that so many teachers were leaving it, she conducted a research review of the field and concluded that "stories provide a depth of ownership and emotion needed to explore important issues in special education that previous studies have not considered" (p. 24).

Each of the five teacher-narrators was described in a detailed profile and participated in two interviews. The first interview lasted 60–90 minutes and provided space for the telling. The second interview occurred a month later and lasted 30–45 minutes. Between the two sessions, the researcher prepared a transcription of the first interview that was handed to each narrator for review and clarification, and as a prompt for what to reconsider in the retelling. In addition, the researcher took field notes and recorded the emotions, nonverbal expressions, and comfort levels of the narrators during each interview. Analysis was a complex process that began with open and axial coding of each transcription and moved back and forth among rereadings, the development of themes and categories, and a review of relevant literature.

DeMilk used member checks to keep her own stories about special education separate from those of the narrators, and she used graphic organizers to triangulate the data. Upon completing her final analysis, the researcher shared her conclusions with the narrators. While her original intent was to uncover through stories the concerns that drove special educators to stay or leave, DeMilk discovered something quite different:

> The same passion that gave these teachers the drive to remain in the job and continue to help students with disabilities also drove some of them out of the field. All five of the teachers in my study spoke passionately about their students with disabilities and the importance of helping them find success. This passion affected their choice to stay or move. [For those who stayed], the passion they felt gave them fuel to continue in the struggle, despite the problem issues they discussed. This passion gave them the energy they need to survive the hours required for completing the paperwork, to stand firm in their advocacy of their students, and to find creative ways to inspire and educate students so desperately in need of help and support. (p. 31)

In reflecting on the study, the author commented on how the stories that lives tell are often not the stories that researchers think they will hear.

Evaluating a Narrative Study

In evaluating a narrative study, the reader should again use the rubric provided in Chapter Three. The guiding question for the trustworthiness of a narrative study is this: Does the study present a coherent story or collection of stories that ring true? In assessing the research stance, the reader should consider whether and how the researcher maintained neutrality during the interviews. In assessing thick descriptions, the reader should take into account the degree to which the voice of each narrator is privileged over that of the researcher. In judging data analysis, the focus should be on the degree of collaboration between researcher and narrator(s).

In terms of trustworthiness, the DeMilk study develops a coherent reading of the five narratives that rings true. The researcher is clear about her research stance, her rationale for using a narrative approach, and her research question. She made special mention of her efforts to maintain neutrality and not to inject her own experiences into the narratives. The narrators' voices are clear and dominant throughout the study. Thick descriptions in the form of individual profiles create a sense of being present in the narratives. The interviews were extensive and allowed for saturation of data. There is strong evidence of triangulation, along with a detailed description of the process of open and axial coding for data analysis. The researcher and the narrators collaborated throughout the study; the narrators received copies of each transcribed interview for reflection and review. The author's final reflection about the disconnection between her original research question and the narratives she collected is particularly worthy of note, because it describes the equality of authority between the researcher and the researched that narrative studies seek to achieve. In terms of transferability, the rich description of the sample and the strong voices of the narrators allow a reader to connect with and learn from the stories.

QUALITATIVE DOCUMENT ANALYSIS   MAP 5.4

> *Qualitative document analysis* (also called *qualitative content analysis*) describes and interprets written materials that are produced by actors and are not solicited by the researcher.

Definition and Characteristics

What distinguishes a qualitative document analysis from other forms of qualitative research is that the documents exist independently of a researcher's instigation. Educational institutions are replete with official and personal written documents that provide information about the institutions themselves and the people who inhabit them. Formal documents (such as curriculum guides, textbooks, policy manuals, memos, minutes of meetings, news releases, student records, and yearbooks) provide insight into the official messages a school or a school district wants to convey about its social world to internal and external audiences. Personal documents (such as journals, letters, notes, and college admission essays) provide insight into the way that actors make sense of their experiences in the various social worlds they inhabit. More recent forms of personal documents include online forums/discussion groups and blogs.

Since documents exist in such large numbers, a researcher has to decide what to include in the sample and has to set clear guidelines for inclusion and exclusion. As in all qualitative research, (1) the reduction of data into themes may involve generative or a priori coding schemes, or a systematic reading and rereading of the documents; and (2) interpretation depends on the stance of the researcher. The following are two examples of qualitative document analysis, one that examined official documents and the other that studied personal documents.

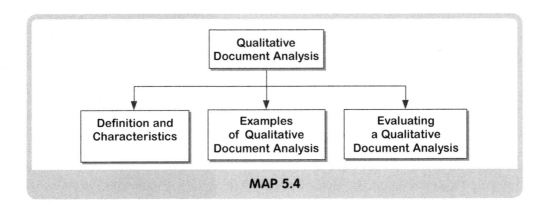

MAP 5.4

Two Examples of Qualitative Document Analysis

1. Analysis of Official Documents

Podeh, E. (2000). History and memory in the Israeli educational system: The portrayal of the Arab–Israeli conflict in history textbooks (1948–2000). *History and Memory,* *12*(1), 65–100.

Podeh conducted a qualitative document analysis of Israeli history textbooks and their portrayals of the events in 1948 that led to the Palestinian exodus and the creation of a refugee problem. His analysis considered three interrelated issues: "(1) the attitudes of historians and education officials toward the role and function of textbooks; (2) the relation between the spirit of the time (zeitgeist) and the content of the textbook; and (3) the impact of historiography on textbooks" (p. 69). The textbooks were divided into three generations, each published during a distinct period in Israel's history. First-generation books were published from 1948 to 1967, when the state of Israel was in its infancy; second-generation books were published from 1975 to 1990, after Israel's victories in the wars of 1967 and 1973; third-generation books appeared after 1990, when a peace process had begun and new historical documents came to light. Both first- and second-generation textbooks were authorized by the state; third-generation books represented a policy shift that allowed schools to select from a wider range of perspectives.

First-generation books placed the blame for the Palestinian exodus exclusively at the feet of the Arab leadership, described it as a voluntary departure, and did not acknowledge that a refugee problem existed. The second-generation texts gave more credence to the Palestinian perspective and corrected false information that had appeared in the first-generation textbooks, but they still blamed the Arab leadership for the events after 1948. They described the movement of whole towns into refugee camps as being voluntary acts, and they painted sanitized versions of the camps. Although the second-generation books presented a more nuanced view of the Arab–Israeli situation, the first two generations of texts provided a unified narrative that was dominated by what Podeh called the "national school of historiography," which strove to promote the current social order, instill values of nationalism, and encourage reverence for Israel's Zionist history and heroes.

While some of the third-generation books continued in the vein of the previous generations, others acknowledged instances of a "deliberate policy of expulsion" (p. 90), admitted to the wretched conditions of the refugee camps, provided accurate data on the number of refugees, and opened discussion about the various ways to interpret history. This generation of textbooks incorporated much of the historiography of what Podeh called the "academic school," which advocated an objective, social-scientific stance and acknowledged "shameful or regrettable episodes in the nation's history" (p. 72).

In the relationship of the textbooks to the spirit of the times, Podeh concluded that the first- and second-generation books served the "goals of a newly emerging society . . . their biased historical narrative can be explained as the need to construct a collective memory and coalesce Israeli society, haunted by a sense of isolation and a siege" (p. 91). The third-generation books reflected "the onset of the peace process in the early 1990s," and, according to Podeh, "the hope that a solution could at last be found to the Arab–Israeli conflict transformed Israeli society's view of the 'enemy' " (p. 84).

2. Analysis of Personal Documents

Pennington, T., Wilkinson, C., & Vance, J. (2004). Physical educators online: What is on the minds of teachers in the trenches? *Physical Educator, 61*(1), 45–56.

The three authors of this article conducted a qualitative document analysis of 333 messages that were posted during 1 month on a listserv that was supported by the National Association for Sport and Physical Education. Since physical educators are often isolated from each other and rarely have the opportunity to talk to each other about their work, the listserv provided a vehicle for communication among peers. The goal of the research was to understand the nature of the messages and what they conveyed about the educators who participated.

The authors analyzed the data by using the constant comparative method; as they explained, "essentially this process consists of comparing and contrasting each unit of information with other units of information to unite those with similar meaning and to separate those with different meaning" (p. 45). Two of the authors assumed responsibility for the actual data analysis, while the third author served as a peer debriefer with whom the other two met weekly during data collection and data analysis.

As a result of their analysis, the authors identified six themes: (1) concerns about professional issues ranging from safety and equipment to salary and professional identity; (2) better ways to implement new lessons and activities that would engage students; (3) instructional strategies for teaching difficult or challenging tasks more effectively; (4) ways in which the use of technology could improve practice; (5) things that listserv participants learned from professional conferences; and (6) ways to advocate for physical education in schools and instruct the public about its importance. Each theme was elaborated with full excerpts from the listserv messages.

The researchers concluded that the postings focused on professional rather than social matters, and that listserv participants were willing to pose and answer questions and to share perspectives and resources with each other. Most important, they found that the listserv alleviated feelings of isolation among members and helped to create a sense of shared responsibility for students and for the profession.

Evaluating a Qualitative Document Analysis

In evaluating a qualitative document analysis, the reader should use the rubric provided in Chapter Three but should omit the quality of engagement, since it is not applicable here. The guiding question for evaluating trustworthiness is this: Does the analysis answer the research question and provide insights into the messages that the documents conveyed? In assessing the research stance, the reader should look for a clear statement of the specific focus of the study and the question(s) it seeks to answer. In making a judgment about sampling, the reader should consider how documents were selected and their appropriateness for the purpose.

In terms of trustworthiness, both of the document analyses described above answer the research questions, provide insights into the messages the documents conveyed, and thus fulfill the purpose of the inquiry. Neither of the studies provides an explicit description of the research stance. However, it is clear that Podeh favors the unfiltered approach advocated by the academic school, and that Pennington and colleagues advocate the use of technology to alleviate the isolation of physical education teachers. Neither article makes explicit reference to triangulation. Both studies reduce data into themes, but again, the authors are not explicit about the methods they used. However, both studies provide clear examples from the documents of each theme they developed. In both cases, the authors reflect on the research, though Podeh's article is much stronger in this regard. In terms of transferability, the selection of documents for examination and the thick descriptions of their contents allow readers to make connections to their own textbooks and electronic messaging.

CRITICAL DISCOURSE ANALYSIS MAP 5.5

Critical discourse analysis applies critical theories to written texts and speech with the aim of identifying underlying ideologies and power relationships.

Definition and Characteristics

By way of analogy, critical discourse analysis is to the study of documents and speech what critical ethnography (see Chapter Four) is to the study of cultures and groups. In educational research, critical discourse analysis looks for the unintended consequences of practices and policies, and examines how they privilege and reproduce existing power relationships and social structures.

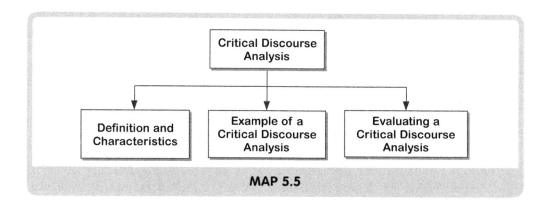

MAP 5.5

Its procedures for analysis are markedly different from those employed in other qualitative designs. Most researchers who use this design use distinctive methods of critical discourse analysis. Fairclough (1993, 1995) proposed three dimensions of this type of analysis: (1) *analysis of text*, which examines language structure; (2) *analysis of discursive practices*, which examines how texts are produced and used; and (3) *analysis of sociocultural practices*, which examines the particular sociocultural context of the discourse. Gee (2004) has made a distinction between "small d" and "large D" discourses. "Small d" discourses have to do with language in use and how it forges social identities, contextualizes meanings, and incorporates cultural models. "Large D" discourses connect language to "other stuff"—the nonlinguistic power relationships and social hierarchies that render some discourses dominant and others marginalized. Gee (2004) explains: "Critical discourse analysis argues that language-in-use is always part and parcel of, and partially constitutive of, specific social practices and that social practices always have implications for inherently political things like status, solidarity, the distribution of social goods, and power" (p. 47). Critical discourse analysis has assumed an increasingly important role in educational research.

Example of a Critical Discourse Analysis

Prins, E., & Toso, B. W. (2008). Defining and measuring parenting for educational success: A critical discourse analysis of the Parent Education Profile. *American Educational Research Journal, 45*(3), 555–596.

This study examined the Even Start Family Literacy Parent Education Profile (Parent Education Profile or PEP), an assessment of parental behaviors that support literacy. The instrument was developed by the New York State Department of Education and uses a scale of 1–5 to rate parental behaviors. The authors located the PEP within two discourses: (1) the discourse on assessment and accountability promoted by the federal government's No Child Left Behind policies and (2) the discourse of parent involvement, which views parents as the first teachers of literacy. Prins and Toso raised three questions for research: (1) How does the text of the PEP construct the ideal parent? (2) What assumptions about parenting and education are evident in the PEP? and (3) What are the ideological effects of these assumptions?

In regard to data collection, the authors explained: "We focused on the scales because they define and categorize more or less desirable literacy-related parenting behaviors and on the support materials because they express how the authors want professionals and parents to use and interpret the PEP" (p. 568). Combining Fairclough's and Gee's analytic frameworks, they analyzed small units of language as well as the larger messages that the text conveys, and clearly explained their analysis in terms of their methods and theoretical stance. They provided numerous examples from the document, linked their analysis to current literatures, and engaged in reflection (or reflexivity) by examining their assumptions as white middle-class educators.

From their analysis, the researchers conclude that the PEP conveys an image of the ideal parent that privileges middle-class values (e.g., independence, self-reliance, and boundary setting), middle-class practices (e.g., reading to children and engaging actively in the school), and middle-class linguistic conventions (e.g., asking open-ended questions and initiating conversation). The authors make the case that the image of the ideal parent conveyed in the documents requires a flexible schedule, disposable income, high-quality child care, and access to social networks that share information about schooling—most or all of which are not available to poor and working-class parents. In their final discussion of findings, the authors state:

> This study illuminates how the PEP discursively constructs the ideal parent and its underlying assumptions about parenting and education, demonstrating how many of its features perpetuate discourses and ideologies that may inadvertently uphold power inequities between poorer and wealthier families, and between participants and professionals. In addition to explicating the content of the ideal parenting model, our analysis shows how the instrument itself, the rating system, standardized format, and instructions for administration serves to rank and normalize parental practices and guide staff and parents toward particular identities, roles, and behaviors. (p. 583)

Evaluating a Critical Discourse Analysis

In evaluating the trustworthiness of a critical discourse analysis, a reader should raise this guiding question: Does the analysis illuminate the norms and power relationships of the dominant culture? A critical research stance should be made explicit and should include specific references to the theoretical commitments of the author. Thick descriptions, in the form of the language used by the speaker or excerpted from the text, should be omnipresent; and a rationale for the selection of the discourse (sampling) should be clearly stated. The process for transforming data into themes should be explained and should refer to methods associated with critical discourse analysis. Reflection, called *reflexivity* in critical discourse analysis, should continue throughout the analysis and should refer specifically to the author's intentions and assumptions. In evaluating transferability, a reader should consider the text selected for analysis and the excerpted language presented in rendering a judgment of applicability. This judgment may also be influenced by the degree to which the reader resonates with the critical perspective.

The Prins and Toso critical discourse analysis meets all of the criteria of trustworthiness described above. Their analysis is successful in illuminating the norms and power relationships embedded in the language of the PEP. They are explicit about their theoretical commitments, their use of critical theory as a lens for analysis, and their rationale for selecting the text. They explain their methods of analysis in some detail, making reference to both the Fairclough and Gee frameworks. They provide lengthy excerpts from PEP and the guide that accompanied it to make the case for their analysis. In terms of transferability, the selection of texts and the use of the language they included make this analysis applicable to other assessment instruments that are used in schools. However, a final judgment about transferability may have more to do with the reader's sympathy with the critical approach than it does with the analysis itself.

CHAPTER SUMMARY   MAP 5.6

✓ Case studies describe and interpret a "phenomenon of some sort occurring in a bounded context" (Miles & Huberman, 1994, p. 25).

✓ There are three kinds of case studies: intrinsic, instrumental, and multiple/collective or cross-case analysis.

✓ The guiding question for judging trustworthiness in a case study is this: Does the study provide an answer to the research question and capture the complexities of the case?

✓ Phenomenological studies investigate human experiences and the meanings these experiences hold for actors.

✓ Bracketing (epoche) separates a researcher's world view from that of an actor in phenomenological studies.

✓ Phenomenological reduction is the process of data analysis in phenomenological research.

✓ The guiding question for evaluating trustworthiness in a phenomenological study is this: Does the study capture the "essence" of the experience?

✓ Narrative studies usually have three stages—telling, transcribing, and analysis—before the actual writing up.

✓ The guiding question for evaluating trustworthiness in a narrative study is this: Does the study present a coherent story or collection of stories that ring true?

✓ Qualitative document analysis examines the content of written products that are not solicited by the researcher.

✓ The guiding question for evaluating trustworthiness in a qualitative document analysis is this: Does the analysis provide insights into the messages that the documents conveyed?

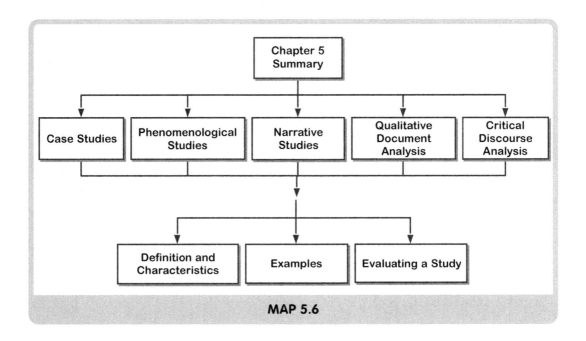

MAP 5.6

✓ Critical discourse analysis applies critical theories to written and oral language with the aim of identifying underlying ideologies and power relationships.

✓ The guiding question for evaluating trustworthiness in a critical discourse analysis is this: Does the analysis illuminate the norms and power relationships of the dominant culture?

KEY TERMS AND CONCEPTS

bracketing/epoche

case study

collective/cross-case analysis

critical discourse analysis

Discourse versus discourse

instrumental case study

intrinsic case study

narrative study

narrator

personal document

phenomenological study

phenomenological/eidetic reduction

qualitative document analysis official document

storying and restorying

REVIEW, CONSOLIDATION, AND EXTENSION OF KNOWLEDGE

1. Describe the similarities and differences in the following pairs of designs:

   ethnography and case study

   phenomenological study and narrative study

   qualitative document analysis and critical discourse analysis

2. Using an electronic database, search for articles using two different qualitative research designs on a single topic or topics (if necessary to find two designs) of interest to you. For each article, fill in the cells on the table below.

	Article 1	Article 2
Title in APA format		
Type of design		
Research questions/purpose		
Research stance		
Data source(s)		
Data analysis		
Guiding question for trustworthiness		

3. Write a short paragraph comparing the two articles you selected and describing how you would evaluate them for trustworthiness.

PART III

Quantitative Research

The Basics

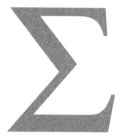

> "If someone separated the art of counting and measuring
> and weighing from all the other arts, what was left of each
> would be, so to speak, insignificant."
>
> —PLATO

Part III marks the transition from the qualitative/postpositivist
paradigm to the quantitative/positivist paradigm. It focuses on
how quantitative researchers select samples and how they collect,
analyze, and display measurable data. This part lays the foundation
for those that follow, which discuss the various designs that come
under the broad umbrella of quantitative research.

CHAPTER SIX

Introduction to Quantitative Research

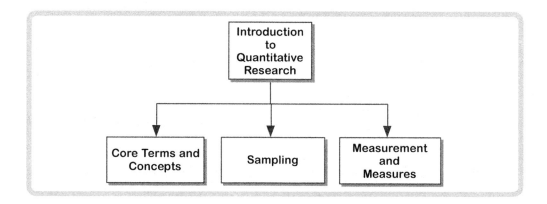

As we shift from qualitative to quantitative research, we shift paradigms from postpositivism (or antipositivism) to positivism. Whereas the goal of the former is to describe and analyze people's subjective states and the meanings they ascribe to their particular life situations, the goal of the latter is to describe and analyze phenomena that can be objectively observed and/or measured and generalized to other people and places. This chapter begins with an introduction to some distinguishing characteristics of quantitative research and then goes into detailed explanations of two more: sampling and measurement.

CHAPTER OBJECTIVES

✓ Define some core quantitative terms and concepts: variables, statistics, and quantitative designs.

✓ Understand sampling, sampling error, and sampling bias.

✓ Understand the difference between a population and a sample, as well as how they are related.

✓ Understand the relationship between the size of a population and the size of a sample.

✓ Understand the difference between random and nonrandom sampling.

✓ Understand the strategies for selecting random and nonrandom samples.

✓ Understand the questions a researcher answers in selecting a measure.

✓ Understand the types of measures and the information they provide.

✓ Understand the response formats used in measures.

✓ Understand how the quality of measures is ensured through procedures for determining validity and reliability.

CORE TERMS AND CONCEPTS   MAP 6.1

Variables

The concept of *variables* is central to developing an understanding of quantitative research.

> *Variables* are those characteristics, attributes, conditions, or qualities of subjects that can be observed and/or measured.

At their most basic level, variables can be classified by their intrinsic characteristics as being either *categorical variables* or *continuous variables.*

> *Categorical (or nominal) variables* can be observed, but not measured.

They are based on some intrinsic trait that can be observed and expressed as a label or category. Because they do not vary in magnitude, categorical variables cannot be assigned a value that can be measured mathematically. For example, occupation, eye color, and religion are categorical variables. You can have only one eye color, religious affiliation, or occupation; you are or you are not a teacher. Categorical variables are reported in terms of the numbers or percentages of subjects who are members of specific categories.

> *Continuous (or quantitative) variables* can be both observed and measured. They are assigned numerical values that place them along a scale from less to more. For instance, height is a continuous variable that is measured in feet and inches; test scores are reported on continuous scales, such as 0–100 for many classroom tests and 200–800 for the SAT. A researcher can calculate the average test scores of a group of subjects and describe how scores are distributed and how they vary within the group.

Statistics

Quantitative researchers use *statistics*, or mathematical calculations and algorithms, to analyze and interpret data. The term *statistics* is also used to describe a field of study:

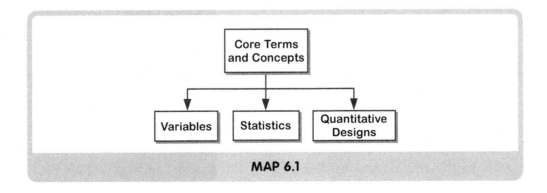

MAP 6.1

"the science of learning from data, and of measuring, controlling, and communicating uncertainty; . . . it thereby provides the navigation essential for controlling the course of scientific and societal advances" (Economic Cooperation Organization, 2013).

Descriptive statistics describe or summarize data at a specific point in time; they provide snapshots of the status of variables. Descriptive statistics include measures of central tendency (mean, median, and mode), measures of distribution and variability, and correlations. Chapter Seven explains these statistics and describes how the data they collect are visually displayed. The calculation of descriptive statistics lays the foundation for inferential statistics.

Inferential statistics allow researchers to make inferences about the data, whether they report true relationships between and among variables, and whether results can be generalized to other subjects, settings, and times. Inferential statistics are based on the probability that there are errors in sampling. A low probability of sampling error makes it more likely that results are true and that they can be generalized to the population the sample represents. Chapters Eight to Twelve explain these statistics, discuss how they are used, and describe how the data they collect are presented.

Quantitative Designs

Quantitative designs are best understood according to the statistics they use to analyze data. Studies that use descriptive statistics include *test reports* and *surveys*. Studies that use inferential statistics investigate relationships between and among variables. *Experiments* investigate causal relationships between and among variables; experiments are highly controlled and investigate the effect of an intervention on subjects. *Nonexperiments* investigate noncausal relationships between and among variables. These designs often serve as proxies for causation when it is difficult to meet the controlled conditions of an experiment.

SAMPLING

MAP 6.2

Subjects, Populations, and Samples

Subjects are the participants in a quantitative study.

A *population* is the universe of people that a researcher wants to know about.

A *sample* is a subset of a population of interest that is meant to represent this population.

In selecting the subjects for a quantitative study, a researcher must first identify the general population he or she wants to know about, and then decide whether the entire population can be accessed or whether it is more feasible to select a sample from the population. The procedures a researcher chooses for selecting a sample has major implications for the generalizability of findings to other people and places.

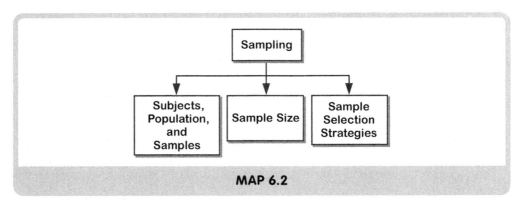

MAP 6.2

Sampling holds a position of utmost importance in quantitative research. As indicated on page 99, a sample is a subset of a population. Researchers may choose to include a whole population or a sample of the population in a quantitative study. Entire populations may vary in size. For example, a population may comprise all graduating seniors in the United States in a certain year who took the SAT, or those students within a particular state, city, school district, or school. In the first instance, the population will be very large; it will be smaller by degrees in the other instances.

Researchers use samples because it is often difficult or impractical to gain access to all members of a population. For example, samples are used to compare student achievement on national and international assessments, such as the National Assessment of Educational Progress (NAEP), the Trends in International Mathematics and Science Study (TIMSS), and the Program for International Student Assessment (PISA). These tests do not collect data for all of the students in all of the states or countries that participate; they are administered to selected samples for data collection and analysis. Similarly, commercial test makers use samples to field-test questions and to establish percentile rankings for standardized assessments. When students receive percentile scores on the SAT, they are not finding out how they did in relation to all students in the population of students who took the test when they did. Rather, they are finding out how they performed against a sample of students who took the test as part of the *norming* procedure.

There are two important considerations in sampling: the size of the sample and how it is selected. A high-quality sample has a low probability of *sampling error* and *sampling bias*.

Sampling error is inherent in sampling and is a result of errors in sampling size and selection.

Sampling bias is not inherent in every sample and is the result of the exclusion of possible subjects from the sample because of errors in sample selection. Sampling bias is discussed further below in connection with nonrandom sampling.

TABLE 6.1. Determining Sample Size from the Size of a Population

N	S	N	S	N	S	N	S	N	S
10	10	100	80	280	162	800	260	2800	338
15	14	110	86	290	165	850	265	3000	341
20	19	120	92	300	169	900	269	3500	246
25	24	130	97	320	175	950	274	4000	351
30	28	140	103	340	181	1000	278	4500	354
35	32	150	108	360	186	1100	285	5000	357
40	36	160	113	380	181	1200	291	6000	361
45	40	180	118	400	196	1300	297	7000	364
50	44	190	123	420	201	1400	302	8000	367
55	48	200	127	440	205	1500	306	9000	368
60	52	210	132	460	210	1600	310	10000	373
65	56	220	136	480	214	1700	313	15000	375
70	59	230	140	500	217	1800	317	20000	377
75	63	240	144	550	225	1900	320	30000	379
80	66	250	148	600	234	2000	322	40000	380
85	70	260	152	650	242	2200	327	50000	381
90	73	270	155	700	248	2400	331	75000	382

Note. Based on Krejcie and Morgan (1970).

Sample Size

Sample size refers to the number of subjects in a sample. In large-scale studies that use samples to represent a larger population, researchers use a table like Table 6.1 as a guide. In reading the table, note that N is population size and S is sample size.

Although it may seem counterintuitive, the rule of thumb for sample size is this: *As the population size increases, the proportion of sample to population decreases.* (See Figure 6.1.) For instance, when the population is only 15, the sample is also 15, or 100% of the population; as the population size increases, the percentage of the population needed for the sample decreases. When we reach a population of 1,400, the sample size is 302 (21.6% of the population); for a population of 750,000, the sample size is 382, only 0.05% of the population. Just remember that any one sample taken with these guidelines has a high likelihood of providing a very good estimate of the population. A table like Table 6.1 is used for making estimates of sample sizes for surveys and polls—for example, on an election day. However, not all studies draw on such a table of sample size. In particular, small classroom experiments usually don't draw samples from a population. In these instances, which are discussed in full in Chapter Eight, a sample size of 30 subjects per group is considered adequate. More specific discussion of sample size and power analysis can be found in Chapter Eight.

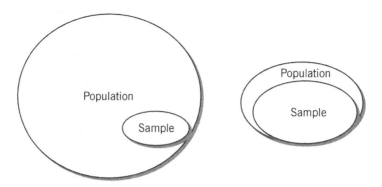

FIGURE 6.1. As the population size increases, the proportion of sample to population decreases.

Sample Selection Strategies   MAP 6.3

Studies that use rigorous sampling strategies can provide accurate and useful estimates of the population. On the other hand, studies that fail to adhere to high-
quality standards of sampling can provide erroneous information, which can be open
to misinterpretation and misuse.

There are two strategies for selecting samples in quantitative research: *random*
and *nonrandom*. Although the common use of the word *random* connotes disorder and
chaos, and that of the word *nonrandom* connotes order and control, the meanings of
the terms in quantitative research are just the opposite. In effect, random sampling
uses orderly and rigorous procedures providing confidence that it represents the population, whereas nonrandom sampling does not.

Random sampling is a set of procedures that use statistical techniques for selecting members of a sample; such techniques ensure that all members of the population will have
equal chances of being chosen.

Nonrandom sampling uses nonstatistical processes, which do not ensure that all members
of the population will have equal chances of being chosen for the sample.

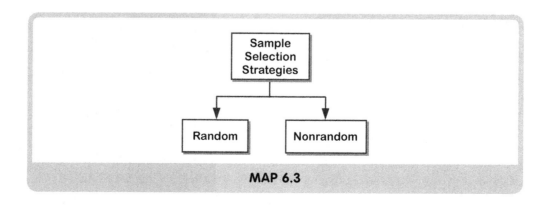

TABLE 6.2. An Example of a Table of Random Numbers

41034	34366	01254	27148	76023	76282	28621	45047	69210
23280	61069	21144	67478	01917	51715	02322	23944	12194
47442	15139	58933	27552	48252	59596	52120	74550	07258
35693	50388	53188	71346	16871	06853	63464	67073	29689
41843	78823	94440	74146	35029	25821	26889	23684	33298
04458	17535	31420	63205	14735	13262	44238	24753	30093
14071	62137	17939	77091	73078	38234	16208	55728	37166
19412	46115	66005	32893	32230	07662	07922	60260	76687
00849	54919	92709	52783	99117	33557	56797	33961	29025
17276	52524	46779	90572	59192	79891	91236	83759	06190
38897	40775	82027	84827	02985	48511	11935	68546	98713

Note. This table was generated by using the Random Number Generator page of the Stat Trek website (*http://stat-trek.com/statistics/random-number-generator.aspx*; Acklam, 2015).

Random sampling is the preferred sampling strategy in quantitative research, because it relies on methods that are more objective than human judgment and because it controls for sampling bias; as all forms of sampling do, it does include the possibility of sampling error. In order to construct a random sample, researchers usually depend on a table of random numbers. The table is generated from a computer program. No two tables that the program generates will be the same. By way of example, a researcher may go to the Random Number Generator page of the Stat Trek website (*http://stattrek.com/statistics/random-number-generator.aspx*; Acklam, 2015) and ask for a table of 100 numbers with values from 0000 to 99999. A table like Table 6.2 will appear on the screen.

Types of Random Samples

MAP 6.4

There are four types of random samples: *simple random samples, stratified random samples, cluster random samples,* and *systematic random samples.*

1. *Simple random samples* are composed of subjects who are independently selected from a population by using a table of random numbers. For example, a researcher who wanted to select a random sample from a population of 100 subjects would (according to a table like Table 6.1) need a sample size of 80. The researcher would begin by assigning each member of the population a number from 1 to 000 (which stands for 100), and then consult a table of random numbers (such as Table 6.2) and match the numbers on the table to the numbers assigned to subjects. To do this, the researcher would go down the first column of the table and match the first two digits of each number with the numbers assigned to subjects. In Table 6.2, the first two digits of the numbers in the first column are 41, 23, 47, 35, 41, 04, 14, 19,

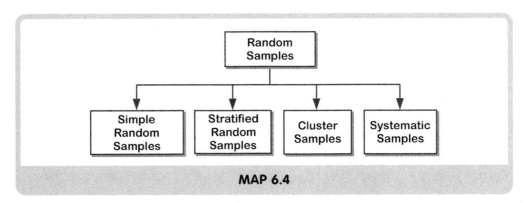

MAP 6.4

00, 17, and 38. Subjects assigned those numbers would be the first 11 members of the sample. The researcher would proceed to the next columns until 80 subjects had been selected for the sample. With larger populations, a researcher would use student ID numbers or telephone numbers as ways to assign numbers to subjects. Once the first two digits of each column were exhausted, the researcher would go back to the first column and use the third and fourth digits to select the sample, and so on.

2. *Stratified random samples* are selected from subgroups within a population, in the same proportion that each subgroup is represented in the population. In order to do this, researchers proceed in two steps: They (a) sort possible subjects into categories according to some characteristics (race, gender, age, income level, etc.) and (b) use simple random sampling to select members from each category.

3. *Cluster random samples* are selected for a sample from natural groupings in a population. In order to select a cluster sample, researchers also follow a two-step process: They (a) randomly select clusters for the sample (by geographic area, type of school, etc.) and (b) use simple random sampling to choose members of each cluster for the study.

4. *Systematic random samples* are selected by what is known as the *Nth name selection technique*, in which subjects are selected at specified intervals on a list of all members of the population. In this method, the first member of the sample is selected randomly from a list of everyone in the population; the rest of the sample is selected by choosing subjects who lie at equal intervals from each other on the list of population members. For example, the interval may be every 10th name or number.

Types of Nonrandom Samples   MAP 6.5

Nonrandom sampling methods do not ensure that everyone in a population has an equal chance of being chosen for a sample. This makes nonrandom samples subject to sampling bias. Like all samples, they are also subject to sampling error. Although nonrandom methods are less rigorous methods of selecting subjects for a sample, they have the advantage of requiring less time and effort and being more easily accessible

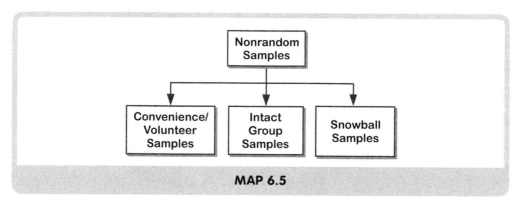

MAP 6.5

to researchers. There are three commonly used strategies for generating nonrandom samples.

1. *Convenience/volunteer samples* are composed of individual subjects who are willing to participate in a study and who are easily available to the researcher.

2. *Intact group samples* are composed of already formed groups, such as classrooms or grade levels. In these samples, all members of a group are included as subjects. Intact groups are used extensively in educational research experiments.

3. *Snowball samples* are composed of subjects who are nominated by other subjects in the population. An initially small number of subjects provide names of possible future subjects, who then provide the names of other possible subjects.

MEASUREMENT AND MEASURES   MAP 6.6

Researchers may choose from existing instruments or create their own. In both instances, they have to answer three questions:

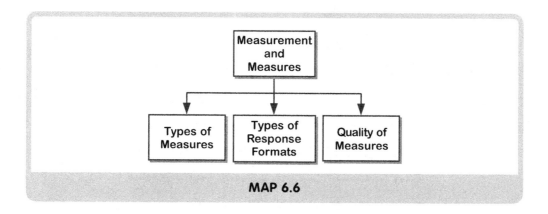

MAP 6.6

1. *Questions about types of measure.* What do researchers want to know about the subjects in the sample? Do they want to know about their skills, aptitudes, and dispositions, or about their attitudes and beliefs, or about their behaviors?

2. *Questions about response format.* How do researchers want subjects to respond? Do they want short written responses? Do they want subjects to choose from a list of possible responses? Do they want a combination of both?

3. *Questions about the quality of the measure.* Does the measure do what it purports to do? Is the measure consistent?

Types of Measures   MAP 6.7

Assessments

Assessments measure academic aptitude and achievement, vocational interests, personality, and emotional or mental states. There is increasing dependence on assessments in both educational and clinical practice, and the use of commercial standardized assessments has grown exponentially. Intended for testing multiple individuals in diverse settings, commercial assessments are uniform in format and questions, and are highly standardized in their conditions for administration, procedures for scoring, and methods of reporting results. Many researchers, however, develop their own assessments or modify existing assessments for specific purposes and contexts. Regardless of how they are developed, assessments must adhere to specific test construction guidelines and procedures for field-testing. Table 6.3 shows some commonly used commercial standardized assessments in education and clinical practice.

Assessments may vary in how they report results.

• A norm-referenced assessment reports results for individuals in terms of how they compare to a sample that had previously taken the assessment. For example, the SAT and most standardized tests are norm-referenced; they compare students' achievement to that of others along a continuum from below to above average.

• A criterion-referenced assessment reports results in terms of the degree to which individuals have mastered a particular content. The Advanced Placement

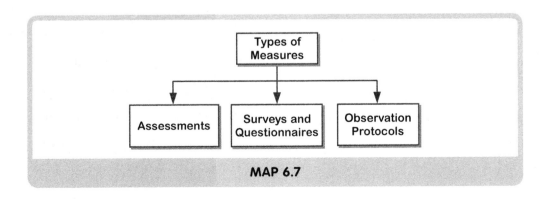

MAP 6.7

TABLE 6.3. Frequently Used Assessments in Education and Clinical Practice

What is measured	Assessment
Academic aptitude	• Stanford–Binet Intelligence Scales (SB) • Wechsler Intelligence Scale for Children (WISC) • Wechsler Adult Intelligence Scale (WAIS) • Armed Forces Qualifying Test (AFQT) • Woodcock–Johnson Tests of Cognitive Abilities
Academic achievement	• Woodcock–Johnson Tests of Achievement • Peabody Individual Achievement Test (PIAT) • Advanced Placement Examinations • NWEA Measures of Academic Progress (MAP) • National Assessment of Educational Progress (NAEP) • No Child Left Behind (NCLB) state tests
Vocational aptitude	• Armed Services Vocational Aptitude Battery (ASVAB) • Strong Interest Inventory
Personality	• Minnesota Multiphasic Personality Inventory (MMPI) • Myers–Briggs Type indicator • Thematic Apperception Test (TAT)
Emotional or mental state	• Beck Depression Inventory (BDI) • Dementia Rating Scale

Exam and most classroom assessments are criterion-referenced; they only report an individual's level of achievement and do not rank students from below to above average.

Surveys and Questionnaires

Surveys and *questionnaires* are familiar instruments for gathering data. They measure the characteristics, perceptions, interpretations, attitudes, preferences, and/or dispositions of a group of subjects. A survey may appear to be a long list of questions, but a high-quality survey has a framework or structure that organizes the information. For example, a survey with a total of 100 questions may be organized into known categories. From 3 to 10–15 related items or questions make up each category. Questions are grouped together in categories to provide multiple data points for the measurement target or concept.

Observation Protocols

Quantitative measures for observing behavior are gaining wide use in educational research. Much of this growth in use is due to the demand for methods associated with observing children on the autism spectrum. Unlike qualitative observation, which depends on a researcher's ability to observe and record events and behaviors in words and images, quantitative observation relies on instruments that identify discrete behaviors specifically enough to enable researchers to observe and measure them with numerical notations marking their frequency and duration. Like assessments, observation protocols may be norm- or criterion-referenced. For example, the Conners Teacher Rating Scale (Conners, 2008) is a norm-referenced checklist of observed student behaviors associated with attention-deficit/hyperactivity disorder (ADHD); it is completed by teachers and is used as part of a general assessment that leads to a diagnosis for students. The Classroom Observation and Analytic Protocol (Horizon Research, 2000) is a criterion-referenced checklist of observed behaviors in K–12 science or math lessons; it is completed by colleagues or supervisors and is used for professional development, evaluation of teaching practice, or program implementation.

Types of Response Formats   MAP 6.8

The types of formats that a measure uses for obtaining responses from subjects can be categorized as *questions* or as *scales*.

Questions

There are two types of questions: *constructed-response* or *selected-response*.

Constructed-response (also called *open-response*) questions provide spaces for writing original answers. Each response is assigned a quantitative score that is aligned with a rubric, as in the assessments used for meeting No Child Left Behind requirements.

Selected-response (also known as *closed-response*) questions provide a given set of responses from which to choose. These questions may be presented as *dichotomous* or *multiple-choice* questions.

> *Dichotomous* questions provide two possible responses from which to choose. True–false and yes–no questions fall into this category. For example, the well-known Minnesota Multiphasic Personality Inventory—Form A has 487 true–false items or questions to be answered.

> *Multiple-choice* questions provide a number of possible responses and ask the respondent to select one answer, or in some cases "all that apply."

Scales

A *scale* assigns numerical values to attitudes, values, and interests. In social-scientific research, the most commonly used types of scales are *nominal*, *ordinal*, *interval*, and *ratio* scales.

Nominal scales ask respondents to place themselves into categories such as race, ethnicity, first language, and gender. Nominal scales usually code responses by using numbers. These numbers serve as placeholders for the categorical/nominal variable; they have no arithmetic value and cannot be calculated mathematically or represented statistically.

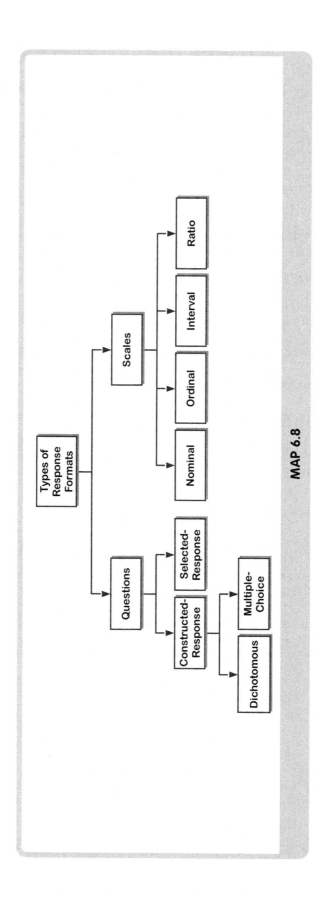

MAP 6.8

Ordinal scales ask respondents to rank-order a set of given responses from highest to lowest.

Interval scales ask respondents to place their responses on a continuum of answers that are located at intervals of equal value. The *Likert scale* is the most frequently used type of interval scale. It is used in surveys and questionnaires to ask for the degree of agreement with a statement; responses range from, for example, 1 = "strongly agree" to 5 = "strongly disagree."

Ratio scales have all the properties of interval scales, but include 0 as the starting point.

Quality of Measures   MAP 6.9

Quantitative researchers must take great care in choosing high-quality measures. Quantitative measures have to meet two criteria for quality: *validity* and *reliability*.

Validity means that an instrument measures what it purports to measure.

Reliability means that a measure yields consistent results.

It is the responsibility of those who develop measures to provide evidence of validity and reliability. If researchers use measures that have been developed by others, they look to see whether the developers have provided evidence of validity and reliability. If they are developing their own instruments, they have to provide similar evidence.

Validity of Measures   MAP 6.10

Validity answers this question: "Can I trust this instrument to measure what it purports to measure?" Determining validity is the responsibility of the developer(s) of an instrument or measure. There are four types of validity: *content validity*, *construct validity*, *concurrent validity*, and *predictive validity*.

Content validity is a nonstatistical determination of how well an instrument matches what is being measured. Content validity may be determined by aligning the measure to a table

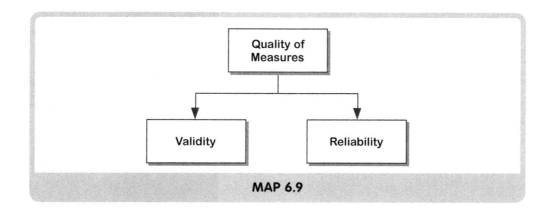

MAP 6.9

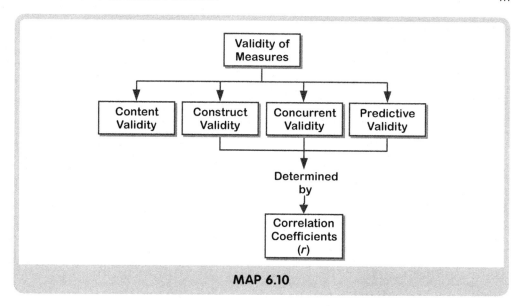

MAP 6.10

of specifications and/or by convening a panel of experts in a given content area (e.g., U.S. history) to review all of the items and make a judgment whether they measure what they claim to measure. Content validity is often used with achievement tests. Content validity is often confused with *face validity*, which is less theoretically based and can be judged by a person less experienced or qualified in a content area. Face validity has to do with the format and organization of the measure.

Construct, concurrent, and predictive validity are determined by comparing one measure to another. For all of these, a statistic known as the *coefficient of correlation* (*r*) is used to show how closely one measure aligns with another. This coefficient has a value from 0 to 1, and *r* = .70 is considered a good threshold for determining validity of measures. (The coefficient of correlation is discussed more fully in Chapters Seven and Eleven.)

Construct validity is a statistical determination of how well an instrument or measure matches an already validated instrument that measures the same thing. Construct validity is often used with constructs that are not observable, such as compassion or working memory.

Concurrent validity is a statistical determination of how well an instrument or measure matches another measure that is administered to a sample at or near the same time, and that purports to measure the same thing.

Predictive validity is a statistical determination of how well a measure will be able to predict an outcome on another measure that it theoretically should be able to predict.

The four types of validity are summarized in Table 6.4.

TABLE 6.4. Types of Validity

	Definition	Method	How determined
Content validity	How well a measure matches what is being measured	Aligning the measure to a table of specifications, or accepting the judgment of an expert panel	Nonstatistical determination of validity, using judgment
Construct validity	How well a measure matches an already validated measure that measures the same thing	Comparing how a sample performs on a measure to how it performs on a previously validated measure	Statistical determination of validity, using the coefficient of correlation (r)
Concurrent validity	How well a measure matches another measure that purports to measure the same thing	Comparing how a sample performs on a measure to how it performs on another measure administered to the same sample at or near the same time	Statistical determination of validity, using the coefficient of correlation (r)
Predictive validity	How well a measure will be able to predict an outcome on another measure that it theoretically should be able to predict	Comparing how a sample performs on a measure with its future performance	Statistical determination of validity, using the coefficient of correlation (r)

Reliability of Measures   MAP 6.11

Reliability answers these questions: "Can I trust the scores or values that are reported? Are they consistent and stable?" Reliability may refer to either the consistency of the scores from a measure itself, or the consistency of raters who are using the measure and who determine scores. As with three of the four types of validity, the first three types of reliability are calculated with the *coefficient of correlation* (r), and r may be used to calculate the fourth type as well (see below). In determining reliability of measures, we look for a moderately strong correlation ($r = .75$ or greater). There are four types of reliability: *test–retest reliability*, *equivalent/alternate forms reliability*, *split-half/internal consistency reliability*, and *interrater reliability*.

Test–retest reliability compares the pattern of scores on the same selected response measure given twice. It is conducted when the developer of the measure administers a measure to a sample. After a sufficient time interval, the developer administers the same measure to the same sample and computes r to determine whether there is a similar pattern of responses.

Equivalent/alternate forms reliability compares the pattern of scores on two selected response measures that purport to measure the same thing. The developer randomly assigns one half of a sample to one group and the other half to another group, and then administers a different version of the same measure to each group.

Split-half/internal consistency reliability compares the pattern of scores on two halves of the same selected response measure. The developer administers a measure to a sample.

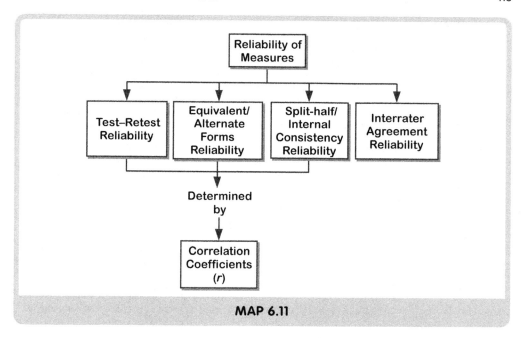

MAP 6.11

The developer then compares the responses of the sample on one half of the measure to the sample's responses on the other half of the measure, the two halves having been randomly assigned.

Interrater reliability compares the consistency of raters, not measures. To determine interrater reliability, individual raters are trained to score responses according to a rubric or scoring guide. After the training, two raters are given a sample of written responses to score with the rubric. In some cases, the correlation coefficient is calculated to examine the agreement between the two raters' scores; in other cases, a simple percentage of agreement is used.

Table 6.5 summarizes the types of reliability.

CHAPTER SUMMARY

MAP 6.12

✓ Some core terms and concepts in quantitative research are variables, statistics, and quantitative designs.

✓ Variables are central to measurement in quantitative research and are classified as categorical or continuous.

✓ Researchers study a whole population or a sample of a population.

✓ As the size of a population increases, the proportion of the sample to the total population decreases.

✓ Of the two major sampling strategies, random samples are preferred over nonrandom samples. Data collection depends on valid and reliable measures, and the most frequently used measures in educational research are assessments, surveys/questionnaires, and observation protocols.

TABLE 6.5. Types of Reliability

	Type of measure with which used	Method	How determined
Test–retest reliability	Selected-response questions	Compares the pattern of performance of a sample on the same measure given at two different times	Statistical determination of reliability, using the coefficient of correlation (r)
Equivalent/alternate forms reliability	Selected-response questions	Compares the pattern of performance of a randomly divided sample on two different, but equivalent, forms of a measure	Statistical determination of reliability, using the coefficient of correlation (r)
Split-half/internal consistency reliability	Selected-response questions	Compares the pattern of performance of a sample on two halves of the same measure	Statistical determination of reliability, using the coefficient of correlation (r)
Interrater reliability	Constructed-response questions	Compares the ways that individual raters score or code responses on a measure according to a rubric, scoring guide, or coding sheet	Statistical determination of reliability, using either the coefficient of correlation (r) or percentage of agreement

✓ Response formats use questions that require constructed and selected responses (dichotomous or multiple-choice) and scales (nominal, ordinal, interval, and ratio).

✓ There are four kinds of validity: content, construct, concurrent, and predictive. The coefficient of correlation (r) is used to establish all of these kinds except content validity.

✓ There are four kinds of reliability: test–retest, equivalent/alternate forms, split-half/internal consistency, and interrater. The first three of these use the coefficient of correlation (r) to establish reliability. Interrater reliability may use either r or percentage of agreement for this purpose.

KEY TERMS AND CONCEPTS

assessments	descriptive statistics
categorical variable	descriptive studies
cluster random sample	dichotomous question
coefficient of correlation (r)	equivalent forms
concurrent validity	experiments
construct validity	inferential statistics
constructed-response question	inferential studies
content validity	intact group sample
continuous variable	interrater reliability
convenience/volunteer sample	interval scale

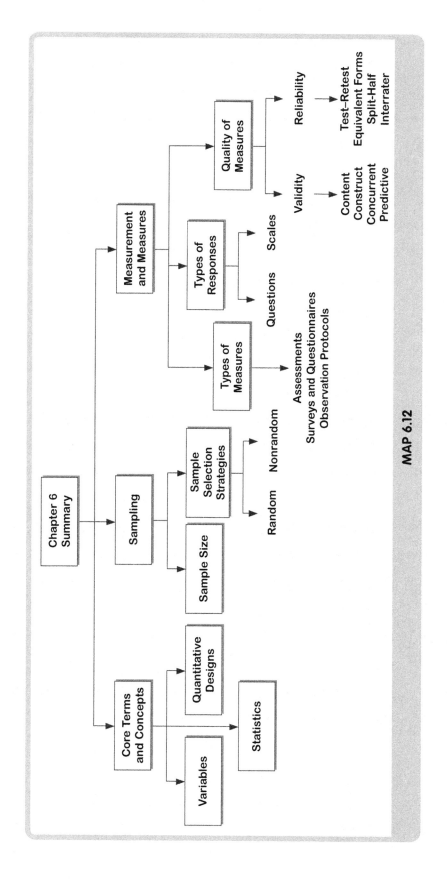

MAP 6.12

115

multiple-choice question

nominal scale

nonexperiments

nonrandom sample

observation protocol

ordinal scale

population

predictive validity

random sample

ratio scale

reliability

sample

sampling bias

sampling error

scale

selected-response question

simple random sample

snowball sample

split-half reliability

statistics

stratified random sample

subjects

surveys/questionnaires

systematic random sample

test–retest reliability

validity

variables

REVIEW, CONSOLIDATION, AND EXTENSION OF KNOWLEDGE

1. In what ways do quantitative sampling and data collection methods differ from those used in qualitative research? Use the list of key terms and concepts above to illustrate your answer.

2. What can you find out about the sampling strategies of the NAEP, TIMSS, or PISA? Do you think that these samples are good representations of the populations to which these assessments are administered?

3. What can you find out about the SAT and ACT in regard to the following:

   a. The sample size and sampling strategy used in developing norms?
   b. The response formats for questions?
   c. Indications of validity and reliability?

4. The Annual Phi Delta Kappa (PDK)/Gallup Poll of the Public's Attitudes Toward the Public Schools is a well-known and often quoted survey. What can you find out about the following:

   a. The sample size and sampling strategy?
   b. The response formats for questions?
   c. Indications of validity and reliability of the poll?

5. Using a professional commercial database, search for a primary, peer-reviewed, quantitative research article. Scan the article and look for the sections on sampling and measurement; they may be under the heading "Methodology" or "Methods."

   a. What does the article say about the sample? What was the sample size? What was the strategy for selecting the sample? Is there any reference to "randomization"? What are the subject characteristics?

   b. What measures were used? Are there indications of validity and reliability?

6. Answer the following questions about an assessment that you or your workplace uses, and write a review of about 500 words of the assessment you have selected.

   a. What is the name of the assessment? Who is the publisher?

   b. Is the assessment norm- or criterion-referenced? If norm-referenced, how were norms developed? If criterion-referenced, how were standards established?

   c. What skills, knowledge, or depositions/moods are being assessed?

   d. How many questions are asked? What types of questions and response formats are used?

   e. Are there indications of validity and reliability?

CHAPTER SEVEN

Descriptive Statistics and Data Displays

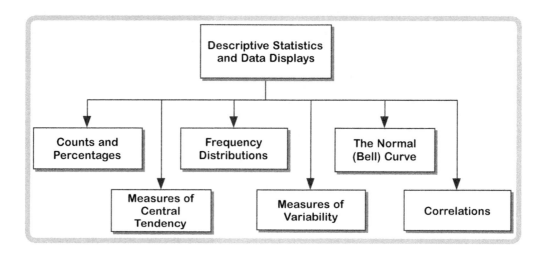

As indicated in Chapter Six, descriptive statistics report on the status of variables at a point in time. They report on data that a researcher collects in several ways: as counts and percentages; as measures of central tendency (means, medians, and modes); and as frequency distributions and measures of variability. They also play a vital role in inferential statistics. This chapter explains the various descriptive statistics and provides examples of how descriptive statistical data are displayed graphically and visually.

CHAPTER OBJECTIVES

✓ Understand what descriptive statistics do.

✓ Understand counts and percentages, and how both of these are displayed.

✓ Understand measures of central tendency and how they are displayed.

✓ Understand frequency distributions and how they are displayed.

✓ Understand measures of variability (range, spread, variance, and standard deviation) and how they are displayed.

✓ Understand what the normal (bell) curve represents and how it is used.

✓ Understand correlations and how they are displayed.

COUNTS AND PERCENTAGES

Counts and percentages are the most basic descriptive statistics. They are used primarily to describe categorical data that are visually displayed in pie charts and in line and bar graphs.

  Counts describe how many subjects within a group fall within a specific category.

  Percentages describe counts as a fraction of the total number of subjects.

Pie Charts

Pie charts compare how many or what percentage of subjects or grouped values in a sample fall within a particular category. They organize data into circular charts to represent the comparison. For example, the pie chart in Figure 7.1 shows the percentage of students from each category who took the SAT in 2012. The variable in this pie chart is "type of high school," and the categories are public, religious, and independent schools.

Bar Graphs

Like pie charts, *bar graphs* compare how many or what percentage of subjects fall within a particular category on a single variable. However, they do so by organizing data into either horizontal or vertical bars. On one axis of the graph are the labels

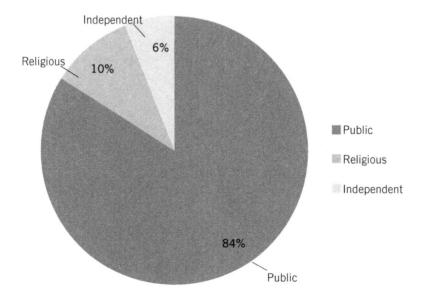

FIGURE 7.1. Pie chart showing SAT participation (percent) by type of high school, SAT 2012 national sample (*n* = 1,664,479). Data from the College Board (2012).

(or categories) that are being compared; on the other axis are the values (counts, percentages, raw scores).

Simple bar graphs display comparisons of categories on a single variable. For example, the vertical bar graph in Figure 7.2 presents the same data as those in the Figure 7.1 pie chart.

Stacked bar graphs also display comparisons of categories on a single variable. In this case, the graph shows all of the categories on one graph that is divided into segments that represent the proportion of subjects in each category. Figure 7.3 shows a vertical stacked bar graph presenting the same data as those in the Figure 7.1 pie chart and the Figure 7.2 simple bar graph.

Grouped bar graphs display more complex comparisons by adding subcategories (e.g., gender). The graph in Figure 7.4 compares the percentages of students falling into one of seven categories of courses within the single variable "type of computer courses," and further compares the percentage of males and females in each category, in a horizontal display.

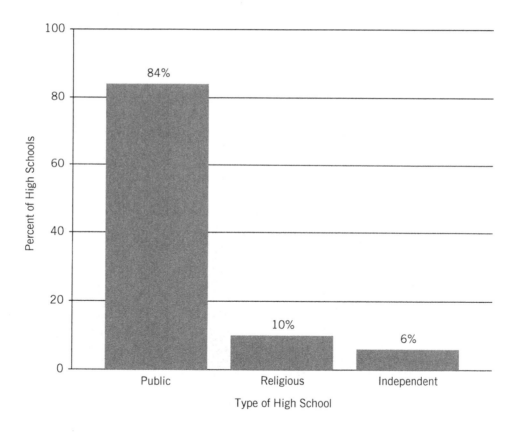

FIGURE 7.2. Simple bar graph showing SAT participation (percent) by type of high school, SAT 2012 national sample (*n* = 1,664,479). Data from the College Board (2012).

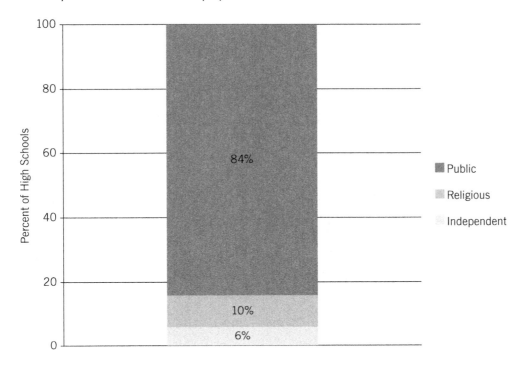

FIGURE 7.3. Stacked bar graph showing SAT participation (percent) by type of high school, SAT 2012 national sample (n = 1,664,479). Data from the College Board (2012).

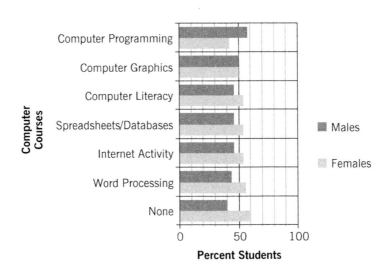

FIGURE 7.4. Grouped bar graph showing computer course-taking patterns by gender, SAT 2012 national sample (n = 1,664,479). Data from the College Board (2012).

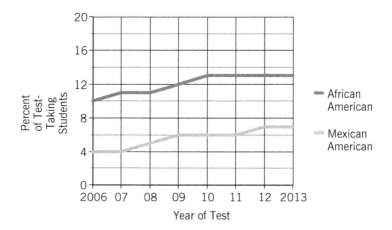

FIGURE 7.5. Line graph showing percentages of African American and Mexican American test takers, SAT national samples (approximately 1.5 million total per year). Data from the College Board (2012).

Line Graphs

Line graphs display change in a categorical variable over time. Each data point on a line represents a count or a percentage of subjects falling into a category over a period of time. Line graphs are used to look at trends for groups and itndividuals. Figure 7.5 shows the trend in percentages of African Americans and Mexican Americans taking the SAT.

MEASURES OF CENTRAL TENDENCY   MAP 7.1

The term *measures of central tendency* refers to calculations that determine a value or values that are representative of all values within a dataset. There are three measures of central tendency: *mean, median,* and *mode.*

Mean is the measure of central tendency that is the arithmetic average: the sum of values divided by the number in the sample or population. Means are usually displayed in line and bar graphs.

Median is the measure of central tendency that is the midpoint in a distribution of values scores; that is, it denotes the point below which and above which 50% of values scores occur.

Mode is the measure of central tendency that represents the most commonly occurring values or scores.

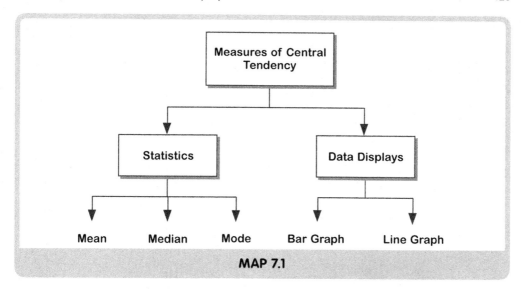

MAP 7.1

Of the three measures of central tendency, the mean is the most widely reported; computing means is an important step in more complex statistical reasoning. For example, SAT reports show the mean scaled scores for the total number of test takers, and also for different groups (e.g., females and males). Teachers usually average grades to determine a final grade for a student. Survey researchers average responses on numerical scales in reporting results. However, the mean does not always provide a full picture. For example, consider one classroom's math scores, which are represented below.

98, 94, 94, 90, 88, 88, 88, 88, 88, 86, 86, 86, 86, 86,
84, 84, 82, 82, 82, 80, 80, 80, 78, 76, 70, 58

The mean score for Room 115's data = 83.9, while the median score = 86.0. According to the mean, we could conclude that a student scoring 84 is at the average of the class, but according to the median, that same student is in the lower half of the class scores.

The median is higher than the mean because it is not as sensitive to outliers (high and low scores). In this case, the low score of 58 is a definite outlier, falling a full 12 points below the next lowest score. A median reduces the effect of outliers. It provides information about how scores are distributed within a group and is used extensively in demographic studies and census reports, especially in regard to income distribution. What about the mode? The mode score in this class is 88; 5 out of 26 (or almost 25% of) students earned this grade. The mode only focuses on the most frequent scores. In some ways, it points to the "typical" score. All this is to say that while the mean, median, and mode all report on central tendency, they may represent it differently. Taken together, they provide a more accurate representation of a dataset.

Line Graphs

Line graphs can be used to display changes in means over time. The line graph in Figure 7.6 displays changes in means on a single variable (SAT Writing scores) for a span of 6 years. The line graph in Figure 7.7 displays mean scores for Critical Reading and Mathematics for a span of 30 years.

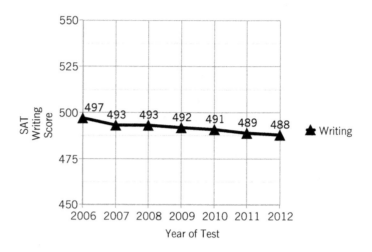

FIGURE 7.6. Line graph showing SAT mean Writing scores over time (2006–2012), SAT national samples (approximately 1.5 million total per year). Data from the College Board (2012).

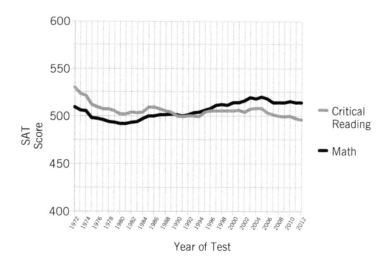

FIGURE 7.7. Line graph showing SAT Critical Reading and Mathematics scores over time (1972–2012), SAT national samples (approximately 1.5 million total per year). Data from the College Board (2012).

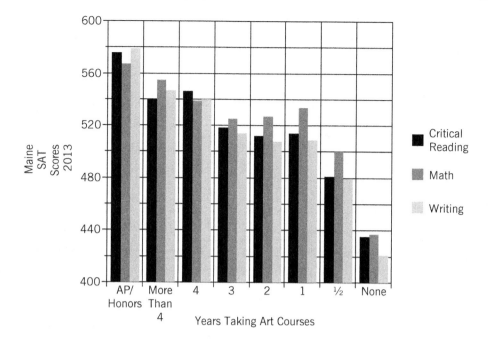

FIGURE 7.8. Maine SAT 2013 average scores (sample = 14,501 students), by number of years students took high school visual/performing arts courses.

Bar Graphs

Bar graphs can also be used to display means. The bar graph in Figure 7.8 depicts the mean SAT Critical Writing, Reading, and Mathematics scores of Maine students in 2013 (y-axis) according to the number of years these students took high school courses in visual and performing arts (x-axis).

FREQUENCY DISTRIBUTIONS   MAP 7.2

Frequency distributions describe the number of times that grouped continuous variables occur within a sample. Frequency distributions are displayed in *stem-and-leaf plots*, *frequency tables*, and *histograms*.

Stem-and-Leaf Plots

A *stem-and-leaf plot* converts continuous variables into categories. For example, given the set of math scores presented earlier for one classroom, Room 115—

98, 94, 94, 90, 88, 88, 88, 88, 88, 86, 86, 86, 86, 86,
84, 84, 82, 82, 82, 80, 80, 80, 78, 76, 70, 58

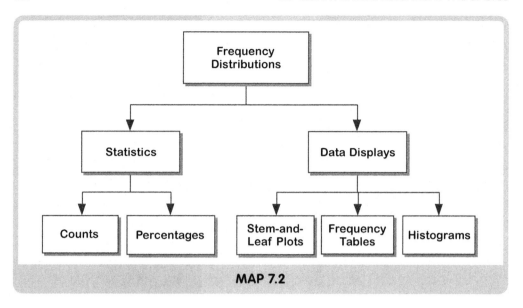

MAP 7.2

—a researcher can divide the scores into groups according to the tens digits of the scores and plot them as in Figure 7.9. To read the plot, the numbers on the left side are the first digits of scores; these are called the *stems*. The numbers on the right side are the second digits of the scores within each leaf; these are called the *leaves*. In the plot in Figure 7.9, <u>5 | 8</u> represents a score of 58, and <u>8 | 0 0 0</u> shows that three students in Room 115 achieved a score of <u>80</u>.

Frequency Tables

In a *frequency table*, the grouped data are presented as categories in three columns. The first column on the left shows the categories; the second column shows the number of times each category appears in the data; the third column shows the same information as percentages.

Table 7.1 shows how a researcher presents the frequency of occurrences of the categories of free, reduced-pay, and full-pay lunch in a class of 24 students. Table 7.2 shows how a researcher groups the 26 scores for Room 115, represented by the

Stem	Leaf
5	8
7	068
8	000222446666688888
9	0448

FIGURE 7.9. Stem-and-leaf plot for math scores, Room 115.

TABLE 7.1. Frequency of Occurrences of Lunch Status Categories

Lunch status	Frequency	%
Free lunch	8	33.3
Reduced-pay lunch	10	41.7
Full-pay lunch	6	25.0
Total	24	100.0

TABLE 7.2. Frequency of Occurrences of Math Scores in Room 115

Score	Frequency	%
90–100	4	15.38
80–89	18	69.23
70–79	3	11.54
60–69	0	0
50–59	1	3.85
Total	26	100.00

stem-and-leaf plot in Figure 7.9, into five categories by ranges of scores: 90–100, 80–89, 70–79, 60–69, and 50–59.

Histograms

In a *histogram*, continuous test score data that have been grouped into categories are represented in bar graphs. For instance, the histogram in Figure 7.10 depicts the same five categories of Room 115 data as in Table 7.2.

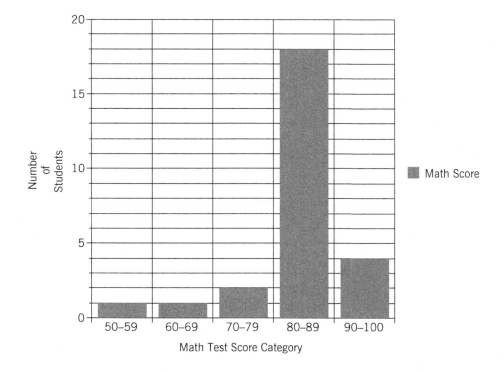

FIGURE 7.10. Histogram depicting math test score distribution, Room 115.

MEASURES OF VARIABILITY   `MAP 7.3`

Measures of variability describe to what degree the values of continuous data in a sample diverge from the average or mean of values in a sample. *Variability* also refers to the extent to which data points differ from each other. Measures of variability provide a more complete description of the data than do measures of central tendency or frequency distributions. High variability indicates that scores or values are widely scattered and that the sample is heterogeneous. Low variability indicates that scores and values are tightly clustered around the mean and that the sample is homogeneous. The most common measures of variability are *spread, range, quartiles, variance,* and *standard deviation.*

Spread simply reports the highest and lowest score. The spread of scores in Room 115 is from a low score of 58 to a high score of 98.

Range is the arithmetic difference between the highest and lowest scores. The range of scores in Room 115 is 40 (98 minus 58).

Quartiles divide ranked data into four equal parts.

Standard deviation (often abbreviated as *SD*, especially in equations) is a calculation that determines the average variability of all scores from the mean.

Variance is the standard deviation squared and is very important in many more complex calculations.

The formula for calculating standard deviation is presented in Figure 7.11. Although this may seem daunting, it is not so difficult to understand. The key elements in the calculation include each score value, the *deviation score* (which is the difference in each score from the mean), and the sample size. The first step is to calculate the mean; the next step is to determine a deviation score for each value $(x_i - \mu)$; the next step is to square each deviation score. Then the squared deviation scores are added together, and the sum (Σ) is divided by the sample size $(1/N)$. The final step is to take the square root $(\sqrt{})$ of that figure; the result is the standard deviation (*SD* or σ). It is not necessary to calculate *SD* by hand; this can be done with a computer program like SPSS or SAS, with a scientific calculator, or with a web-based calculator (e.g., *www.easycalculation.com/statistics/standard-deviation.php*). The important things to understand are what standard deviation means and how it is used. Measures of variability are displayed in box-and-whisker plots and in tables that include both means and standard deviations.

Box-and-Whisker Plots

Box-and-whisker plots (also known simply as *box plots*) use the median and quartiles to summarize variability of data. The ends of the box are the lowest and highest quartiles; the whiskers, or error bars, extend to the extreme lowest and highest scores in

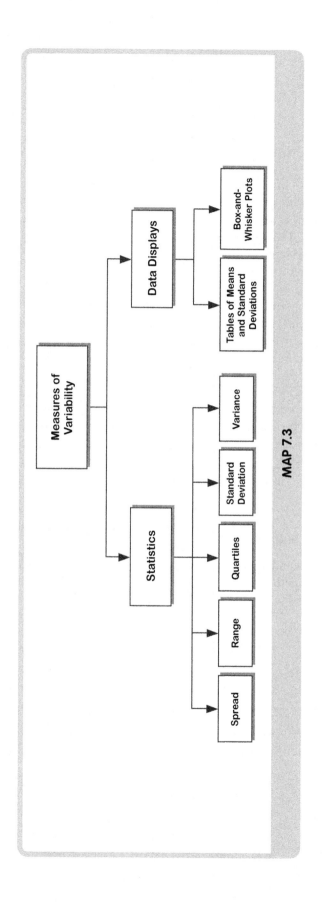

MAP 7.3

129

$$\sigma = \sqrt{\frac{1}{N}\sum_{i=1}^{N}(x_i - \mu)^2}$$

FIGURE 7.11. Formula for calculating standard deviation.

the distribution. The central line in the box is the median. Box-and-whisker plots provide a succinct visual summary of the spread, the central tendency, and the shape of the distribution. The following are examples of how data counts, percentages, and measures of central tendency can be represented in the various visual formats. The box-and-whisker plot in Figure 7.12 shows a hypothetical normal distribution of test scores of students at one point in time with a range of scores from 2 to 14, showing a summary of data on an interval scale. The plot shows the symmetry of this distribution, the range, shape, and median.

The box plot in Figure 7.13 shows a hypothetical, positively skewed distribution of the same scores as in Figure 7.12, this time with a range of 3 to 14. In both examples, the box contains the middle 50% (median) of the data. The upper edge (hinge) of the box indicates the 75th percentile of the dataset, and the lower hinge indicates the 25th percentile. The range of the middle two quartiles is known as the *interquartile range*. The line in the box indicates the median value of the data. The ends of the vertical lines or whiskers indicate the minimum and maximum data values. The points outside the ends of the whiskers are *outliers* or suspected outliers. In both cases, the boxes are equal, but the whiskers are different, indicating that the range of scores is different.

Tables of Means and Standard Deviations

In quantitative research studies, tables report means and standard deviations alongside each other and thus provide rich data about the characteristics of groups. For example, look at Table 7.3, which presents mean math scores and standard deviations

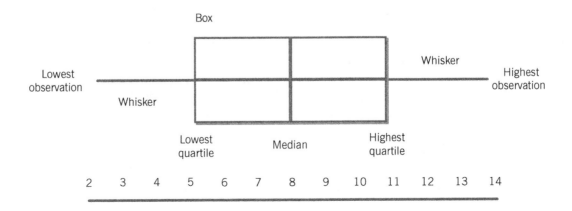

FIGURE 7.12. Box-and-whisker plot model.

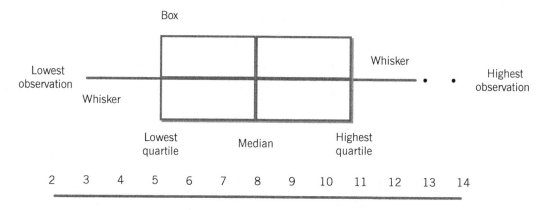

FIGURE 7.13. Box-and-whisker plot showing test scores of students receiving free and reduced-pay lunch. Note outliers at right.

TABLE 7.3. Math Scores in Rooms 115 and 120		
Class	Mean	SD
Room 115	83.9	7.9
Room 120	84.1	3.3

for two classrooms, Rooms 115 and 120. If we look only at means (Room 115 M = 83.8; Room 120 M = 84.1), the two classes appear very similar. However, the different standard deviations (Room 115 SD = 7.9; Room 120 SD = 3.3) tell a different story. They indicate that Room 115 has more variability in scores and is more heterogeneous than Room 120.

THE BELL CURVE

The *bell curve* (also known as the *normal* or *Gaussian distribution curve*; see Figure 7.14) displays the distribution of naturally occurring phenomena and values as they normally appear in nature. The values that occur most frequently are clustered around the midpoint of the curve, and the least frequently occurring values (lowest and highest) values are located at the two ends, or tails. The bell curve has the following characteristics:

- The mean, median, and mode are the same.
- The curve is smooth and symmetrical.

Of the values, 68.2% fall within the first SD plus or minus (±) 1 SD, and 95.4% fall within the second SD plus or minus (±) 1 SD.

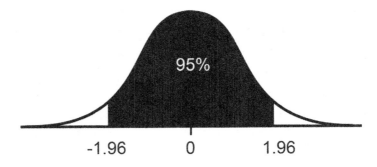

FIGURE 7.14. The normal (bell) curve.

Figure 7.15 illustrates the normal distribution of IQ scores. Note that the mean and median = 100, and the *SD* = 15. When IQ scores are reported for a random sample of subjects, about 68% of IQ scores will fall within the first standard deviation; this is considered the normal range and consists of scores from 85 to 115 (100 ± 15). About 95% of scores will fall within two standard deviations of 70 (which has traditionally been used as the cutoff score for a diagnosis of intellectual disability); this range will include scores from 70 to 130. At the other end of the curve are scores that are above 130, the traditional cutoff for a designation as "gifted."

The bell curve is used not only to report data on scores, but also to establish norms. For example, in establishing norms for IQ tests, researchers field-test items with a random sample of subjects, and then select items that about 68% of the sample answered correctly and items that only 2% answered correctly. Figure 7.16 shows the curve for SAT scores, where the mean score is 500 and the standard deviation is 100 points. About 68% of scores fall between 400 and 600, and scores below 300 and over 700 will each account for 2.28% of test takers. As in the IQ test, and all other norm-referenced measures, test developers select items so that correct answers will reflect the bell curve.

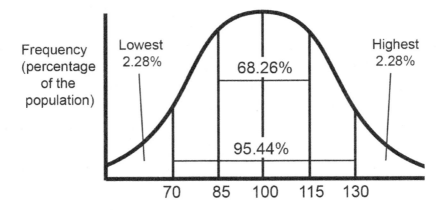

FIGURE 7.15. Normal distribution curve for IQ.

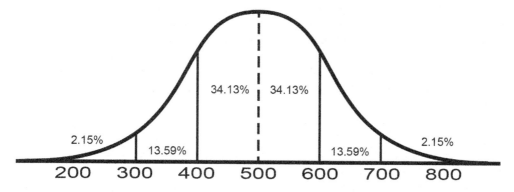

FIGURE 7.16. Normal distribution curve for SAT scores (mean = 500, *SD* = 100).

Percentiles are also derived from the bell curve and are reported to show how scores stand in relation to each other. Percentiles are not equal intervals along the curve. For instance, a 30-point difference in SAT scores at the middle of the curve (between scores of 570 and 600) yields an 8-point difference in percentile rank, from the 71st to the 79th percentile, while a 30-point difference at the tail of the curve (between scores of 770 and 800) yields no difference at all in percentile rank; both are at the 99th percentile.

CORRELATIONS   MAP 7.4

A *correlation* describes a noncausal relationship between and among variables in terms of the direction and strength of the relationship. In terms of direction, a correlation may be positive (+) or negative (−).

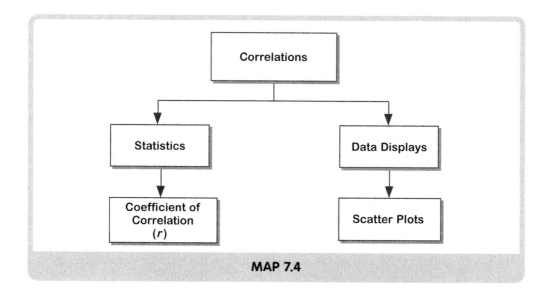

MAP 7.4

A *positive correlation* means that as one variable increases in value, so does the other. For example, as caloric intake increases, so does weight.

A *negative correlation* means that as one variable increases in value, the other decreases in value. For example, as hours of exercise increase and caloric intake remains constant, weight decreases.

The *coefficient of correlation* (*r*) is the statistic that describes the direction and strength of a correlation.

The coefficient of correlation uses a range of values from +1.00 to −1.00, where the plus sign indicates a positive correlation and the minus sign indicates a negative correlation. A perfect positive correlation is represented as *r* = 1.00; a perfect negative correlation is represented as *r* = −1.00. Chapter Six has introduced the coefficient of correlation as a way to determine the reliability and validity of measures. In empirical research studies, the strength of a correlation is judged by the following criteria (based on Cohen, 1988, and Salkind, 2004):

Weak correlations: *r* = ±.24 or less

Moderate correlations: *r* = ±.25 to .49

Moderately strong correlations: *r* = ±.50 to .74

Strong correlations: *r* = ±.75 to .99

The coefficient of correlation is a very handy statistic that is used for a variety of purposes in educational research. It can also be misused and misunderstood. It is important to remember that *r* describes the direction and strength of a relationship; it does not tell whether the relationship between variables is one of actual cause and effect. Correlations are visually represented in scatter plots.

Scatter Plots

A *scatter plot* expresses the direction and strength of a correlation. The scatter plot in Figure 7.17 shows the relationship between two variables: female median income in each state and the percentage of people in that state who have a bachelor's degree. The *x*-axis provides data about the median income of female workers in each state, and the *y*-axis provides the data on the percentage of people who have bachelor's degrees. Notice that the two variables move in the same direction: As the percentage of women in a state with bachelor's degrees goes up, so does the median wage for all people in the state, and vice versa. This indicates a positive correlation. The scatter plot also demonstrates a strong correlation. The way to judge this is by examining how close the values of the variables are to a straight line. The stronger the relationship, the closer it will be to the straight line. A perfect correlation is called the *line of best fit*. A visual examination of the scatter plot in Figure 7.17 shows that most of the values of the two variables cluster moderately close to the straight line. In fact, in this case, *r* = .61; this is a moderately strong, positive correlation.

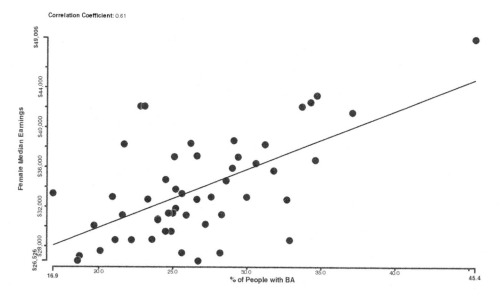

FIGURE 7.17. Scatter plot showing the relationship between female workers' median income and the percentage of people with bachelor's degrees in each state.

CHAPTER SUMMARY

MAP 7.5

✓ Descriptive statistics describe the status of variables at a point in time.

✓ Descriptive statistics include counts and percentages, measures of central tendency, frequency distributions, measures of variability, and correlations.

✓ Counts and percentages describe categorical data and are visually displayed in pie charts and in bar and line graphs.

✓ Measures of central tendency (the mean, median, and mode) describe the midpoint of continuous variables within a sample and are visually displayed in bar and line graphs.

✓ Frequency distributions describe the number of times that categorical variables and grouped continuous variables occur within a sample and are displayed in stem-and-leaf plots, frequency tables, and histograms.

✓ Measures of variability include range, spread, quartiles, variance, and standard deviations, and are displayed in box-and-whisker plots and in tables.

✓ The bell curve is a visual representation of the normal distribution of naturally occurring phenomena and their standard deviations.

✓ Correlations show the strength and direction of a relationship, are calculated by the coefficient of correlation (r), and are displayed in scatter plots.

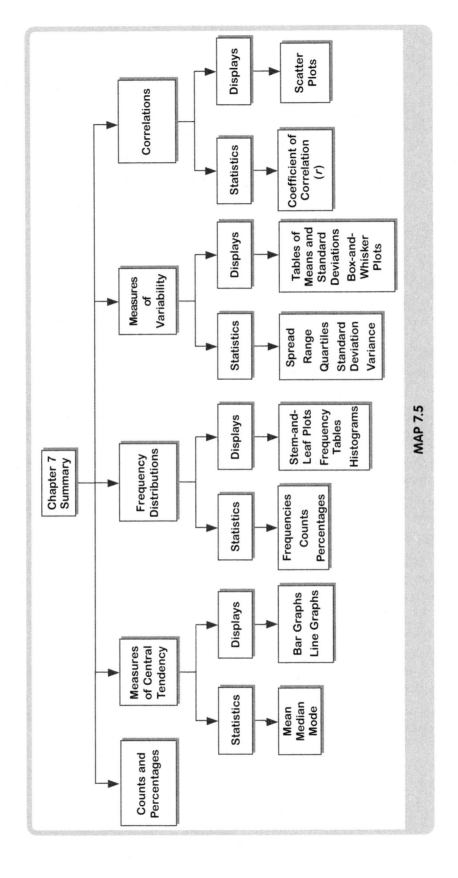

MAP 7.5

KEY TERMS AND CONCEPTS

bar graph

bell curve

box-and-whisker plot

coefficient of correlation (r)

correlation

counts

descriptive statistics

frequency distribution

frequency table

grouped bar graph

histogram

line graph

mean

measures of central tendency

measures of variability

median

mode

normal distribution

percentages

pie chart

quartile

range

scatter plot

spread

stacked bar graph

standard deviation (SD)

stem-and-leaf plot

table of means and SDs

variance

REVIEW, CONSOLIDATION, AND EXTENSION OF KNOWLEDGE

1. Explain the difference between *mean* and *median*, and indicate how this might have an impact on decision making.

2. Go to this URL (*nces.ed.gov/nceskids/createagraph*), and follow the instructions to create a pie graph, bar graph, and line graph of any data that are available to you or that you can access on the Internet.

3. Construct a frequency table of any data that are available to you or that you can access on the Internet.

4. Construct a stem-and-leaf plot of any data that are available to you or that you can access on the Internet.

5. Go to this URL (*www.easycalculation.com/statistics/standard-deviation.php*), and compute the mean and standard deviation of any set of values or scores you can access.

PART IV
Experimental Research

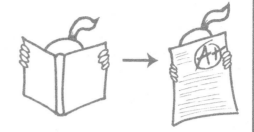

"Our actions run as causes and return to us as results."
—HERMAN MELVILLE

Part IV focuses on experimental research, the only kind of research that can demonstrate causal relationships. It replicates with human subjects, as much as possible, the conditions of a laboratory experiment in which the researcher measures the effect of an intervention on measured outcomes. In education, an intervention may be something like a new teaching approach, a program, a curriculum, or a behavioral intervention; an outcome may be academic achievement, engagement in learning, an acquired behavior, or the like.

CHAPTER EIGHT

Introduction to Experimental Research

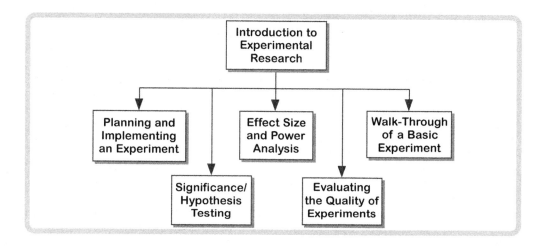

Experimental research depends on a researcher to control all aspects of a study from start to finish. This chapter describes how this is done in experimental research in general, and it explains the most basic experimental design.

CHAPTER OBJECTIVES

✓ Understand that the purpose of an experiment is to investigate a causal relationship.
✓ Understand the role of the researcher: to control all aspects of the experiment from start to finish.
✓ Understand the research review and how it identifies a theory that supports a research hypothesis.
✓ Understand independent and dependent variables.
✓ Understand the unit of analysis, sampling, data collection, and data analysis in experiments.
✓ Understand the difference between a true experiment and a quasi-experiment.
✓ Understand treatment and control groups and how they are used in between-group experiments.
✓ Understand inferential statistics in significance and hypothesis testing.
✓ Understand one- and two-tailed tests.
✓ Understand the *t*-test and how it is used in between-group experiments.
✓ Understand Type I and Type II errors in making decisions about hypotheses. Understand effect size estimates and power analysis.
✓ Understand the concept of validity.
✓ Understand how to evaluate an experiment.

PLANNING AND IMPLEMENTING AN EXPERIMENT   MAP 8.1

In planning an experiment, researchers have to (1) review relevant research to support the experiment, and (2) make decisions about elements of design.

Researchers review relevant and recent research in order to make a case for the study and to develop a rationale for hypothesizing that a particular intervention or treatment will effect a desired change in subjects. A well-grounded intervention has a strong explanatory theory that can lead to the identification of variables and the statement of a research hypothesis.

An *independent variable (IV)* represents the causal agent of the theory. Depending on their level of complexity, experimental studies may have one or multiple IVs (see Figure 8.1).

A *dependent variable (DV)* represents the outcome, or the *effect* that the researcher predicts will occur as a result of the intervention (see Figure 8.1).

The *research hypothesis* predicts the effect of the IV(s) on the DV(s). It can be stated as either a directional or a nondirectional hypothesis.

A *directional hypothesis* predicts that the treatment will result in a change, and that the change will be a positive result of the experiment.

A *nondirectional hypothesis* predicts that a treatment will result in a change in outcomes, but does not predict the direction of the change (i.e., whether it will be positive or negative).

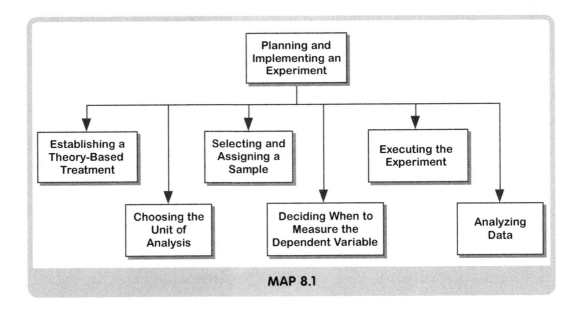

MAP 8.1

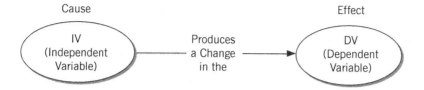

FIGURE 8.1. The relationship of the independent variable (IV) and the dependent variable (DV).

Choosing the Unit of Analysis

Between-group designs compare outcomes between groups after an intervention has occurred.

The *treatment group* receives the theory-based intervention.

The *control group* continues with "business as usual" and serves as a reference point for comparison with the treatment group.

Repeated-measures designs compare outcomes for individual subjects within a group.

Repeated-measures designs, and more complex types of between-group designs, are discussed in Chapter Nine. This chapter focuses on the simplest type of between-group design, with two groups and a single intervention.

Selecting and Assigning a Sample

Ideally, an experimental researcher will randomly select a sample of 60 or more subjects from a population. While randomized selection makes it more likely that findings can be generalized from the sample to the population, it is often not feasible for researchers to do this. In these cases, the researchers will use a convenience sample.

In a between-group design, researchers also have to decide how to assign the sample to control and treatment groups. The method of group assignment is what distinguishes a *true experimental design* from a *quasi-experimental design*.

A *true experimental design* uses a table of random numbers to assign subjects to groups.

A *quasi-experimental design* assigns subjects to groups nonrandomly, and usually assigns different *intact groups* (e.g., classrooms and schools) to treatment and control groups.

Deciding When and How Often to Measure the DV

Data may be collected on the DV before an intervention is introduced *and* after the experiment has concluded, or they may be collected only after an experiment has concluded.

A *pre- and posttest design* measures the DV(s) before the IV is introduced and again at the conclusion of the experiment. The most basic pre- and posttest design has one treatment group and one control group.

A *posttest-only design* measures the DV(s) only at the conclusion of the experiment.

Executing the Experiment

The researcher manipulates the IV so that the theory–based treatment is administered and is compared with a control condition. The researcher tries, as much as possible, to control all conditions of the experiment. However, this is more difficult to do with human subjects in real–life situations than with nonhuman subjects in a laboratory. The experiment concludes with a final measurement of the DV(s).

Analyzing Data

Once researchers have collected data from the posttest, they either calculate the means and standard deviations or the variances on the posttest. When they find changes in the DV, they use a process of statistical reasoning to establish statistical significance and test whether a hypothesis is true.

SIGNIFICANCE/HYPOTHESIS TESTING   MAP 8.2

Basic Terms and Concepts

The purpose of significance/hypothesis testing is to determine the probability (expressed as a statistic, p) that findings are due to an error in sampling. A low p-value indicates that the findings are *not* due to sampling error and are most likely due to the treatment. This allows the researcher to confirm the hypothesis.

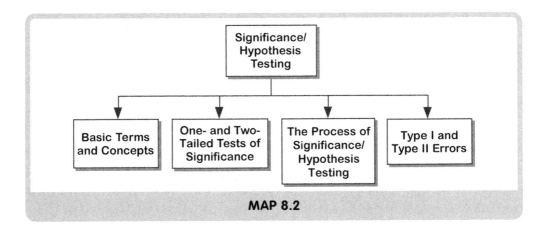

MAP 8.2

Statistical significance means that there is a low probability of the results being due to sampling error. It does not mean that the findings are important. The lower the *p*-value, the better.

Alpha (α) is the term used to indicate the level of *p* the researcher will accept for statistically significant findings. The researcher establishes the alpha before the experiment begins.

p ≤ .05 is the conventional alpha for experiments in education and other social sciences. It means a 5% or lower probability that the results are due to sampling error and a much greater likelihood that they are due to the treatment.

Significance/hypothesis testing in experiments depends on inferential statistics, sometimes referred to as *tests of significance*.

The *t-test* is the simplest way to establish the statistical significance of results between two groups. The *t*-test yields a statistic, *t*, which is then aligned with a *p*-value.

Analysis of variance (ANOVA) is a more robust statistic because it can be used with two or more groups and with additional IVs. *Multiple analysis of variance* (MANOVA) extends ANOVA to combine two or more DVs in the analysis. ANOVA/MANOVA yield a statistic, *F*, which is aligned with a *p*-value.

Analysis of covariance (ANCOVA) adjusts values on the DV when there is reason to think that the groups being compared are not equivalent. Nonequivalence can be detected on a pretest; it may be assumed in quasi-experiments when nonrandom assignment may result in uneven groups; or it may be used to control for another variable. *Multiple analysis of covariance* (MANCOVA) extends ANCOVA to combine two or more DVs in the analysis.

One- and Two-Tailed Tests of Significance

All inferential tests are based on probabilities of there being errors in sampling; these probabilities are derived from the bell curve and from a table of probabilities with the sample size and level of probability to guide the decision. Researchers can choose between using a *one-tailed* or *two-tailed* inferential test.

A *one-tailed test* (Figure 8.2) uses one end, or tail, of the curve to generate *p* ≤ .05.

A *two-tailed test* (Figure 8.3) uses two ends, or tails, with *p* ≤ .025 on each end of the curve, to generate *p* ≤ .05.

A two-tailed test is the more objective type of test. It represents a higher standard and degree of difficulty, because the probability must be distributed to both ends of the curve. Researchers often use a two-tailed test when there is a nondirectional hypothesis. A one-tailed test is more lenient, because all of the probability for the hypothesis test is on one side of the distribution curve.

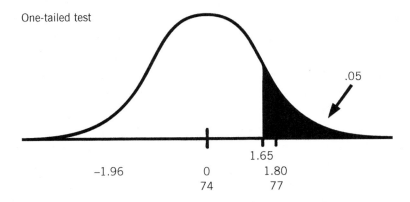

FIGURE 8.2. One–tailed test.

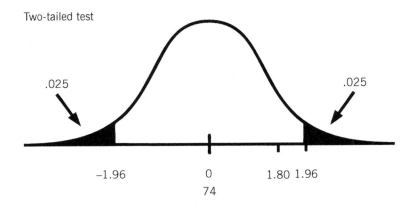

FIGURE 8.3. Two–tailed test.

The Process of Significance/Hypothesis Testing

Significance/hypothesis testing is a multistep statistical reasoning process that involves the *null hypothesis*.

The *null hypothesis* restates the hypothesis in negative terms *and* predicts that there will be no significant difference on the DV between the treatment and control groups.

To confirm that a hypothesis is true, a researcher has to demonstrate there is a low probability that the null hypothesis is true and that results are due to sampling error. In effect, the null hypothesis is set up as a "straw man"; it is easier to prove something false than it is to prove something true. This is where inferential statistics come in. The *p*-value represents the probability that results are due to error and that the null is true.

Before the experiment begins, the researcher establishes an *alpha* (α), which identifies the level of error the researcher will accept (see p. 145). For instance, if the researcher establishes an alpha of $p \leq .05$ and significance testing yields $p \leq .05$, the researcher can conclude that there is a 5% or lower probability that the null hypothesis is true. In other words, when $p \leq .05$, the researcher can reject the null hypothesis and confirm the research hypothesis.

Type I and Type II Errors

Despite all of this attention to statistical reasoning, there is still no guarantee that the decision about the hypothesis is correct; this is an admission of research fallibility. The possibility of making a wrong decision is known as a *Type I* or *Type II* error (see Figure 8.4).

> *Type I error*, also known as the *alpha-level error*, occurs when the researcher rejects the null hypothesis even though this hypothesis is true.

> *Type II error*, also known as the *beta-level error*, occurs when the researcher accepts the null hypothesis even though this hypothesis is false.

A researcher can control for Type I error by simply adjusting the alpha level for hypothesis testing to $p \leq .025$, thus making it more difficult to reject the null hypothesis. Correcting for a Type II error is more complicated and requires strengthening the theory, increasing the sample size, or improving the measurement.

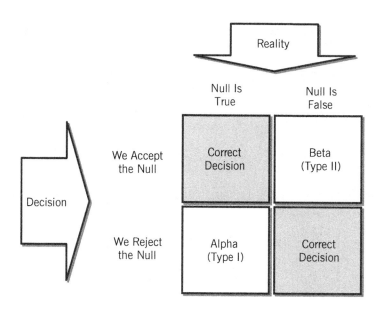

FIGURE 8.4. Decision making about the null hypothesis (with Type I and Type II errors).

EFFECT SIZE AND POWER ANALYSIS   MAP 8.3

While inferential statistical significance testing can indicate the probability that differences are due to treatments and not to chance or sampling error, it cannot indicate the magnitude of differences or the strength of an intervention. This is left to another statistic, known as the *effect size*.

Effect Size

> *Effect size* (often abbreviated as ES, especially in equations) is a standardized number that describes the overall strength of an experimental intervention in terms of changes in the standard deviation that result from the IV.

For example, ES = 0.5 means there has been a one-half standard deviation increase in values due to the treatment.

There are several formulas for determining effect size. For instance, the simplest delta (Δ) formula, developed by Glass (1976), is shown below. More advanced and sophisticated formulae are also used.

$$\Delta \text{ (delta)} = \frac{\text{Mean (experimental group)} - \text{mean (control group)}}{SD \text{ of the control group}}$$

There are also *Cohen's d* and *Hedges's g*. The following guidelines for judging ES are recommended:

<0.1 = trivial effect
$0.1–0.3$ = small effect
$0.3–0.5$ = moderate effect
>0.5 = large effect

In most cases, ES = 0.5 is desired.

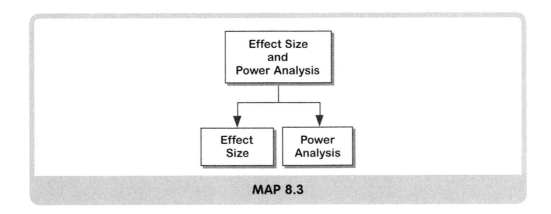

MAP 8.3

An analogy for effect size is the *signal-to-noise ratio*, which compares the size of the desired signal to extraneous or competing noise (Bickman & Rog, 2009). In addition to reporting on the strength of an intervention in an experiment, effect size estimates can be used to calculate the overall impact of an intervention across multiple studies, called *meta-analyses*. The use of effect size in meta-analysis is discussed in detail in Chapter Sixteen.

Power Analysis

Just as a researcher sets an acceptable level for *p* (i.e., alpha) before the experiment begins, the researcher may also set an estimated effect size. Taken together, the estimated effect size and the alpha can be used to address the age-old issue of sample size and help avoid a Type II error. This is done through the process of *power analysis*, which the researcher conducts before deciding on the final sample size for the study. An adequate sample size will yield a power = .80. To conduct a power analysis, the researcher uses a power software package and enters the following information:

- The inferential test that will be used to analyze data.
- The alpha for significance that will be used.
- The expected effect size (again, ES = 0.5 is recommended).
- The planned sample size for the study.

The software will then generate a power value between 0 and 1. If power is less than .80, the researcher will have to increase the sample size in order to avoid a Type II error. If the sample cannot be increased, the researcher may continue with the study and acknowledge that the study has less power.

EVALUATING THE QUALITY OF EXPERIMENTS `MAP 8.4`

An evaluation of the quality of an experimental study focuses on its validity and the importance of theory and treatment, sample and sampling, and data collection and analysis.

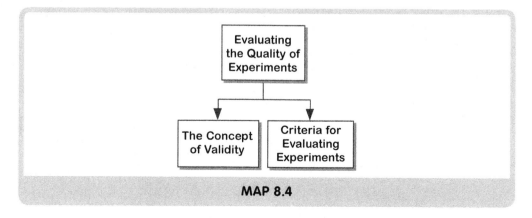

MAP 8.4

The Concept of Validity   MAP 8.5

The concept of *validity* was introduced in Chapter Seven in relation to measures and the degree to which they measure what they purport to measure. In evaluating an experimental study, validity concerns the degree to which the experiment is well planned and executed, establishes a causal relationship between and among variables, and allows the researcher to generalize the results to other populations and settings. Campbell and Stanley (1963) developed the first model of validity; they identified two types of validity (*internal* and *external*) and the threats that could undermine them.

> *Internal validity* is concerned with the strength of causality: whether the changes in the DV are due to the treatment or to alternative explanations or threats that might account for the differences.

Threats to internal validity include (1) maturation (normal developmental processes); (2) history (an unexpected event that affects the relationship between the IV and DV); (3) statistical regression (a sample that includes extremes, such as all "gifted" students); (4) selection (nonrandomized assignment of subjects, mortality, attrition of subjects); (5) testing (unintended sensitizing of subjects during pretesting); (6) design contamination (subjects' comparing notes or having motivations for the experiment to succeed or fail); and (7) compensatory rivalry (for example, teachers in a control modifying their behavior in order to compete with the treatment group).

> *External validity* is concerned with the strength of generalizability: the degree to which findings can be applied to other individuals, settings, and times (*population validity*) or to other settings (*ecological validity*).

Threats to population validity include (1) nonrandom samples and nonrandom group assignments; (2) the Hawthorn effect (the reaction of subjects to being studied); (3) the experimental conditions effect (the way the experiment is arranged); and (4) the experimenter effect (the characteristics of the person[s] conducting the study). Threats to ecological validity include the second, third, and fourth threats to population validity.

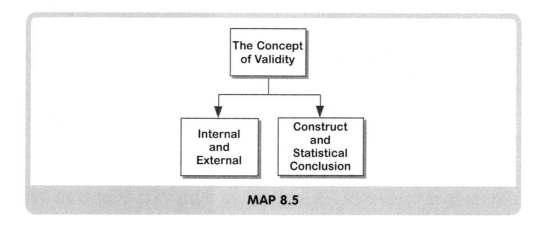

MAP 8.5

The concept of validity was elaborated 16 years later by Cook and Campbell (1979), who added *construct validity* and *statistical conclusion validity* to the mix.

Construct validity (also known as *theoretical validity*) concerns the strength of the theory—its ability to support the choice of treatment, the operationalization of variables, and the development of a hypothesis suitable for hypothesis testing.

Statistical conclusion validity concerns the strength and precision of statistical reasoning to make inferences from the data.

Threats to statistical conclusion validity include (1) "fishing" (reanalyzing data in order to find possible significant results); (2) invalid or unreliable measures; and (3) inadequate sample size or sampling error.

Criteria for Evaluating Experiments   MAP 8.6

We recommend that readers evaluate experimental studies in terms of their theory and treatment, their samples and sampling, and their collection and analysis of data. We believe that these three criteria are reasonable ways to capture the complexity of validity and threats to validity.

Theory and Treatment

The primary considerations for theory and treatment are the quality of the literature review, how well the authors derived operational definitions for the independent and dependent variables, how well the treatment matches the theory, and how well the treatment was implemented.

1. How well does the research review support a theory?
2. How well is the theory operationalized? How adequate is the operationalization of the IV and DV?
3. How well does the treatment match the theory?
4. How well is the treatment implemented?

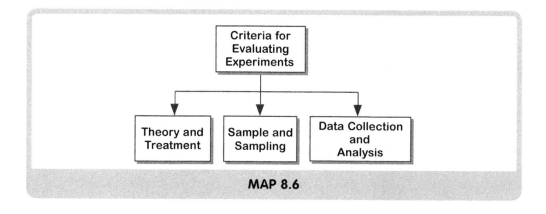

MAP 8.6

Sample and Sampling

The key elements in sampling are the procedures for selecting the sample and assigning subjects to the treatment condition, as well as the size of the sample and the characteristics of the subjects.

1. Is randomization used in selection and/or assignment to the treatment condition?

2. Is there adequate sample size? (Was there a power analysis? Does the sample include a minimum of 30 subjects?)

Collection and Analysis of Data

The key elements in evaluating collection and analysis of data are the validity and reliability of the measures, as well as the appropriateness of the statistical analysis and the process of statistical reasoning. Figure 8.5 shows a rubric for evaluating the quality of experiments.

Criterion	Strong	Moderate	Weak
Theory and treatment	Clear, current, and sufficient literature review, including 10 or more references; clearly defined IV and DV.	Literature review may not make a clear connection to the research question or has fewer than 10 references; IV and DV definitions missing or unclear.	Unclear literature review; fewer than 5 references; no reference to or definitions of IV and DV.
Sample and sampling	Clear description of the sample characteristics and the population; clear description of sample; evidence of sufficient size (60 or more, or use of power analysis); random assignment of subjects to control conditions. The sample allows for the generalization of findings to other subjects and settings.	Description of sample is present, but lacking in details about characteristics and the population; insufficient sample size; nonrandom assignment to control condition; unclear description of sample size. The sample does not allow for generalization of findings.	No description of the sample; total lack of details about the population; nonrandom assignment to control condition; insufficient sample size. The sample does not allow for generalization of findings.
Data collection and analysis	Clear description of measures selected to collect data on DV and evidence of validity and reliability (r); clear description of statistical significance (p) and of the inferential tests used; clear reporting on hypothesis testing; clear indication of whether ES was calculated; and clear reporting of results. Researcher stays close to data and does not overconclude.	Mention of measurement, but lacking in details about validity and reliability (r); mention of statistical significance (p), but without including inferential tests used; no reporting on hypothesis testing or indication of ES. Researcher avoids overconcluding.	Minimal or no mention of measurement; no mention of validity or reliability; no mention of significance, hypothesis testing, or use of ES. Researcher may overconclude.

FIGURE 8.5. Rubric for evaluating quality of experiments.

1. How good are the validity and reliability of the measures?
2. How well are the measured data reported and analyzed?
3. Are appropriate statistics applied? Statistical significance? Effect size?
4. Are hypotheses adequately tested and evaluated? Is the alpha set too high?
5. Are there alternative explanations due to extraneous and confounding factors, or threats that affect the conclusion?

WALK-THROUGH OF A BASIC EXPERIMENT

The most basic experimental designs are between-group designs with one IV, one control group, and one treatment group, as illustrated in Figures 8.6 and 8.7. This section describes the step-by-step process in a basic posttest-only experiment that a researcher used to investigate the effects of verbal praise on graduate students.

Hancock, D. R. (2002). Influencing graduate students' classroom achievement, homework habits and motivation to learn with verbal praise. *Educational Research, 44*(1), 83–95.

Research Review

An extensive research review of more than 35 studies established the efficacy of well-constructed verbal praise in improving student achievement, home preparedness, and motivation. This led to the development of three research hypotheses:

1. Postsecondary students exposed to well-administered verbal praise by a professor would demonstrate higher achievement levels on a professor-made examination than would students who received no well-administered verbal praise.
2. Postsecondary students exposed to well-administered verbal praise by a professor would spend significantly more time preparing at home (i.e., doing homework) for each lesson than would students who received no well-administered verbal praise.
3. Postsecondary students exposed to well-administered verbal praise by a professor would demonstrate higher motivation levels to learn in the classroom than would students who received no well-administered verbal praise.

The IV was feedback to students (verbal praise vs. no verbal praise). The DVs were as follows: DV 1, achievement; DV 2, homework preparation; DV 3, motivation to learn. There were three separate statistical analyses.

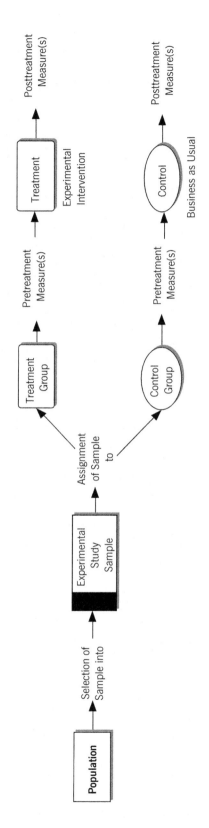

FIGURE 8.6. Basic pre– and posttest design.

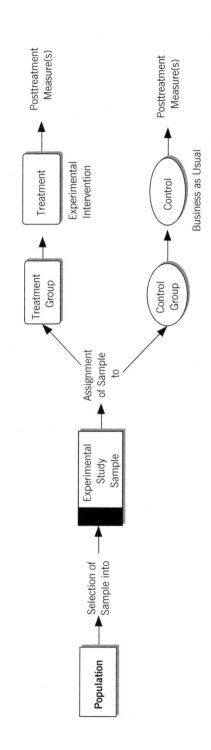

FIGURE 8.7. Basic posttest-only design.

Sampling

The sample consisted of 54 graduate students (49 females and 5 males) who were enrolled in two sections of a graduate-level course that the researcher taught. One intact class was designated as the control group; the other intact class was designated as the treatment group. This procedure for group assignment marks the study as a quasi-experiment; however, the matching of the subjects in the groups increased the likelihood that the groups were equivalent.

Data Collection

The measures for the DVs were as follows. Achievement was measured with an instructor-made examination that was vetted for validity and reliability; homework preparation was measured with a student-reported homework log of hours spent in homework; and motivation was measured with the Motivated Strategies for Learning Questionnaire (MSLQ), a standardized questionnaire that showed adequate validity and reliability. The measures were administered and scored at the end of the experiment.

Purpose and Design

For the purpose of investigating the effect of verbal praise on the three DVs, the researcher used a posttest-only design (see Figure 8.8). At five randomly selected class meetings, he viewed the homework logs of students in both groups, and he verbally praised subjects in the treatment group who had met the expectation of 180 minutes per week of home preparation. Subjects in the control group received a neutral response of "Thank you." During the last class, the instructor collected the homework logs, administered the MSLQ, and gave the final exam.

Data Analysis, Interpretation, and Conclusions

The t-test is often used with a randomized posttest-only design; here the researcher used three two-tailed t-tests, one for each DV. There were three steps involved in arriving at p-values: (1) calculation of the means and standard deviations for the posttest scores; (2) calculation of the t-values; and (3) consulting a table of critical t-values to see whether the calculated t-values met the alpha level the researcher had set.

Table 8.1 shows the results of the t-test analysis. The table presents the mean and standard deviation for control and treatment groups on each of the three DVs. The t-values are also indicated. The number in parentheses (52) before each t-value is the *degree of freedom* (often abbreviated as *df*, especially in equations), which is used to determine the p-value. The *df* is simply the number of subjects minus the number of groups (in this case, $54 - 2 = 52$). The asterisk ($\star$) that appears next to each t-value indicates that $p \leq .05$ has been achieved; this is explained in the footnote at the bottom of the table.

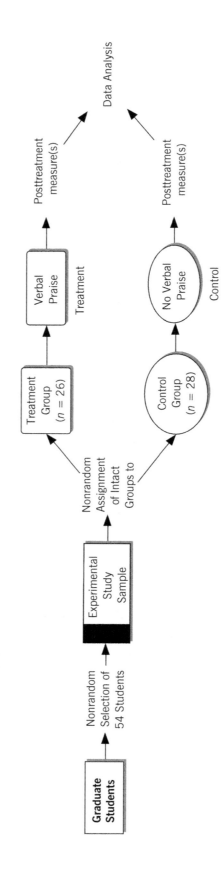

FIGURE 8.8. Design for the Hancock (2002) experiment.

TABLE 8.1. Results of the Hancock (2002) *t*-Test Analysis

	Teacher test		Homework hours		MSLQ	
	Control	Treatment	Control	Treatment	Control	Treatment
Mean	81.86	85.11	137.14	149.38	4.97	5.11
SD	6.06	5.49	15.17	22.16	0.251	0.221
	t (52) = 2.065*		*t* (52) = 2.38*		*t* (52) = 2.170*	

*$p \leq .05$.

In order to generate the *p*-value, the researcher consulted a table of critical *t*-values, illustrated in Table 8.2. At the top are the alpha levels for one- and two-tailed tests. The first column on the left lists degrees of freedom. The next six columns present the critical *t*-values for each type of test and at each alpha for each degree of freedom. Results are considered significant when the *t*-values from an experiment are higher than the critical *t*-value. Looking across the *df* = 52 row and down the column for a two-tailed test at alpha = .05, we can see that the critical *t*-value = 2.007 (underlined). Since the Hancock article reported higher *t*-values for differences in each of the three DVs, the three differences were judged to be statistically significant at $p \leq .05$. This also meant that the null hypotheses were rejected and the research hypotheses were confirmed.

In addition, the researcher reported effect sizes for the three DVs as follows: achievement, ES = 0.54; homework, ES = 0.80; motivation, ES = 0.56. In other words, the administration of verbal praise led to a one-half standard deviation increase

TABLE 8.2. Table of Critical *t*-Values for Hancock (2002)

	Alphas					
	Significance for a directional (one-tailed) test					
	.05	.025	.01	.005	.0025	.001
	Significance for a nondirectional (two-tailed) test					
df	.10	.05	.02	.01	.005	.002
50	1.676	2.009	2.403	2.678	2.937	3.261
51	1.675	2.008	2.402	2.676	2.934	3.258
52	1.675	2.007	2.400	2.674	2.932	3.254
53	1.674	2.006	2.399	2.672	2.929	3.251
54	1.674	2.005	2.397	2.670	2.927	3.248
55	1.673	2.004	2.396	2.668	2.925	3.245
60	1.671	2.000	2.390	2.660	2.915	2.232

Note. df = 50–60.

in achievement and in motivation, and a four-fifths standard deviation increase in hours of home preparation. These are substantial gains.

The researcher concluded that the three research hypotheses were confirmed, and that there were significant and ample differences in change on the DVs between the control and treatment groups.

Evaluation

The overall rating of this study is moderate, based on three criteria:

1. Theory and treatment were strong; construct validity was demonstrated; and the researcher controlled for threats to internal validity. The author begins the article with a review of more than 35 previous studies, to establish the theoretical foundation for the experiment. The IV and DVs were clearly defined, as were the three hypotheses.

2. Sampling was weak to moderate and threatened external validity. The author provides some detail about sample characteristics. The sample size was a bit smaller than 60 and was disproportionately female. Intact groups were assigned to control and treatment groups; however, the matching of the subjects in the groups increased the likelihood that the groups were equivalent.

3. Collection and analysis of data were strong, and statistical conclusion validity was demonstrated. The measures of achievement and motivation are clearly described, and the measures for achievement and motivation were vetted for validity and reliability. Analysis included significance/hypothesis testing (with an appropriate alpha) and effect size estimates. In describing results, the researcher stays close to the data and does not overconclude.

CHAPTER SUMMARY   MAP 8.7

✓ The purpose of an experiment is to investigate a predicted causal relationship when an intervention is introduced and manipulated by a researcher.

✓ The research review makes a case for the study and establishes a theory that guides the development of a hypothesis and the selection of variables.

✓ Hypotheses may be directional or nondirectional.

✓ Independent variables (IVs) = causes; dependent variables (DVs)= effects.

✓ Researchers make the design decisions about (1) the unit of analysis (group or individuals); (2) sampling (size, selection, assignment); and (3) data collection (when and how often to measure the DV).

✓ Between-group designs have a control group and a treatment group.

✓ Experiments use randomized samples from a population or convenience samples; sample size should be at least 60.

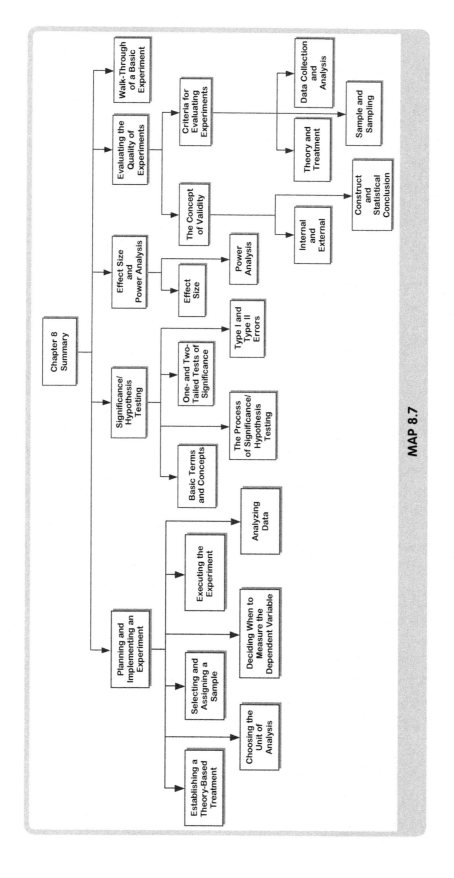

MAP 8.7

✓ True experiments randomly assign subjects to groups; quasi-experiments do not use random-ized group assignment.

✓ Analysis of data always involves significance testing and hypothesis testing; they may also include effect size estimates and power analysis.

✓ Statistical significance means a low probability (p) that a difference between groups is due to sampling error, and a high likelihood that it is due to the treatment.

✓ The t-test is the simplest way to establish the statistical significance of the difference in results between one control and one treatment group.

✓ $p \le .05$ is the threshold (alpha or α) conventionally used for statistical significance.

✓ Inferential/significance tests are based on the normal (bell) curve and may be one- or two-tailed.

✓ Hypothesis testing uses alpha (α) to determine the probability that the null hypothesis is false.

✓ Type I error, also known as the alpha-level error, occurs when the researcher rejects the null hypothesis even though this hypothesis is true; Type II error, also known as the beta-level error, occurs when the researcher accepts the null hypothesis even though this hypothesis is false.

✓ Effect size (ES) is a standardized number that describes the overall strength of an experimental intervention; ES = 0.5 is considered adequate.

✓ Statistical power tells the likelihood that the researcher has established an adequate sample size and will thus avoid making a Type II error. Power = .80 is desired.

✓ Validity of a study refers to the strength of the inferences and conclusions that can be drawn, and the level of confidence in results.

✓ Internal validity answers this question: Are the changes in the DV due to the treatment, or are there alternative explanations (threats to internal validity) that might account for the differ-ences?

✓ External validity answers this question: Can the findings be generalized to other individuals, settings, and times? There are two types of external validity: population validity and ecological validity.

✓ Construct or theoretical validity answers this question: How well does the research review sup-port the operational definitions used in the research question and hypotheses?

✓ Statistical conclusion validity answers this question: Do the measurement and statistical argu-ment support the relationship between the IV and DV?

✓ Threats to validity are alternative explanations that can account for results.

✓ Evaluating an experiment depends on three sets of criteria: theory and treatment, sample and sampling, and collection and analysis of data.

KEY TERMS AND CONCEPTS

alpha	population validity
construct/theoretical validity	power/power analysis
control group	p-value
degree of freedom (df)	quasi-experiment
dependent variable (DV)	research hypothesis
directional hypothesis	statistical conclusion validity
ecological validity	statistical significance
effect size (ES)	table of critical t-values
external validity	threats to validity
hypothesis testing	treatment group
independent variable (IV)	true experiment
internal validity	two-tailed test
nondirectional hypothesis	Type I (alpha-level) error
null hypothesis	Type II (beta-level) error
one-tailed test	validity

REVIEW, CONSOLIDATION, AND EXTENSION OF KNOWLEDGE

1. Match the terms in Column A to the definitions in Column B.

Column A	Column B
independent variable	magnitude of difference
true experiment	the causal variable
alpha	rejects the null hypothesis when it is true
null hypothesis	effect is due to the cause
effect size	random assignment to groups
Type I error	test for significance
Internal validity	$p \leq .05$, used in hypothesis testing
t-test	predicts no difference in outcomes

2. Using an electronic database, search for an article describing an experiment on a topic of interest to you. Follow the Guide to Reading below as you work through the article. Then, with the Guide as a template, write a critique of the article you have selected.

Guide to Reading

Research Review: Does the review establish a theoretical foundation for the experiment? How current is the review? Are more than 10 studies reviewed? What hypothesis/hypotheses or research questions are generated from the research review?

Purpose and Design: What was the purpose of the study? What were the IV and DV(s)? How were they operationalized? What was the design of the study?

Sampling: What was the sample size? How was the sample selected (randomly or nonrandomly)? What were the characteristics of the sample? How was the sample assigned to groups (randomly or nonrandomly)?

Data Collection: What specific data collection strategies were used? Do the authors give indications of the measures' validity and reliability? If so, what are they? How well did the data collection strategies match the research question or purpose?

Data Analysis, Interpretation, and Conclusions: How were the data analyzed? What statistical tests were used? What were the results? Were the results significant or nonsignificant? How well does the data analysis match the research question or purpose? To what degree do the analysis, interpretation, and conclusions stay close to the data? Have the researchers overconcluded?

Evaluation: How do you rate the overall quality of the study? Strong? Moderate? Weak? How do you rate the categories below, and what is your reason for each rating?

Theory and treatment: Strong, moderate, weak

Sample and sampling: Strong, moderate, weak

Data collection and analysis: Strong, moderate, weak

Sample Critique

This sample critique is a review of the same article covered in the "Walk-Through of a Basic Experiment" section of this chapter, with more details included.

Hancock, D. R. (2002). Influencing graduate students' classroom achievement, homework habits and motivation to learn with verbal praise. *Educational Research, 44*(1), 83–95.

Research Review

The article begins with a review of more than 35 previous studies to establish a theoretical framework for the study. The articles reviewed focused on the relationship between verbal praise and "motivation to learn, classroom achievement, homework habits, and graduate education" (p. 83), as well as developing a detailed description of well-constructed verbal praise. The researcher developed three hypotheses from the review (pp. 88–89):

1. Postsecondary students exposed to well-administered verbal praise by a professor would demonstrate higher achievement levels on a professor-made examination than would students who received no well-administered verbal praise.
2. Postsecondary students exposed to well-administered verbal praise by a professor would spend significantly more time preparing at home (i.e., doing homework) for each lesson than would students who received no well-administered verbal praise.
3. Postsecondary students exposed to well-administered verbal praise by a professor would demonstrate higher motivation levels to learn in the classroom than would students who received no well-administered verbal praise.

Purpose and Design

The purpose of the study was to investigate the effect of well-constructed verbal praise on student outcomes. The IV was well-constructed verbal praise. The DVs were as follows:

DV 1 = achievement

DV 2 = homework preparation

DV 3 = motivation to learn, measured by the Motivated Strategies for Learning Questionnaire (MSLQ)

Sampling

The convenience sample consisted of "54 graduate students in a one-semester course in Educational Research Methods that the researcher taught at a middle-size[d], state-supported university in the southeastern United States" (p. 86). The 49 female and 5 male students were enrolled in one of two relatively equal-sized sections. The researcher designated one section as the treatment group and the other as the control group. This intact groups sampling strategy is indicative of a quasi-experiment. The researcher noted that the sections were matched with respect to age, gender, degree program, GPA, and socioeconomic status.

Data Collection

The measure of home preparation was a self-reported homework log. The measure for motivations was a portion of the MSLQ, a 7-point Likert scale questionnaire that was administered during the 15th class session. The MSLQ assesses motivational tendencies, self-efficacy, and success expectancy. Its predictive validity was reported as .29; internal consistency ranged from .62 to .93. The measure of achievement was an instructor-created final examination administered during the final classes. Content validity was established by having two experts review the test's alignment to lesson objectives; the split-half reliability coefficient was .76.

Students were told that there was an expectation for homework of about 180 minutes weekly. The instructor viewed the logs during five randomly selected classes. In the treatment group, the instructor verbally praised students who had met the expectations. Students in the control group received a neutral response of "Thank you." An independent observer checked the fidelity of the treatment.

Data Analysis, Interpretation, and Conclusions

Data were analyzed with three t-tests, one for each measure. Results for the three DVs were as follows: for achievement, $t = 2.065$; for homework, $t = 2.38$; for motivation (MSLQ), $t = 2.170$. Each finding was significant at $p \leq .05$. The results indicated that the effects were most likely due to the treatment and not to chance or error. The researcher rejected the null hypotheses and accepted the research hypotheses as listed. In addition, the researcher conduced an effect size estimate that yielded these results: ES = 0.54 for achievement; ES = 0.80 for homework; and ES = 0.56 for motivation.

Evaluation

Using the criteria of theory and treatment, sample and sampling, and data collection and analysis, I give this study an overall rating of moderate.

- *Theory and treatment* merit a rating of strong. The article begins with a review of more than 35 previous articles to establish the theoretical foundation for the experiment. The researcher clearly defined the IV and DVs at the start of the research.

- *Sample and sampling* merit a rating of only weak to moderate. The author has provided a description of the sample size and some details about sample characteristics. However, the sample size was below 60; the sample was disproportionately female; and there was nonrandom group assignment. As a result, the sample does not lead to the generalization of findings.

- *Data collection and analysis* are rated as strong. The measures of achievement and motivation are clearly described, and the measures for achievement and motivation were vetted for validity and reliability. Hypothesis testing may be assumed from the alpha level and t-values. The researcher stays close to the data and does not overconclude.

CHAPTER NINE

Factorial Designs
Between-Group and Repeated-Measures Designs

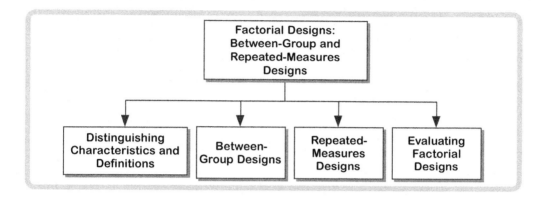

Chapter Eight introduced experimental research and demonstrated its key elements by focusing on the basic design, which includes one treatment and one control group and a pre- and posttest or posttest only, and which uses a *t*-test to establish statistical significance and to conduct hypothesis testing. This chapter introduces more complex experiments that use multistep statistical procedures.

CHAPTER OBJECTIVES
✓ Understand between-group and repeated-measures factorial designs.
✓ Understand how levels of a treatment are used in these designs.
✓ Understand the analysis of main effects, interactions, and covariates.
✓ Understand how to evaluate the quality of factorial designs.

DISTINGUISHING CHARACTERISTICS AND DEFINITIONS MAP 9.1

Factorial designs investigate the influence of two or more treatments (IVs) and/or levels of treatment in a single study. In addition, they can examine the influence of other variables.

Factors, Levels, and Effects

Factor is the term applied to the main treatment or treatments (IVs), and is also used to refer to modifying or intervening variables that may influence the DV(s) in a factorial study.

Levels are the varying categories within a factor.

Factorial designs allow researchers to investigate both main effects and interaction effects.

A *main effect* is the effect of each factor on the DV(s).

An *interaction effect* is the uneven impact of the levels on the DV(s).

Designs

There are several factorial designs that fall within the following two broad categories:

Between-group designs investigate differences between groups that receive varying treatments and/or levels of treatment

Repeated-measures designs investigate differences within individuals who receive varying treatments and/or levels of treatment.

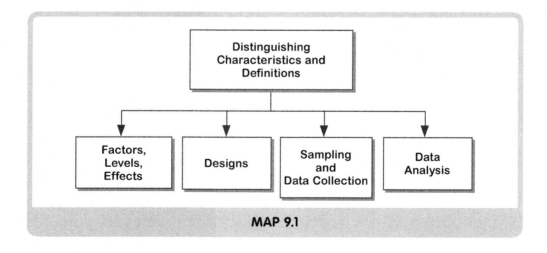

MAP 9.1

Sampling and Data Collection

In factorial studies, sampling and data collection are very similar to the procedures used in other experimental designs. (See Chapter Eight.)

Data Analysis

Because factorial designs consider the effect of one or more factors (IVs) and levels (and often involve two or more groups), they require inferential tests for significance and hypothesis testing that are more powerful than the *t*-test, which can only compare two groups with the same IV. The ANOVA/MANOVA and ANCOVA/MANCOVA, described in Chapter Eight, are used extensively in factorial designs to determine the statistical significance of the main and interaction effects of factors.

In factorial designs, the ANOVA and MANOVA calculate the main effect of (1) one factor with more than one level or (2) two or more factors, each with one or more levels. The ANOVA is used when there is one DV; the MANOVA is used when there are two or more DVs.

- In a between-group design with a single factor, the *one-way ANOVA* is used to analyze the data.
- In a between-group design with two or more factors, the *factorial ANOVA* is used to test all of the group differences with a single *F*-test.
- In a repeated-measures design, the *repeated-measures ANOVA* is used.

Both the ANOVA/MANOVA and ANCOVA/MANCOVA yield an *F*-value, which leads to a *p*-value that determines the overall main effects of the factors. The ANCOVA and MANCOVA calculate main effects when there is a *covariate*. The covariate may be (1) a difference in groups or individuals before the experiment begins and (2) the influence of another IV that the researchers seek to remove. They function in the same way as ANOVA/MANOVA, in that they calculate main effects and interaction effects by incorporating the covariate adjustments.

Because it may be the case that the main effect is significant and not all levels of treatment are significant, researchers want to know which treatment level or levels are the precise source(s) of the main effect. In order to do this, they perform a series of *t*-tests to isolate the source(s) of the effect. Statistical reasoning for the ANOVA/MANOVA and ANCOVA/MANCOVA procedures involves a three-step process: (1) determination of the overall main effects with a calculated *F*-score and *p*-value, (2) additional statistical tests to see whether there are interaction effects, and (3) follow-up *t*-tests and *p*-values for each of the possible combinations of treatment and control.

BETWEEN-GROUP DESIGNS   MAP 9.2

Between-group designs investigate the differences in two or more groups that (1) receive a treatment, (2) have multiple levels of one treatment, or (3) have more than one treatment with one or more levels. Between-group designs are classified as either *single-factor designs* or *factorial (multifactor) designs.*

Single-Factor Designs

Single-factor designs have one factor (IV) and two or more levels of the factor.

For example, a researcher could examine the effect of feedback to students on achievement and decide to have three levels of factors:

Single factor (IV) = feedback
    Level 1 = feedback as comments
    Level 2 = feedback as comments plus grades
    Level 3 = feedback as grades only

The researcher would assign the subjects in the sample to one of three groups:

    Group 1 would receive comments as feedback.
    Group 2 would receive comments plus grades as feedback.
    Group 3 would receive grades only.

The researcher would analyze the findings by using a one-way ANOVA to calculate F- and p-values, followed by individual t-tests to determine which of the three levels had statistically significant results.

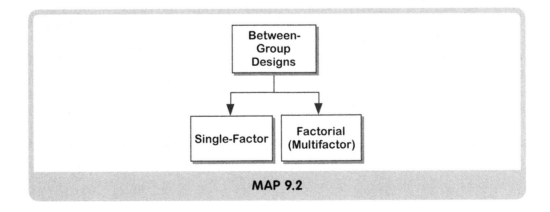

MAP 9.2

Factorial (Multifactor) Designs

Factorial designs (multifactor designs) have two or more factors and one or more levels for each factor.

For example, a researcher may decide to expand on the single-factor design described above by introducing the additional factor of gender. In this case, the design is called a 3 × 2 factorial design, because it has one factor with three levels and another factor with two levels. Factorial designs are always identified by the number of factors and the number of levels in each factor.

In the 3 × 2 factorial design of the effect of feedback, the researcher would assign subjects in the sample to one of six groups, each representing a different combination of factors and levels:

Group 1: Males/comments only

Group 2: Females/comments only

Group 3: Males/comments and grades

Group 4: Females/comments and grades

Group 5: Males/grades only

Group 6: Females/grades only

The researcher would use a factorial ANOVA to calculate *F*- and *p*-values, followed by individual *t*-tests to determine which of the three levels had statistically significant results. The advantage of a 3 × 2 factorial design is that it allows a researcher to test more than one hypothesis, to build additional variables into the design as factors, and to test interaction effects. The disadvantage is that it requires a large sample.

Below are four examples of between-group designs, with increasing levels of complexity.

1. Single-Factor Design with One-Way ANOVA

Gencosman, T., & Dogru, M. (2012). Effect of student teams–achievement divisions technique used in science and technology on self-efficacy, anxiety and academic achievement. *Journal of Baltic Science Education, 11*(1), 43–54.

This study examined one factor with one treatment group and two control groups. The experiment was designed to compare one treatment approach (cooperative learning strategies) against two comparable learning strategies deemed to be control conditions. Students were randomly assigned to all three conditions, and each group completed a curriculum unit in physics on "Force and Motion." Both control conditions contained lectures and whole-group discussions/questioning. In addition, the Control 2 condition used a constructivist approach, which encouraged individual development of conceptual knowledge. (The researchers considered their design to have two control groups, but the Control 2 condition may be considered a treatment group.)

    Factor = Teaching strategies

        Treatment group = Cooperative learning (student teams)

        Control 1 = Lectures and whole-group discussions

        Control 2 = Constructivist approach, lectures, and whole-group discussions

There were three DVs:

    DV 1 = achievement

    DV 2 = self-efficacy

    DV 3 = test anxiety

Each DV was measured on a pretest and a posttest. The study's design is illustrated in Figure 9.1.

    The treatment, cooperative learning, was an approach carefully designed to reflect DVs. The results for self-efficacy showed a statistically significant difference among the three groups ($F = 10.37$, $p < .0001$), as did the results for test anxiety ($F = 10.79$, $p < .0001$) and the results for academic achievement ($F = 3.53$, $p < .03$).

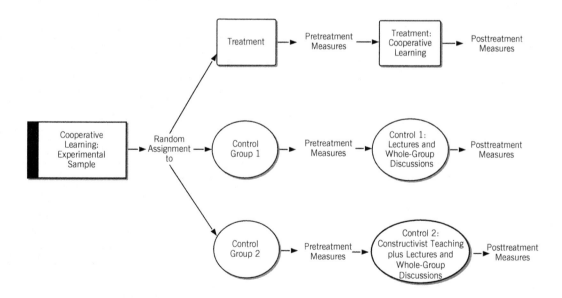

FIGURE 9.1. Design for the Gencosman and Dogru (2012) experiment.

2. Single-Factor Design with One-Way ANCOVA

Nesbit, J., & Adesope, O. (2011). Learning from animated concept maps with concurrent audio narration. *Journal of Experimental Education, 79,* 209–230.

This study investigated a series of hypotheses related to the impact of concept maps on undergraduate students' recall and understanding of the course topic of attribution theory. Three different forms of expert maps were created by the research team: (1) plain, black-and-white concept maps; (2) color-coded concept maps; and (3) animated concept maps, using visual icons. "Each participant was randomly assigned to one of four groups in a single factor, between-subject experimental design" (p. 218). The research hypotheses were as follows: (1) Participants receiving either the plain concept maps or the color-coded concept maps would outperform students who received the plain text only; (2) participants receiving the color-coded maps would outperform the students receiving plain maps; and (3) participants receiving the animated concept maps would outperform the students who received plain text, and students receiving color-coded maps would outperform students who received plain concept maps on measures of the central ideas and supporting details.

Factor = Concept mapping

　　Group 1 = Black-and-white concept maps (plain maps)

　　Group 2 = Color-coded concept maps (color maps)

　　Group 3 = Text-animated concept maps (prior text)

　　Group 4 = Control (plain text)

There were two DVs: free-recall short-term memory and achievement on a knowledge examination. Each DV was measured with a separate ANCOVA. The researchers used an ANCOVA in order to adjust for differences in scores on a midterm examination.

Covariate = Midterm exam scores

DV 1 = Free-recall short-term memory

DV 2 = Knowledge test (multiple-choice test)

Figure 9.2 represents this design visually.

The overall results of the ANCOVA were found to be statistically significant for the main effect of concept mapping on the knowledge measure ($F = 11.06, p < .001$). In addition, the researchers conducted *t*-tests to determine the specific sources of the main effect. There were statistically significant differences for color-coded concept maps versus text, and for plain concept maps versus text. However, they found no statistically significant differences between students who used color-coded concept maps and students who used plain, black-and-white concept maps.

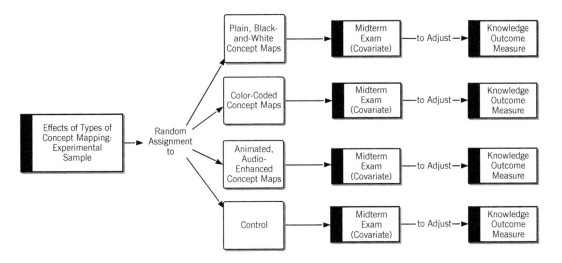

FIGURE 9.2. Design for the Nesbit and Adesope (2011) experiment.

3. Factorial Design with 3 × 2 ANOVA

Lim, K. Y., Lee, H. W., & Grabowski, B. (2009). Does concept-mapping strategy work for everyone?: The levels of generativity and learners' self-regulated learning skills. *British Journal of Educational Technology, 40*(4), 606–618.

The researchers conducted a 3 (treatment) × 2 (self-regulated learning) factorial analysis of concept-mapping strategies. They were interested in the effects of three levels of the concept-mapping treatment on two levels of students' self-reported self-regulated learning, as well as their effects on student knowledge of a topic. The participants were randomly assigned to three groups, each receiving a different concept-generating strategy. The three levels of treatment were these: Level 1 = expert-generated, Level 2 = partially student-generated, and Level 3 = fully student-generated.

The second factor was a categorical variable, student self-regulated learning. The researchers used a survey to divide students in each group into two categories: Level 1 = high self-regulated learning, and Level 2 = low self-regulated learning. In the end, therefore, six groups of students were compared: two groups (high and low self-regulated learning) using expert maps; two groups (high and low self-regulated learning) using partially learner-generated maps; and two groups (high and low self-regulated learning) using fully learner-generated maps.

Factor 1= Type of concept mapping

    Group 1 = Expert-generated concept map

    Group 2 = Partially learner-generated concept map

    Group 3 = Learner-generated concept map

Factor 2 = Self-regulated learning

    Group 1 = Low self-directed learning

    Group 2 = High self-directed learning

DV = Achievement on knowledge and concepts

The design is illustrated in Figure 9.3.

The researchers analyzed the effect of each factor and its levels on knowledge acquisition, as measured by a multiple-choice test. The means and standard deviations for each factor and level are presented in Table 9.1.

The results of the 3×2 ANOVA indicated an overall difference in the level of concept mapping ($F = 4.43$, $p = .014$) and a statistically significant difference for the factor of self-regulated learning ($F = 7.95$, $p = .006$). Both the treatment with concept mapping and the factor of self-regulated learning therefore produced significant effects. Follow-up t-tests isolated these effects. For the concept mapping, the condition in which students fully generated their own concept maps performed better than the other conditions. In addition, the group with higher scores for self-regulated learning outperformed the group with lower scores. The test for the interaction of the IVs was not statistically significant.

4. Factorial Design with 3 × 2 MANOVA with Interaction

Carrier, S. (2009). Environmental education in the schoolyard: Learning styles and gender. *Journal of Environmental Education, 40*(3), 2–12.

The researcher studied the impact of environmental education lessons by comparing "activities conducted in the schoolyard with traditional classroom activities involving elementary school boys and girls" (p. 2). In this study, the overall statistical test was a MANOVA, because four DVs were measured and analyzed: (1) achievement, (2) attitudes toward the lesson, (3) behaviors, and (4) comfort level with learning outdoors. The experiment examined the treatment variable (classes conducted in the schoolyard on environmental activities) versus the traditional classroom instruction, and added the mediating variable of gender (boys vs. girls).

IV = Treatment (outdoor learning included or not)

    Group 1 = Use of outdoors (schoolyard) for instruction

    Group 2 = Control (indoor, classroom only)

IV = Gender

    Group 1 = Girls

    Group 2 = Boys

DV = measures of knowledge, understanding, and attitudes

    DV 1 = Achievement

    DV 2 = Attitudes toward the lesson

174

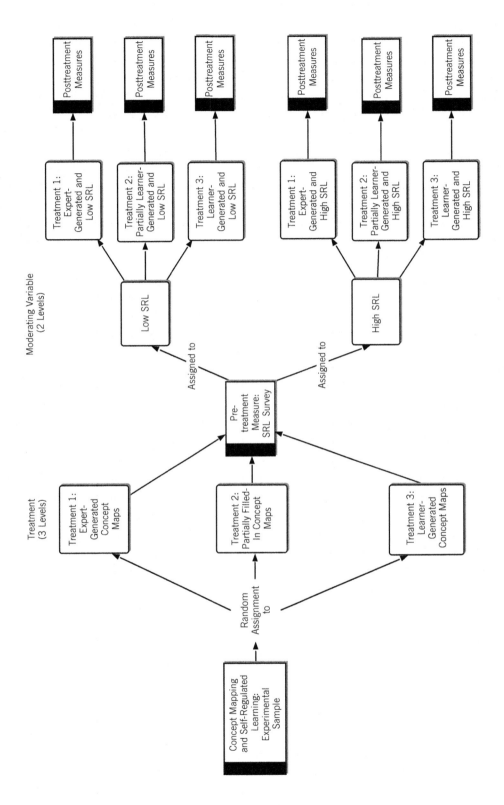

FIGURE 9.3. Design for the Lim, Lee, and Grabowski (2009) study.

TABLE 9.1. Means and Standard Deviations for Concept-Mapping Study (Lim et al., 2009)

Self-regulated learning skill level	Levels of concept map generativity		
	Expert-generated	Partially generated by learners	Fully learner-generated
Low	20.23 (8.2)	22.53 (8.6)	23.0 (9.7)
High	22.78 (9.4)	24.92 (8.4)	31.0 (5.8)

Note. Standard deviations are in parentheses.

DV 3 = Behaviors

DV 4 = Comfort level with learning outdoors

Figure 9.4 illustrates the design.

The researcher hypothesized the interaction effect that boys and girls would respond differently, and the results showed statistically significant differences for the interaction of treatment with gender ($F = 4.12$, $p < .01$). This means that boys and girls rated their experiences of schoolyard learning activities differently. Follow-up analysis was necessary, and it showed that comparisons of boys' treatment versus control scores on all four DVs were statistically significant, whereas there were no significant differences when girls in the treatment and control groups were compared.

The best way to describe the interaction is with a visual representation of the group means. In Figure 9.5, the scores are disaggregated into male and female groups, and the mean scores are placed on the graph. The graph shows the changes in the boys' scores between experimental and control groups for environmental attitudes,

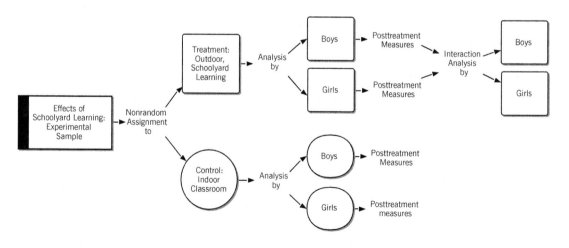

FIGURE 9.4. Design for the Carrier (2009) experiment.

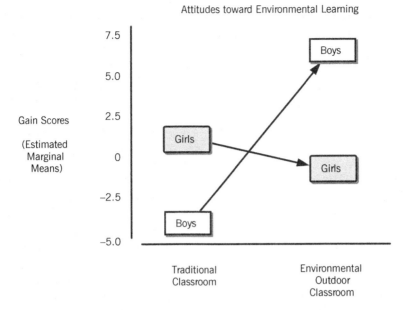

FIGURE 9.5. Interaction effects in the Carrier (2009) study.

but shows little change in the girls' scores. The crossover of lines indicates the incon-sistent effect of the treatment on males and females; this is the interaction effect.

REPEATED-MEASURES DESIGNS

MAP 9.3

Repeated-measures designs investigate differences in individual subjects in a group after treatments are introduced and the outcomes are repeatedly measured over time.

Other terms for repeated-measures designs are *time series designs* and *within-subject designs*. The most common repeated-measures design is the *crossover study*, which is a

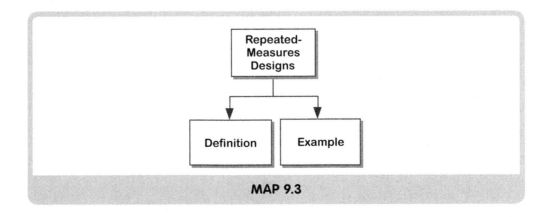

longitudinal study in which every subject in every group receives a series of different, counterbalanced treatments. That is to say, each subject in each group receives the same treatments, but in a different order.

Repeated-measures designs are practical because they can reduce the logistical problems of conducting research in classrooms, and they can be done with limited sample sizes.

Example of a Repeated-Measures Crossover/Counterbalanced Design

Agarwal, P. K., Karpicke, J. D., Kang, S. H. K., Roediger, H. L., & McDermott, K. B. (2008). Examining the testing effect with open- and closed-book tests. *Applied Cognitive Psychology, 22,* 861–876.

This study investigated the effect of open-book and closed-book tests on long-term retention. A random sample of 36 subjects was recruited for the study from a human subjects pool at a university. Each subject experienced four treatment and two control conditions.

Treatment condition = Open-book

Open-book condition 1 = Read passage first and was then tested while rereading passage

Open-book condition 2 = Was tested while reading the text for the first time (simultaneous answering)

Treatment condition = Closed-book

Closed-book condition 1 = Read passage and was tested with book closed

Closed-book condition 2 = Read passage, was tested, and provided feedback on answers

Control condition

Level 1 = Read passage and was not tested

Level 2 = Was tested

The sample was divided into six groups, with six subjects in each group. Each subject in each group received all treatment and control conditions in alternating sequence, as represented in Figure 9.6.

The researchers predicted "that taking a test would enhance long-term retention more than studying the passage once . . . and that providing feedback after an initial test would produce a positive effect on long-term retention" (p. 863). The DV was a short-answer test matched with the reading passages. There were two measurements of achievement; one occurred immediately after the treatment, and the second took place 1 week later. The test questions were graded with a 3-point holistic rubric. "Two raters scored 10% of the tests and the Pearson product moment correlation between their scores was $r = 0.98$" (p. 865). A one-way ANOVA was used as a measurement check, and there was consistency in scoring.

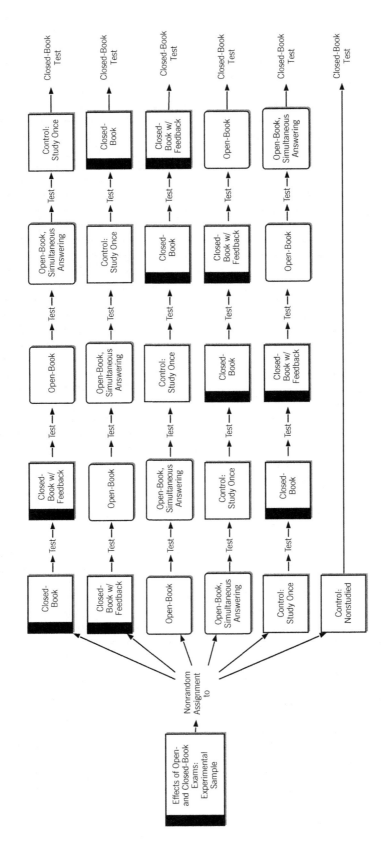

FIGURE 9.6. Design for the Agarwal, Karpicke, Kang, Roediger, and McDermott (2008) study.

The researchers used a repeated-measures ANOVA to calculate the main effect of the four test conditions on the DV of initial recall performance. The results were significant, $F(3, 105) = 11.27$. They then did multiple analyses of the four test conditions, using follow-up ANOVAs and t-tests to analyze the multiple main effects. On final measurement, both the open- and closed-book tests produced ES > 0.87. This repeated-measures study represents an efficient and complex approach to experimental design.

EVALUATING FACTORIAL DESIGNS   MAP 9.4

In evaluating factorial designs, a reader should apply the three categories of (1) theory and treatment; (2) sample and sampling; and (3) data collection and analysis, as first presented in the rubric for evaluating the quality of experimental designs in Chapter Eight (see Figure 8.5 there). Below is a sample evaluation of the Agarwal et al. (2008) repeated-measures study, which is organized according to these three categories.

Example: Evaluation of a Repeated-Measures Experimental Study
Theory and Treatment

The Agarwal et al. (2008) study merits a strong rating in the category of theory and treatment. The theory for the study of open- versus closed-book examinations is stated clearly and is very well supported in the literature review. There are over 40 references in the literature review, with over 40% of the citations very recent (published within the previous 5 years). The researchers state clear research questions concerning the use of testing situations to increase long-term retention of information: "We predicted that taking a test would enhance long-term retention more than studying the passage once. We also expected that providing feedback after an initial test would produce a positive effect on long-term retention" (Agarwal et al., 2008, p. 863). Overall, the IV was the use of open versus closed book in the testing conditions, but the researchers created levels of the IV to examine variations of these

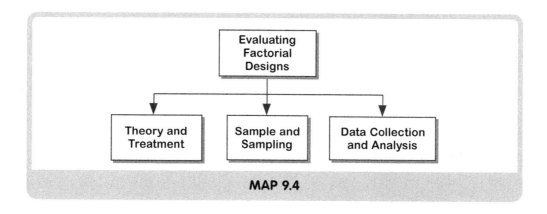

MAP 9.4

conditions. The DV was a short-answer test matched with the reading passages (one each in history, science, and literature).

Sample and Sampling

The study merits only a moderate rating for sample and sampling. The researchers used a nonrandom sample of 36 subjects, who were recruited from the Human Subject Pool of the university's Department of Psychology. The repeated-measures experimental design used each individual participant as his or her own control, and each participant was involved in six treatment conditions. The advantage was that the comparison was the measure of within-subject change, and the sample did double duty as treatment and control. The disadvantage was that there might be some carry-over between treatments. However, it would have been difficult to set power analysis because of the requirements for the design.

Data Collection and Analysis

The study merits a strong rating for data collection and analysis. The DV of major interest was performance on the short-answer tests given to subjects in the open- and closed-book testing conditions. The test questions required reading and grading with a 3-point holistic rubric. "Two raters scored 10% of the tests and the Pearson product moment correlation between their scores was $r = 0.98$. Given the high inter-rater reliability, one rater scored the remaining tests" (Agarwal et al., 2008, p. 865). The inferential tests matched the experimental design, with the use of a repeated-measures ANOVA and a series of follow-up ANOVAs and t-tests. Researchers performed a variety of statistical tests but were careful not to overanalyze, and they avoid overconcluding in their article. Effect sizes were published for all results, indicating the researchers' attention to the practical as well as the statistical significance of their findings.

CHAPTER SUMMARY   MAP 9.5

✓ Complex experimental designs can be organized into between-group and repeated-measures designs.

✓ These designs allow researchers to study and control multiple IVs and DVs.

✓ Factorial designs allow researchers to examine main effects and interactions of variables.

✓ Repeated-measures designs are used to study the changes of a treatment within individuals, who experience all control and treatment conditions.

✓ Theory and treatment, sample and sampling, and data collection and analysis are key elements in evaluating the quality and validity of experiments and quasi-experiments.

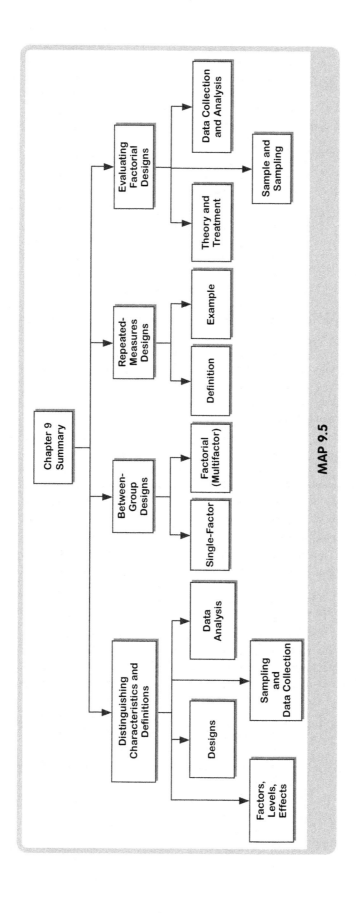

MAP 9.5

KEY TERMS AND CONCEPTS

ANCOVA/MANCOVA

ANOVA/MANOVA

between-group designs

covariate

factorial ANOVA

factors

interaction effects

levels

main effects

one-way ANOVA

repeated-measures ANOVA

repeated-measures designs

t-test

REVIEW, CONSOLIDATION, AND EXTENSION OF KNOWLEDGE

1. Using an electronic database, search for an article describing a factorial analysis on a topic of interest. In doing your search, the first keyword will be *factorial analysis*; the second keyword will be the topic of interest (e.g., *reading*). Follow the Guide to Reading below as you work through the article. Then, with the Guide as a template, write a critique of the article you have selected.

Guide to Reading

Research Review: Does the review establish a theoretical foundation for the experiment? How current is the review? Are more than 10 studies reviewed? What hypothesis/hypotheses or research questions are generated from the research review?

Purpose and Design: What was the purpose of the study? What were the factors and/or levels and DV(s)? How were they operationalized? What was the design of the study (between-group or repeated-measures)?

Sample: What was the sample size? How was the sample selected (randomly or nonrandomly)? What were the characteristics of the sample? How was the sample assigned to groups (randomly or nonrandomly)?

Data Collection: What specific data collection strategies were used? Do the authors give indications of the measures' validity and reliability? How often were outcomes measured? How well did the data collection strategies match the research question or purpose?

Data Analysis, Interpretation, and Conclusions: How were the data analyzed? What statistical tests were used? What were the results for main effects and, if appropriate, interaction effects? Was there a covariate? Were the results for the main effect significant or nonsignificant? Were follow-up *t*-tests performed to isolate sources of significance? If so, what were the results? How well does the data analysis match the research question or purpose? To what degree do the analysis, interpretation, and conclusions stay close to the data? Have the researchers overconcluded?

Evaluation: How do you rate the overall quality of the study? Strong? Moderate? Weak? How do you rate the categories below, and what is your reason for the ratings in each category?

Theory and treatment: Strong, moderate, weak

Sample and sampling: Strong, moderate, weak

Data collection and analysis: Strong, moderate, weak

CHAPTER TEN

Single-Subject Research and Designs

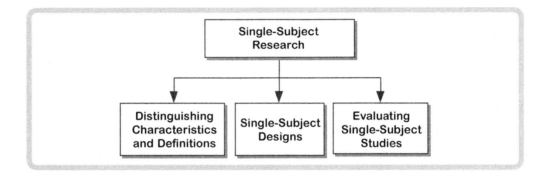

Single-subject research is a type of repeated-measures research that investigates the effects of an empirically based intervention on a specific behavior of individual subjects. Its goal is to identify evidence-based practices that can be used in special education, school psychology, and clinical practice.

CHAPTER OBJECTIVES

✓ Understand the purpose of single-subject research and the reasons why it is quasi-experimental.

✓ Understand sampling and procedures in single-subject research.

✓ Understand single-subject designs.

✓ Understand how data are collected, analyzed, and reported in single-subject research.

✓ Understand how single-subject studies are evaluated for validity.

DISTINGUISHING CHARACTERISTICS AND DEFINITIONS   MAP 10.1

Behaviorism

Single-subject research is grounded in B. F. Skinner's theory of radical behaviorism.

> *Radical behaviorism* is based on the premise that social investigation should follow the methods of natural science and focus on behavior rather than on consciousness.

As Skinner (1974) explained, "The present argument is this: mental life and the world in which it is lived are inventions. . . . Thinking is behaving. The mistake is in allocating the behavior to the mind" (p. 115). Like all experiments, single-subject studies begin with a research review. In this case the review identifies an intervention that has been documented as having a positive effect on behaviors. The hypothesis states that the intervention (IV) will bring about positive change in a target behavior (DV) in individual subjects. The targeted behavior is determined by observations of problematic past behaviors in the subjects. A single-subject study may involve one subject or a small number of subjects. In the latter case, each subject receives the same intervention (IV), but has a different target behavior (DV). Single-subject research is similar to repeated-measures designs, the difference being that the treatments and measures are administered to single subjects rather than to a group of subjects.

> *Applied behavior analysis* is "the process of systematically applying interventions based upon the principles of learning theory to improve socially significant behaviors to a meaningful degree, and to demonstrate that the interventions employed are responsible for the improvement in behavior" (Baer, Wolf, & Risley, 1968, p. 91).

Social Validity and Replication

Single-subject research focuses on outcomes of social importance and aims to produce findings that will be of use to practitioners who work with similar subjects in other settings. Because of this, external validity is defined in this type of research as having two distinctive qualities: *social validity* and *replication*.

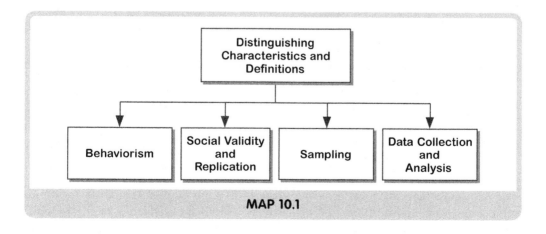

MAP 10.1

Social validity is the perceived importance of the target behavior for the participant, for those who know and interact with the participant, and for society in general.

This concept is central to single-subject research. Bailey and Burch (2002, p. 16) explained its importance this way: "The field of applied behavior analysis stresses the study of socially important behavior that can be readily observed, and it uses research designs that demonstrate functional control usually at the level of the individual performer." Social validity is usually assessed with an interview or questionnaire at the end of a study.

Replication occurs when the effects of an intervention are reproduced "across participants, conditions, and/or different measures" (Horner et al., 2005, p. 171).

Replication allows practitioners to adopt interventions that have been found to be effective with multiple subjects and in multiple settings.

Sampling

Most single-subject studies in education are conducted with children who are on the autism spectrum or who have behavioral disorders. Because of the limited population from which subjects are drawn, the sample is not selected through random sampling, and it is not possible to use random assignment to the treatment condition. These characteristics mark single-subject research as being quasi-experimental research. As noted above, the sample size is small as well; a study may include as few as one subject and as many as nine.

Data Collection and Analysis

Measurement is crucial in single-subject research. Each DV is observed and measured repeatedly for each subject with a validated observational instrument that is vetted for reliability through interobserver agreement. Measured observations are conducted at two critical points in the experiment, designated by letters of the alphabet (A and B, plus more as needed).

A (or the *baseline measurement*) refers to the phase of the experiment when observations of the target behavior are recorded before the intervention is introduced and at points when it is withdrawn. It is the measurement of the DV under control conditions, making each subject his or her own control in the experiment.

B refers to the phase of the experiment when observations of the target behavior are recorded immediately after the intervention has been administered. It is the measurement of the DV under treatment conditions. In cases where other interventions are added, the interventions are labeled as C, D, and so on.

Although there have been recent attempts to apply statistical analysis to single-subject research, most studies rely exclusively on *visual examination* of the graphed observational data. This "allows viewers to see regression or progression in behavior, assess setting events, and draw a conclusion from the interventions on whether or not they are applicable to the individual" (McCormick, 1995, p. 18). In general, a researcher should include repeated baseline measurements and changes in target behavior at three or more baseline points in time for a visual examination to represent the elements of *level*, *trend*, and *slope*.

> *Level* is the value of the dependent variable at different points of the experiment. It is recommended that a researcher collect data at a minimum of three data points during treatment phases to establish changes in level.

> *Trend* is the direction of change in patterns of data. A positive trend line provides evidence of effective treatment.

> *Slope* is the gradient or steepness of the line drawn between two data points. A pronounced slope provides evidence of the magnitude of the effect.

The underlying assumption of single-subject research is that the levels of measurements taken at baseline and during treatment will be the same if the treatment has not been effective. Conversely, if the levels are different at baseline and at least three points of treatment and show a positive trend, then the researcher can conclude that the IV has caused a change in the DV. In order to draw conclusions about the magnitude of the effect, the researcher examines the slope of the line of best fit. Because this analysis depends so much on the interpretation of the researcher conducting the study, a peer review of the visual examination is highly recommended.

SINGLE-SUBJECT DESIGNS   MAP 10.2

As explained above, single-subject designs have two phases: a *baseline* phase and an *intervention/treatment* phase. In the baseline phase, or A, there is no intervention; in this way, each subject serves as his or her own control. In the intervention/treatment phase, or B, the subject receives the treatment. Single-subject experiments always include multiple baseline observations of the target behavior before the intervention is introduced, followed by multiple observations of the targeted behavior soon after the intervention

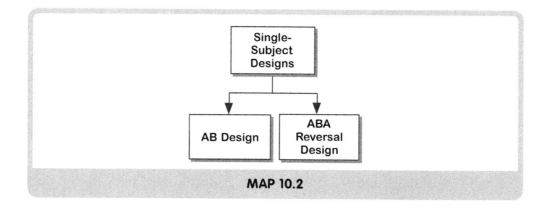

MAP 10.2

has been administered. This process of "A-then-B" may occur only once, or it may be repeated several times. The two major designs are the *AB design* and the *ABA design*.

AB Design

In the AB design, the process of A-then-B occurs once. There is one set of multiple observations at baseline (A), followed by one set of multiple observations when the intervention is administered (B). Figure 10.1 shows an AB design. This type of design is subject to various alternative hypotheses, which make it difficult for the researcher to make solid conclusions about internal validity and leave the research open to speculation that the outcome behavior is due to an alternative explanation.

Example of an AB Design

Foxx, R., & Meindl, J. (2007). The long-term successful treatment of the aggressive/ destructive behaviors of a preadolescent with autism. *Behavioral Interventions, 22*(1), 83–97.

The subject of this study was Johnny, a 13-year-old boy with autism who had exhibited aggressive and destructive behaviors that had not responded to previous treatments. Multiple staff members conducted the first observations (A) of Johnny in his self-contained classroom at a school for children with special needs. This initial observation, which established the baseline, occurred over the course of one school day that was divided into 5-minute segments.

After that, a detailed intervention (B) was developed that consisted of "a token economy system, differential reinforcement of other behaviors (DRO), response cost, over-correction, and physical restraint. A number of classroom rules such as 'No loud talking' were also created" (pp. 88–89). The researchers obtained parental permission for the treatments, which continued for 8 months. The intervention phase "was characterized with response costs for negative behaviors and reinforcement of positive behaviors" (p. 90) and consisted of rewarding Johnny with five tokens for each 5-minute segment in which he exhibited no negative behaviors. Negative behaviors resulted in having the tokens taken away. Johnny's negative behaviors, which were graphed at the baseline, were reduced to near zero at intervention points, and this result was maintained for over a year. Figure 10.2 illustrates the recorded observations at A and B that support the researchers' conclusions.

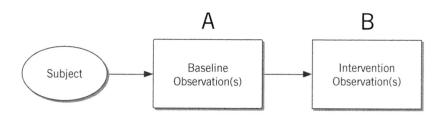

FIGURE 10.1. An AB design.

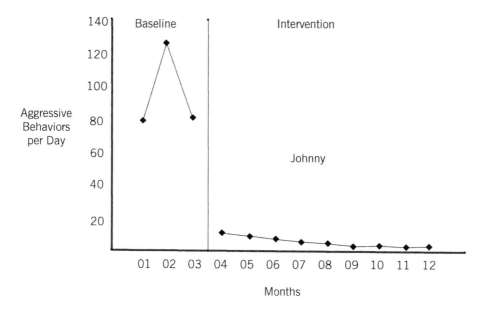

FIGURE 10.2. Observations of aggressive behaviors for Johnny, a 13-year-old boy with autism, at baseline and intervention points. Adapted from Foxx and Meindl (2007, p. 91). Copyright 2007 by John Wiley & Sons, Ltd. Adapted by permission.

ABA Reversal Design

In the ABA reversal design, the process of A-then-B is repeated at least once. There are multiple observations of the target behavior at baseline (A), followed by multiple observations after the intervention has been administered (B), followed by a second set of observations when the intervention is withdrawn (A). This ABA process may be repeated several times, always concluding with a baseline observation when no intervention is present (A). This final A is often referred to as a measure of *maintenance,* which provides data about the degree to which the subject has been able to generalize the behavior to new settings. Figure 10.3 shows an ABA single-subject design. This is the more powerful design of the two discussed here because the use of more than a single set of A-then-B observations provides stronger evidence of internal validity and demonstrates that changes in the target behavior are due to the intervention and not to alternative explanations.

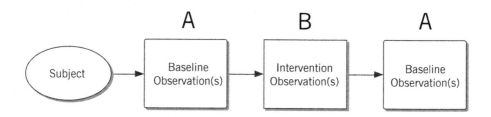

FIGURE 10.3. An ABA reversal design.

Example of an ABA Reversal Design (with an Extension)

Crozier, S., & Tincani, M. J. (2007). Effects of social stories on prosocial behavior of preschool children with autism spectrum disorders. *Journal of Autism and Developmental Disorders, 37*(9), 1803–1814.

The subjects of this study were three children with autism, who were between 3 and 5 years old and who attended an inclusive preschool. Each had a different target behavior, based on prior observations. For Thomas, the target behavior was sitting still during circle time; for Daniel, it was speaking appropriately with peers during snack time; and for James, it was appropriate behavior in the block area. As the result of a research review, the authors decided on social stories as the appropriate intervention for these three subjects and their target behaviors. *Social stories* are short stories that are specifically written for each child, and that describe the target behavior to be observed and recorded. The researchers wrote stories for each child that described the child by name and portrayed him as demonstrating the desired behavior in a school activity. Thomas's social story described him sitting still for 10 minutes during circle time; Daniel's social story described him using specific prompts to talk with other children during snack time; and James's social story described him sharing in the block area. The authors hypothesized that these social stories would improve the children's target behaviors.

The original design was an ABA design, and both James (whose data are not shown here) and Thomas responded to the original design. However, Daniel did not. The researchers added a second intervention for Daniel, making his an ABACBC design. At the end of the experiment and through a process of visual examination, the researchers saw an increase in appropriate behaviors and a decrease in inappropriate behaviors for each subject. The researchers displayed their data for each subject in graphs to support their conclusions about the effectiveness of the intervention (see Figure 10.4 for Thomas's data and Figure 10.5 for Daniel's).

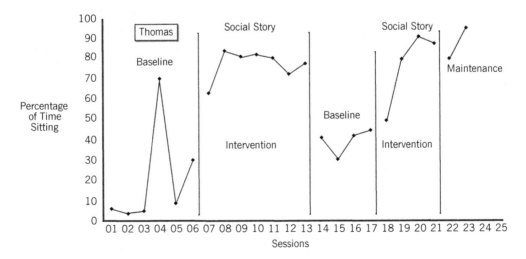

FIGURE 10.4. Data display for Thomas: Percentage of time sitting during circle time. Adapted from Crozier and Tincani (2007, p. 1809). Copyright 2007 by Springer Science+Business Media. Adapted by permission.

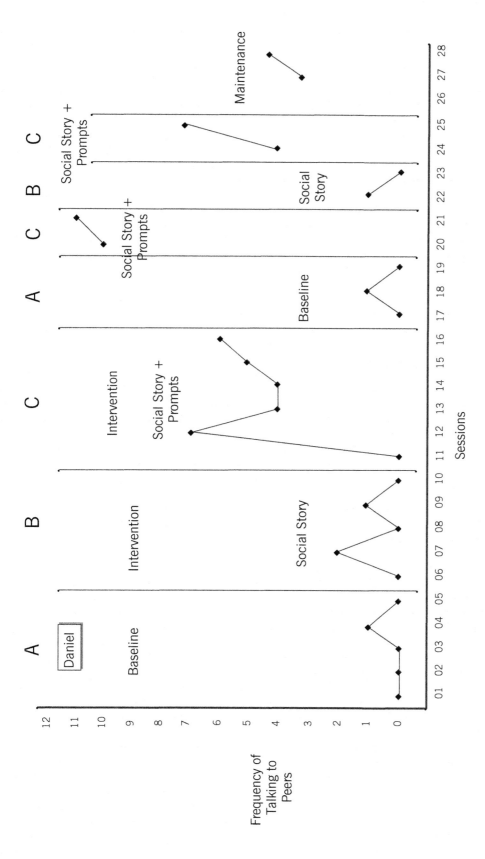

FIGURE 10.5. Data display for Daniel: Frequency of talking with peers at snack time. Adapted from Crozier and Tincani (2007, p. 1809). Copyright 2007 by Springer Science+Business Media. Adapted by permission.

EVALUATING SINGLE-SUBJECT STUDIES   MAP 10.3

As we do with other types of experiments, we evaluate single-subject studies by using the criteria of theory and treatment, sample and sampling, and data collection and analysis.

Theory and Treatment

The primary considerations for theory and treatment are (1) the quality of the research review and the empirical evidence of replication it provides for the intervention; (2) the usefulness, or social validity, of the experiment; and (3) its potential for replication in other settings with similar subjects. The questions to ask about theory and treatment are as follows:

1. How well does the research review support the appropriateness of the treatment for the target behavior and for the subjects?
2. Does the researcher cite replicable studies in the review?
3. How adequate was the operationalization of IV and DV?
4. Is there a precise description of the intervention and manipulation of the IV by the researcher? How well was the intervention implemented? How well can it be replicated?
5. Was there a social validity interview or survey at the conclusion of the study?

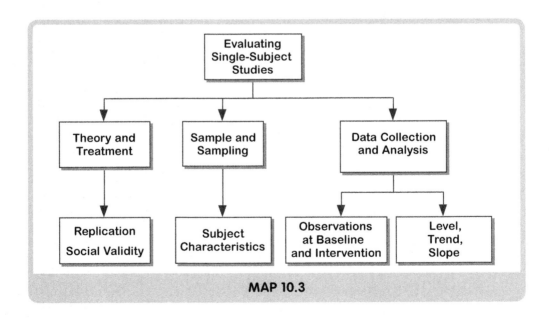

MAP 10.3

Sample and Sampling

The key elements to consider in regard to sample and sampling are the size of the sample, the match between subjects and target behaviors, and the match between subjects and interventions. The questions to ask about sample and sampling are these:

1. Was the sample size appropriate? Did the sample include from one to nine subjects?
2. Is there an adequate description of why and how subjects were selected?
3. Is there a detailed description of subjects and setting?
4. Was there a good match between the subjects and the interventions?
5. Was there a good match between the subjects and the target behaviors?
6. Are there detailed descriptions of subjects' characteristics and backgrounds?

Data Collection and Analysis

The key criteria to apply in evaluating data collection are the quality of the measures and the number of times baseline measurements are taken. The key criteria for data analysis are the quality of the visual display of data, as well as the rigor of visual examination. The questions to ask about data collection and analysis are these:

1. How good are the measures? Is evidence of validity and reliability provided? Are there indications of how interrater reliability was achieved?
2. Was the DV precisely defined in terms of desired behavior?
3. Were baseline measures adequately used as the control condition?
4. Are descriptions of baseline conditions provided?
5. Were there repeated measurements at a baseline, and was there change in target behavior at three or more baseline points in time?
6. Are the recording and graphing of data consistent?
7. How well does the visual display depict level, trend, and slope?
8. Did the researcher consult with others in conducting visual examination of the data?

Figure 10.6 provides a rubric for evaluating single-subject studies.

Example: Evaluation of the Social Stories Article

Crozier and Tincani's (2007) study of the effects of social stories on three preschool children with autism merits a strong rating in all three categories. In terms of theory and treatment, the authors have completed a thorough review of replicated empirical

Criterion	Strong	Moderate	Weak
Theory and treatment	An intervention (IV) that is supported by a research review of at least 5–10 recent, replicable studies, as well as other publications. Precise description of the intervention (IV) and how it was manipulated by the researcher. Precise description of the target behavior (DV), as well as its importance/evidence of its social validity.	An intervention (IV) that lacks clarity and is supported by research review of fewer than five recent, replicable studies. Problems with the clarity of the description. Possible questions about the target behavior (DV) and weak connection with social validity.	Unclear or missing research review; no recent, replicable studies or supporting publications. Missing description of how the intervention was implemented. Poor connection to, or no reference to, social validity.
Sample and sampling	Adequate sample size ($n = 1$–9). Detailed description of subject characteristics and setting. Appropriateness of subjects and of target behaviors for treatment.	Adequate sample size ($n = 1$–9). Unclear description of subject characteristics and setting. Questions about the appropriateness of subjects and of target behaviors for treatment.	Adequate sample size ($n = 1$–9). Unclear or no description of subject characteristics and setting. Subjects and/or target behaviors not appropriate for treatment.
Data collection and analysis	Precise description of a socially important target behavior (DV) for each subject; description of valid and reliable measurement of DV and its interrater reliability. Clear description of baseline observations and use of baseline as the control condition. Repeated measurements at baseline, and evidence of change in DV at three or more baselines. Consistent recording and graphing of data and depiction of level, trend, and slope. Peer consultation in visual examination of the data.	Partial or unclear description of important target behaviors; partial description of valid and reliable measurement of DV; unclear or questionable interrater agreement. Unclear or partial description of the baseline conditions. Questions about repeated measurements. Possible inconsistencies in the recording and graphing of data, with questions about level, trend, and slope. Questions about or partial information about peer audit.	Unclear or missing descriptions of target behaviors; no information about valid and reliable measures; no mention of interrater agreement. No description of baseline conditions. No mention of repeated measurements. Graphs of data missing, or level, trend, and slope unreadable and very difficult to interpret. No peer audit.

FIGURE 10.6. Rubric for evaluating single-subject studies.

studies demonstrating the effectiveness of social stories with similar subjects. The authors also provide a precise description of the intervention and how it was manipulated for each subject. This is further illuminated in the appendix to the article, which includes the texts of the three social stories that were used. The target behaviors for each subject were clearly identified and operationalized. The authors used a survey to collect evidence of social validity. There was sufficient evidence of the treatment for the study to be replicable.

In regard to sample and sampling, the sample of three subjects fell within the suggested parameters for sample size. The authors have provided detailed descriptions of each subject and of the setting. These descriptions justify the selection of the sample and the appropriateness of the intervention and target behavior for each subject.

In the category of data collection and analysis, the authors have provided detailed descriptions of socially important target behaviors, of the validity and reliability of measurement, and of baseline conditions and their use as experimental controls. They conducted frequent and numerous observations during the baseline and intervention phases; the ABA design provided opportunities to demonstrate change in targeted behaviors at three or more baseline measurements. The graphing of data is very clear and visually displays level, trend, and slope. The two authors served as peer consultants in the visual examination of data.

CHAPTER SUMMARY   MAP 10.4

✓ Single-subject research is based on the theory of radical behaviorism and implements a process of applied behavior analysis to establish the effects of an intervention on an individual subject.

✓ Social validity and replication are key elements in single-subject studies.

✓ Single-subject research uses a repeated-measures design applied to individuals rather than to groups.

✓ Single-subject studies focus on individuals as subjects, use the subjects as their own controls, and conduct repeated and frequent observations of the subjects' target behaviors with and without the intervention.

✓ Single-subject studies use small sample sizes ($n = 1–9$), and they are quasi-experiments because they do not randomly assign subjects to the treatment condition.

✓ The most common single-subject designs are AB and ABA reversal designs.

✓ Single-subject designs include one or more subjects. Subjects experience the same intervention (IV) but have different identified target behaviors (DVs).

✓ Single-subject research depends on valid and reliable observations that are vetted for interrater agreement.

✓ Researchers conduct observations before an intervention is introduced (called *baseline* and indicated by the letter A) and after an intervention is introduced (indicated by the letter B).

✓ If additional interventions are introduced, they are labeled C, D, and so on.

✓ Single-subject researchers record and report data studies on graphs that show changes in the DV.

✓ In order to infer causality, a researcher must show evidence of repeated baseline measurements and changes in target behavior at three or more baseline points.

✓ Data analysis depends on visual examination of the graphs rather than on statistical analysis.

✓ Visual examination involves looking at level, trend, and slope, and should involve peer consultation.

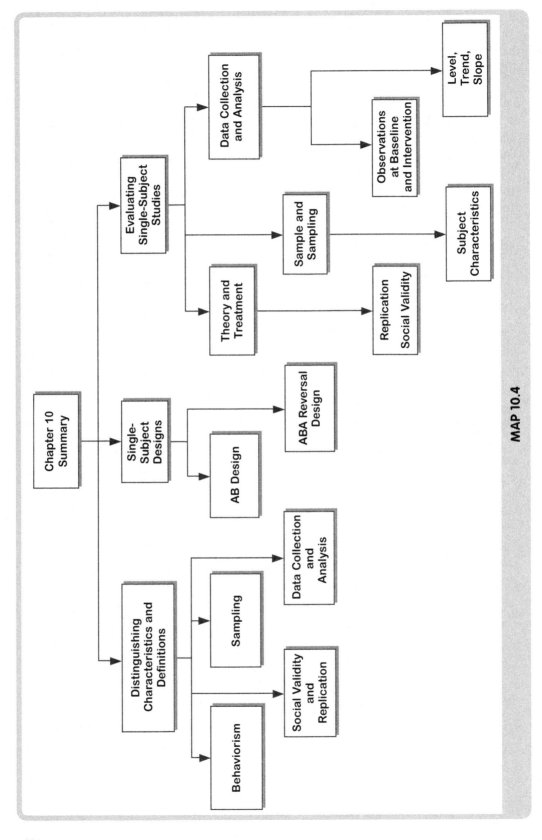

MAP 10.4

KEY TERMS AND CONCEPTS

AB design

ABA design

applied behavior analysis

baseline

intervention

level

observations

radical behaviorism

repeated measures

replication

slope

social validity

target behavior

trend

REVIEW, CONSOLIDATION, AND EXTENSION OF KNOWLEDGE

1. In your own words, describe the purpose of single-subject research and explain why it is quasi-experimental.

2. Using an electronic database, search for a single-subject study. Follow the Guide to Reading below as you work through the article. Then, with the Guide as a template, write a critique of the study you have selected.

Guide to Reading

Research Review: Does the review establish an empirically based intervention for the identified target behavior? How current is the review? Are more than 10 empirical studies reviewed? What hypothesis has been generated from the research review?

Purpose, Design, and Sample: What was the purpose of the study? What was the design of the study? What was the intervention (IV)? Who were the subjects? How many were there? How was the sample selected? Was this an appropriate sample? What were the target behaviors (DV) for each subject? How was the intervention implemented?

Data Collection, Analysis, Interpretation, and Conclusions: How were observations conducted? Were the observational protocols vetted for interrater reliability? If so, how? When and how often did observations (A) and treatment (B) occur? Under what conditions did maintenance occur? How were data analyzed, and how are they displayed? Was there evidence of change in the DV at three baseline measurements? What conclusions does the researcher draw? Does the researcher overconclude?

Evaluation: How do you rate the overall quality of the study? Strong? Moderate? Weak? How do you rate the categories below, and what is your reason for the ratings in each category?

Theory and treatment: Strong, moderate, weak

Sample and sampling: Strong, moderate, weak

Data collection and analysis: Strong, moderate, weak

Sample Critique

This sample critique is a review of the same social stories article covered earlier in this chapter, with more details included.

Crozier, S., & Tincani, M. J. (2007). Effects of social stories on prosocial behavior of preschool children with autism spectrum disorders. *Journal of Autism and Developmental Disorders, 37*(9), 1803–1814.

Research Review

The review provides a synthesis of the social stories literature and makes a strong case for using social stories to change inappropriate behaviors of children with autism spectrum disorders (ASD). The review includes numerous studies published since 1990 that informed this view. The authors explain that social stories are short narratives written for an individual that describe the appropriate behavior for that individual in a particular setting. In addition, the authors make a case for the social validity of social stories as an intervention.

Purpose, Design, and Sample

The purpose of the experiment was to investigate the effect of social stories (IV) on the target behaviors of three children with autism (Thomas, Daniel, and James); the children were between 3 and 5 years old and attended an inclusive preschool. Participants were recruited through the preschool director's and classroom teachers' nominations of children who were diagnosed as having ASD. Each student had an identified and clearly defined target behavior (DV) based on prior observations. For Thomas, it was sitting still during circle time; for Daniel, it was speaking appropriately with peers during snack time; and for James, it was appropriate behavior in the block area. Thomas's social story described him sitting still for 10 minutes during circle time; Daniel's social story described him using specific prompts to talk with other children during snack time; and James's social story described him sharing in the block area. The authors hypothesized that social stories would improve the target behaviors for each individual subject.

The original design was an ABA reversal design, and both Thomas and James responded to the original design. However, Daniel did not. The researchers added a second intervention for Daniel, making his an ABACBC design. An individual observational checklist was developed for each child. The measures were vetted for interrater agreement (at 100%) and for treatment validity as well. Multiple (over 20) observations were conducted and graphed at baseline and during treatment.

Data Collection, Analysis, Interpretation, and Conclusions

The graphs of the data show an increase in the appropriate target behaviors for each subject. Thomas and James responded to the social story alone, while Daniel required an additional prompt to change his behavior in a positive direction. The authors conducted a social validity survey with the teachers, who indicated the usefulness of social stories as a behavioral intervention; however, the teachers did not report that they actually used this intervention once the experiment was completed. The authors indicate some limitations to the study, but conclude that the experiment replicates previous research.

Evaluation

Crozier and Tincani's study of the effects of social stories on three preschool children with autism merits a strong rating in all three categories. In terms of theory and treatment, the authors have completed a thorough review of empirical studies that demonstrated the effectiveness of social stories with similar subjects. There is a precise description of the intervention and how it was manipulated for each subject. This was further illuminated in the appendix to the article, which includes the texts of the three social stories that were used. The target behaviors for each subject were clearly identified and operationalized. The authors used a survey to collect evidence of social validity. There was sufficient detail about the treatment for the study to be replicable.

In terms of sampling, the sample of three subjects fell within the suggested parameters for sample size. The authors have provided detailed descriptions of each subject and of the setting. These descriptions justified the selection of the sample, as well as the appropriateness of the intervention and target behavior for each subject.

In terms of data collection and analysis, the authors have provided detailed descriptions of socially important target behaviors, of the validity and reliability of measurement, and of baseline conditions and their use as experimental controls. They conducted frequent and numerous observations during the baseline and intervention phases; the ABA design provided opportunities to demonstrate change in targeted behaviors at three or more baseline measurements. The graphing of data is very clear and visually displays level, trend, and slope. The two authors served as peer consultants to each other in the visual examination of data.

PART V

Nonexperimental Research

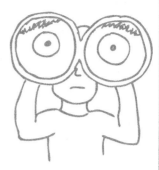

"Where the telescope ends, the microscope begins. Which of the two has the grander view?"

—VICTOR HUGO

Part V introduces nonexperimental research. Unlike experimental research, which manipulates groups and variables and examines the results close up as if through a microscope, nonexperimental research takes a different tack: It takes as given existing groups and variables and looks at the results from a distance, as if through a telescope. Although this approach cannot establish causality, it can make inferences about the extent of group differences and the nature of the relationship between/among variables, and it can predict future outcomes.

CHAPTER ELEVEN

Nonexperimental Group Comparisons

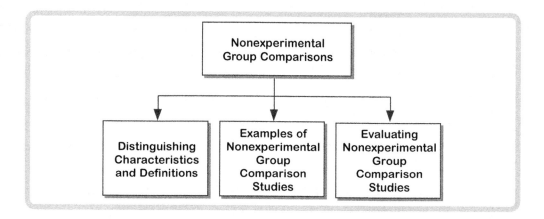

Nonexperimental group comparisons investigate differences that are inherent in groups and are not due to the introduction and implementation of a researcher-controlled treatment or intervention. As a result, these studies can explore the complexity of groups and their members, but cannot offer causal explanations of the differences.

CHAPTER OBJECTIVES

✓ Understand the key elements in a group comparison research article.

✓ Understand what makes nonexperimental group comparisons similar to and different from between-group experiments.

✓ Understand that nonexperimental group comparisons explore differences that might exist between/among existing groups when there is no intervention or treatment present.

✓ Understand that in nonexperimental group comparisons, the dependent variable may be continuous or categorical.

✓ Understand methods of data collection in nonexperimental group comparisons.

✓ Understand the procedures for conducting nonexperimental group comparisons.

✓ Understand inferential tests of significance used for continuous and categorical dependent variables.

✓ Understand how to evaluate nonexperimental group comparisons.

DISTINGUISHING CHARACTERISTICS AND DEFINITIONS   MAP 11.1

> *Nonexperimental group comparisons* investigate differences that exist between or among existing groups when there is no intervention or treatment present.

What distinguishes nonexperimental group comparisons from between–group experiments is that they lack the conditions of control that can lead to conclusions about causal relationships between or among variables. Due to the noncausal nature of these comparisons, researchers may not state a hypothesis, but may instead conduct an exploratory study. Numerous labels have been applied to this form of research, including *ex post facto research, causal comparative studies*, and *preexperimental studies*. This text uses the term *nonexperimental group comparisons* to distinguish this type of research from experimental designs, which can make claims about causal relationships. The distinguishing characteristics of nonexperimental group comparisons have to do with the nature of the sample/sampling, data collection and measurement of the DV, and data analysis. The research review in a nonexperimental groups comparison may—as in experimental research—serve to develop a theory, but it may also serve to establish a framing contruct or to raise research questions that guide the inquiry.

Sample and Sampling

The sample for a nonexperimental group comparison study always includes subjects who are part of an existing membership group that is based on a shared, immutable

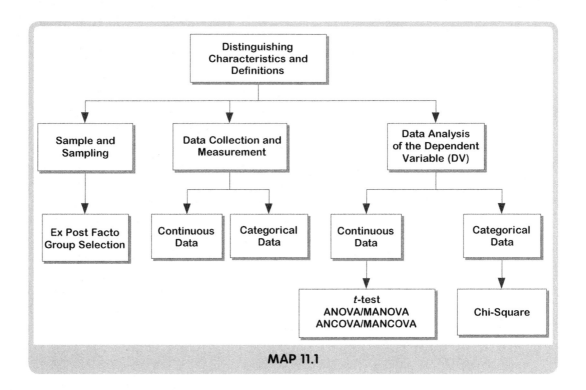

MAP 11.1

characteristic (gender, ethnicity, grade level, etc.). For this reason, the researcher does not control group assignment; the groups already exist and are, in effect, ex post facto. The sample may be randomly or nonrandomly selected. A randomly selected sample is preferred because it controls for the variability of subjects within each group. However, researchers often use a nonrandom sample and control for variability by matching the groups according to other subject characteristics.

Data Collection and Measurement of the DV

The measures used for data collection are most commonly surveys and achievement assessments, which also ask demographic questions about subject characteristics and allow the researcher to sort responses into the relevant categories for later analysis. Unlike experiments, which only collect data on continuous DVs, nonexperimental group comparisons may collect data on both continuous and categorical variables. To review:

A *continuous variable* can be measured and quantified.

Continuous variables may include scaled scores on assessments of achievement or aptitude or responses on a Likert scale survey or questionnaire—all of which can be quantified and described statistically as *means* and *standard deviations*.

A *categorical variable* is an attribute that cannot be measured or quantified.

A categorical variable may be a characteristic that is identified in the demographic section of a measure, or it may be generated by a series of questions that ask respondents to place themselves in categories or to answer dichotomous yes–no questions.

For example, a researcher may want to explore whether there are gender differences in math achievement. The DV in this study is a continuous variable that can be measured by scores on a math test. In this case,

IV = gender differences

DV = math achievement (a continuous variable)

On the other hand, a researcher may want to investigate whether there are differences in how males and females experience bullying: Are they more often victims or perpetrators? In this study, the DV is a categorical variable. That is, a person is or is not a victim of bullying, depending on the answer to a dichotomous question such as "Have you ever been bullied?" In this case,

IV = gender differences

DV = bullying status (categorical variable): bully or victim

The nature of the DV becomes crucial in both data collection and data analysis.

Data Analysis

After administering the measure, the researcher will sort data into the identified groups. For instance, in a study of gender differences, one group will include data from the responses from the males in the sample; the other group will include data from the responses from the females in the sample. Another approach is to use the data from a test or survey to define groups, such as low, medium, and high achievers. The procedures for data analysis differ when the dependent variable is continuous or categorical.

- When the DV is a continuous variable, the researcher follows the same procedures as in experiments: The researcher first calculates means and standard deviations for each group, and then conducts a test of significance (*t*-test, ANOVA, MANOVA, ANCOVA, or MANCOVA).
- When the DV is a categorical variable, the researcher follows a different set of procedures and uses a test of significance called the chi-square. Here, the researcher calculates the percentages or frequencies of responses for each categorical DV and then uses the chi-square (χ^2) test to analyze the differences in these percentages or frequencies.

Both types of analyses yield *p*-levels. As noted in earlier chapters, $p \leq .05$ means a low (5% or lower) probability that the differences between the groups are due to chance or sampling error; in other words, the differences between groups are likely to be genuine differences. In studies where a hypothesis is stated, $p \leq .05$ means a 5% or lower probability that that the null hypothesis is confirmed; in other words, the research hypothesis is confirmed. Table 11.1 summarizes the statistical tests that are used for continuous and categorical variables in nonexperimental group comparisons.

EXAMPLES OF NONEXPERIMENTAL GROUP COMPARISON STUDIES

1. Group Comparison with Continuous DVs

Slate, J. R., Jones, C. H., Sloas, S., & Blake, P. C. (1997–1998). Scores on the Stanford Achievement Test–8 as a function of sex: Where have the sex differences gone? *High School Journal, 81*(2), 82–86.

TABLE 11.1. Tests of Significance Used in Nonexperimental Group Comparison Studies

Type of DV	Significance test
Continuous	*t*-test *F*-test: ANOVA/MANOVA, ANCOVA/MANCOVA
Categorical	Chi-square (χ^2)

This study investigated gender differences in academic achievement. The authors reviewed previous studies of gender differences in achievement and discovered inconsistent findings. Not having a strong theory to work from, the authors conducted an exploratory study that investigated gender differences in math achievement. They selected a convenience sample of 165 students (93 females and 72 males) in grades 7–12 in a rural Arkansas school district.

The researchers chose as their measure the Stanford Achievement Test–8, which was administered by the school system as part of state-mandated testing. Because this is a standardized measure, the authors assumed it had high levels of validity and reliability. The test reports quantifiable scores as a Composite Battery score and as scores for the following subtests: Reading, Mathematics, Spelling, Science, and Social Studies. The composite and subtest scores were each treated as separate, continuous DVs. Therefore, gender difference was the IV, and the DVs were as follows:

DV 1 = Composite Battery
DV 2 = Reading
DV 3 = Mathematics
DV 4 = Spelling
DV 5 = Science
DV 6 = Social Studies

Because the DVs were all continuous variables, the researchers began the analysis by computing means and standard deviations for each variable, and then used an ANOVA to establish statistical significance. They found no significant gender differences at the .05 level on the Composite Battery ($p = .09$), or in Reading ($p = .28$), Math ($p = .44$), or Social Studies ($p = .275$). They did find significant differences in Spelling, where girls outperformed boys ($p = .02$), and in Science, where boys outperformed girls ($p = .01$).

2. Group Comparison with Categorical DVs

Li, Q. (2006). Cyberbullying in schools: A research of gender differences. *School Psychology International, 27*(2), 157–170.

This study investigated whether there were gender differences in occurrences and types of bullying among middle school students. The research review considered articles about bullying in general and cyberbullying in particular, as well as studies that focused on gender differences in the experience of bullying. The original sample of 264 students in grades 7–9 (130 males and 134 females) was randomly selected from three urban middle schools in Canada. Eight surveys were later disqualified.

The researcher administered a survey she had developed that asked for demographic data (e.g., gender) and also asked students to report on their status in the bullying culture of the school, using a yes–no response format. The researcher provided no evidence for the validity or reliability of the measure. Sample questions are listed below.

1. I have been bullied during school: Yes   No
2. I have bullied others: Yes   No
3. I have been cyberbullied (e.g., via email, chat room, cell phone):   Yes   No
4. I have cyberbullied others: Yes   No

Student responses allowed the researcher to create five categorical variables for comparison, each serving as a separate DV. As in the Slate et al. (1997–1998) study, gender difference was the IV.

DV 1 = bully (perpetrator)
DV 2 = bullying victim
DV 3 = cyberbully (perpetrator)
DV 4 = cyberbullying victim
DV 5 = aware of bullying behavior

The researcher began the analysis of data by reporting the percentages of students who fell into each category by gender, as shown in Table 11.2. By looking at these percentages, one might conclude that there are gender differences in several areas. However, as we know from previous chapters, descriptive data like percentages are not sufficient to make inferences about the degree of difference or whether the difference is statistically significant. Because the variables against which the two groups were being compared were categorical, Li used chi-square as the statistical tool to determine whether gender makes a significant difference in bullying.

The chi-square (χ^2) values and p-values are reported in Table 11.3.

TABLE 11.2. Percentages of Students Experiencing Bullying and Cyberbullying		
	Males	Females
Bullying	40.8%	27.8%
Bullying victim	53.7%	44.4%
Cyberbullying	22.3%	11.6%
Cyberbullying victim	25.0%	25.6%
Aware of bullying behavior	55.6%	54.5%
Note. n = 256. Data from Li (2006).		

TABLE 11.3. Results of Cyberbullying Study

IV	DV	(χ^2)	*p*-value
Male vs. female	Traditional bully victim	3.50	0.17
Male vs. female	Cyberbully victim	0.101	0.91
Male vs. female	Being a traditional bully	4.83	0.028*
Male vs. female	Being a cyberbully	4.82	0.021*

*Note. *$p \leq p$ .05. Data from Li (2006).

The results showed significant differences between girls and boys in terms of being a bully and being a cyberbully, but showed no significant differences between girls and boys in terms of being a bully or victim. The inference would be that gender significantly influences being both a bully and a cyberbully, but that it does not significantly influence being a victim of either bullying or cyberbullying.

EVALUATING NONEXPERIMENTAL GROUP COMPARISON STUDIES

MAP 11.2

In evaluating nonexperimental group comparisons, a reader uses two of the same categories as in experiments: sample and sampling, and data collection and analysis. However, since nonexperiments do not introduce an intervention that is supported by a causal theory, the category of *theory and treatment* does not apply here. Instead, we use *theory or framing construct* to describe what guides the study. In some instances, researchers establish a theory to guide the comparison of existing groups, and they state a research hypothesis and conduct hypothesis testing. In other instances, researchers will conduct group comparisons that are more exploratory in nature and develop a framing construct to guide the study.

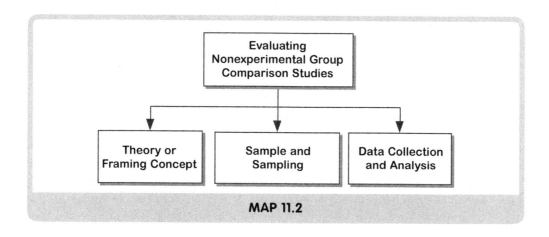

MAP 11.2

Theory or Framing Construct

The primary considerations in evaluating the first category are the quality of the literature review and how well it develops the theory or construct to guide the research.

1. How well does the research review establish a theory or generate a construct to guide the study? For a theory, does the review support a research hypothesis that can be tested? For a framing construct, does the review link various ideas to develop the framing construct?
2. Are relevant and adequate (10 or more) research studies reviewed?
3. Are the IV and DV identified? How well is the DV operationalized?

Sample and Sampling

The key elements in evaluating sample and sampling are the procedures for selecting the sample and controlling for variability among subjects.

1. How was the sample selected? Was randomization used in selecting the sample? If not, was there sample matching?
2. Was the sample of adequate size? Did the sample include a minimum of 60 subjects?

Data Collection and Analysis

The key elements in evaluating data collection and analysis are the validity and reliability of the measures and the appropriateness of both the statistical analysis and the process of statistical reasoning.

1. How good are the validity and reliability of the measure(s)?
2. How well were the measured data reported and analyzed?
3. Were appropriate statistics applied for continuous and categorical DVs? What was the alpha established for statistical significance?
4. Does the author stay close to the data and not overconclude?

Figure 11.1 is a rubric for evaluating nonexperimental group comparisons.

Example: Evaluation of the Cyberbullying Article

A framing construct was used in the Li (2006) cyberbullying study, and this aspect of the study is strong. The research review is clear and current. It links ideas to develop a framing construct of gender and bullying versus cyberbullying. More than 10 references are cited. Specific research questions are generated from the review.

The study also merits a strong rating for sample/sampling. The sample was randomly selected, of ample size, and equally divided by gender. The author provides a

Criterion	Strong	Moderate	Weak
Theory or framing construct	Clear, current, and sufficient literature review that either establishes a theory or links ideas to develop a framing construct, and that includes 10 or more references; strong support for the IV and DV; clear identification of hypothesis or research questions and the DV.	Literature review may not adequately develop a theory or framing construct, or may include fewer than 10 references; research questions implied; adequate support for the IV and DV.	Unclear literature review that fails to link ideas to a framing concept; fewer than five references; no research questions or hypothesis evident; inadequate support for the IV and DV.
Sample and sampling	Clear description of the sample characteristics and the population; clear description of sample; evidence of sufficient size (60 or more); random selection of sample or sample matching.	Description of sample is present, but lacks details about characteristics and the population; scant detail about variability of sample; insufficient sample size.	No description of the sample; total lack of details about the population; sample neither randomly selected or matched.
Data collection and analysis	Clear description of measures selected to collect data on DV and evidence of validity and reliability (r); correct use of tests for DV clear; description of statistical significance (p) and alpha level, as well as of the inferential tests used; researcher stays close to data and does not overconclude; article includes explanatory charts and narratives.	Mention of measurement, but lacking in details about validity and reliability (r); mention of statistical significance (p) without including inferential tests used; researcher avoids overconcluding; article includes explanatory charts and/or narratives.	Minimal or no mention of measurement; no mention of validity or reliability; no mention of significance; researcher may overconclude; article does not include adequate visual or narrative explanations.

FIGURE 11.1. Rubric for evaluating quality of nonexperimental group comparison studies.

clear description of subject characteristics and the population from which the sample was drawn.

Data collection and analysis merit a strong rating as well. The author provides a clear description of the survey instrument used for data collection, and samples of questions are included in the article. Although the survey instrument was not vetted for reliability and validity, its simple yes–no format seemed appropriate for the purpose of the study and not in need of further analysis. The author correctly used the chi-square test for significance for categorical data, with an appropriate alpha level. She stays close to the data and does not overconclude. All data are displayed in tables and charts, and are explained verbally as well.

CHAPTER SUMMARY

MAP 11.3

✓ Nonexperimental group comparisons are similar to group experiments in several ways; they differ in purpose and in how variables are used.

✓ Nonexperimental group comparisons investigate differences that are inherent in groups before the investigation begins.

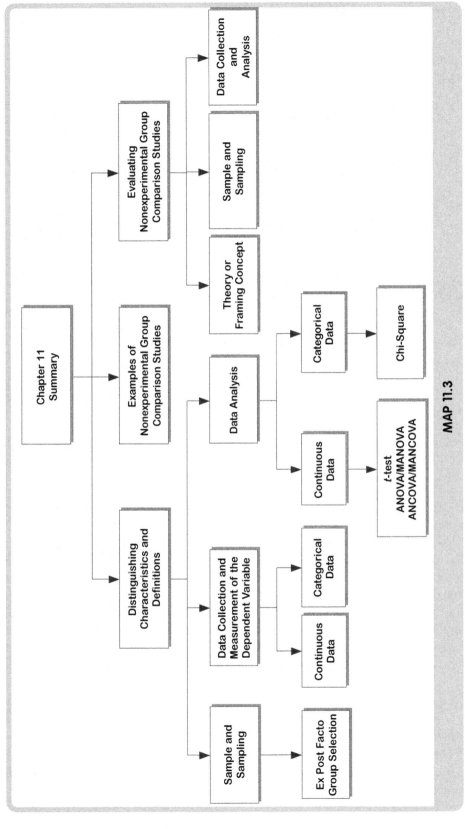

MAP 11.3

✓ Nonexperimental group comparisons do not involve a treatment for intervention manipulated by the researcher; they do not demonstrate causal relationships.

✓ Nonexperimental group comparisons may have continuous or categorical DVs.

✓ Data are commonly collected through surveys, questionnaires, and achievement and aptitude measures that ask for demographic information as well as for responses.

✓ Categorical DVs are tested for significance with the chi-square (χ^2) test.

✓ Continuous DVs may be tested for significance with the *t*-test or with the ANOVA/MANOVA or ANCOVA/MANCOVA (*F*).

✓ Nonexperimental group comparisons are evaluated in terms of theory or framing construct, sample and sampling, and data collection and analysis.

KEY TERMS AND CONCEPTS

categorical variable

chi–square (χ^2) statistic

continuous variable

dependent variable (DV)

framing construct

independent variable (IV)

matched sampling

REVIEW, CONSOLIDATION, AND EXTENSION OF KNOWLEDGE

1. In your own words,

   a. Describe how nonexperimental group comparisons are similar to and different from between-group experiments.

   b. Explain the different tests of significance for continuous and categorical DVs and how they proceed.

2. Using an electronic database, search for a nonexperimental group comparison study (look for *ex post facto* and *causal comparative* as keywords in your search) on a topic of interest. Follow the Guide to Reading below as you work through the article. Then, with the guide as a template, write a critique of about 750 words of the study you have selected. A sample critique is provided after the Guide.

Guide to Reading

   Research Review: What is the purpose of the research review: to establish a theory or to frame a construct? Does the review support the theory or framing construct?

Purpose and Design: What is the purpose of the study? Is a hypothesis stated? If so, what is it? Are there research questions? If so, what are they? What groups were studied for differences? What were the IV and DVs? Were the DVs continuous or categorical?

Sample and Sampling: How was the sample selected, randomly or nonrandomly? If nonrandomly, were the groups matched on characteristics other than their defining characteristics? If so, how? Who was in the sample? What were the characteristics of the sample? What was the sample size?

Data Collection: How were data collected (survey, questionnaire, test report, other)? Are there indications of validity and reliability for each measure? What information does the instrument collect? What is the response format of the questions?

Data Analysis, Interpretation, and Conclusions: What statistical tests were used to analyze the data? Were the results (*p*-values) significant or nonsignificant? What does the researcher conclude about the findings through significance testing and/or hypothesis testing? Does the researcher avoid overconcluding?

Evaluation: How do you rate the overall quality of the study? Strong? Moderate? Weak? How do you rate the categories below, and what is your reason for the rating in each category?

Theory or framing construct: Strong, moderate, weak

Sample and sampling: Strong, moderate, weak

Data collection and analysis: Strong, moderate, weak

Sample Critique

This is a complete critique of the bullying article that was covered earlier in the chapter.

Li, Q. (2006). Cyberbullying in schools: A research of gender differences. *School Psychology International, 27*(2), 157–170.

Research Review

The research review establishes a framing construct for the study: the interaction of gender and cyberbullying. The author reviews a wide range of studies—well over 40 articles—linking the ideas about bullying, cyberbullying, and the relation of gender and bullying.

Purpose and Design

The purpose of the study was to explore the differences between males and females in the experience of bullying, by types of bullying (cyberbullying or regular bullying) and by bullying status (victim or perpetrator). These were all categorical variables. The author raised three questions for research:

1. Do male and female students have different experiences in relation to cyberbullying?

2. Are there gender differences in student beliefs about adults' prevention of cyberbullying?

3. When cyberbullying occurs, do male and female students behave differently in terms of informing adults?

The IV was gender differences. There were five identified DVs: being a bully (perpetrator), being a bullying victim, being a cyberbully (perpetrator), being a cyberbullying victim, and being aware of bullying behavior. All the DVs were categorical variables.

Sample and Sampling

The sample was randomly selected from three middle schools in Canada and originally included 264 subjects (130 males and 134 females) in grades 7–9. The final sample size was $n = 256$. The sample was described in terms of ethnicity and self-reports of achievement.

Data Collection

Data were collected with an anonymous questionnaire that asked questions requiring yes–no responses like the following:

1. I have been bullied during school: Yes No
2. I have bullied others: Yes No
3. I have been cyberbullied (e.g., via email, chat room, cell phone): Yes No
4. I have cyberbullied others: Yes No

The questionnaire had been developed and used by the author previously. However, there was no indication of the measure's validity and reliability.

Data Analysis

The data analysis process involved sorting the responses into male and female groups, and then calculating the percentage of male and female responses for each of the dependent variables. A chi-square test found significant gender differences in two categories; both had to do with being a bully, and both found boys to be significantly different from girls. More specifically, the analysis showed the following gender differences:

1. Boys were more likely than girls to bully ($p = .027$) and to cyberbully ($p = .021$).

2. There was no significant gender difference in who reported being bullied ($p = .17$) or cyberbullied ($p = .91$).

3. Girls who were cyberbullying victims were significantly more likely than boys to inform adults ($p = .012$).

The analysis found no significant gender differences in three other areas:

4. There was no significant gender differences in being the victim of bullying ($p =$ .17) or in being cyberbullied ($p = $ .91).

5. There were no significant gender differences in beliefs about the ability of adults to stop cyberbullying ($p = $ .54). In fact, only 64.1% of the students believed that adults in schools even tried to stop cyberbullying when informed.

6. There were no gender differences in who reported witnessing bullying episodes ($p = $ .72). Across genders, only 30.1% reported witnessing bullying.

In concluding the article, the author highlights issues that the study uncovered and deemed worthy of action on the part of school officials. These included recognizing that cyberbullying is "a bullying problem occurring in a new territory," focusing on adolescence as a pivotal moment in efforts to prevent cyberbullying, and developing systematic educational strategies to prevent cyberbullying at an early age.

Evaluation

The study's framing construct is strong. The research review is clear and current. It links ideas to develop a framing construct of gender and bullying versus cyberbullying. More than 10 references are cited. Specific research questions are generated from the review.

The study also merits a strong rating for sample and sampling. The sample was randomly selected, of ample size, and equally divided by gender. The author provides a clear description of subject characteristics and the population from which the sample was drawn, as well as a detailed description of the sample.

The study merits a strong rating for data collection and analysis as well. There is a clear description of the survey instrument used for data collection, and samples of questions are included in the article. Though the survey instrument was not vetted for reliability and validity, its simple yes–no format seemed appropriate for the purpose of the study and not in need of further analysis. The author correctly used the chi-square test for significance for categorical data, with an appropriate alpha level. She stays close to the data and does not overconclude. All data are displayed in tables and charts, and are explained verbally as well.

The overall rating is strong.

CHAPTER TWELVE

Correlations Research

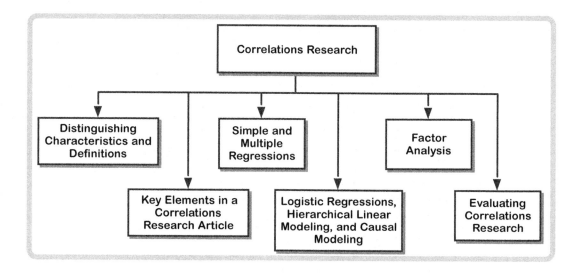

Correlations research is an umbrella term for nonexperimental research that uses correlations to predict the extent to which one variable can predict the outcome of another variable or to explore theoretical concepts within a measure.

CHAPTER OBJECTIVES

✓ Understand that correlation does not mean causation.

✓ Understand the elements of a correlations research article.

✓ Understand the difference between bivariate and multivariate analysis.

✓ Understand the purposes of bivariate and multivariate analyses, regressions, and factor analysis in research.

✓ Understand what statistical tests are used in data analysis in the various forms of correlations research.

DISTINGUISHING CHARACTERISTICS AND DEFINITIONS   MAP 12.1

The purpose of correlations research is "to determine relationships between variables or to use those relationships" (Kerlinger, 1986, pp. 321–322). There are several designs that come under the umbrella of correlations research, each with a specific purpose.

Bivariate analysis (*r*) describes the direction and strength of the relationship between two variables (simple correlation).

Multivariate analysis (*R*) describes the direction and strength of the relationship of a combination of variables to a single DV (multiple correlation).

Regressions predict that a change in one variable will account for a change in another variable.

  Simple regressions predict that one predictor variable will influence the outcome on a criterion variable (see below for definitions of these variables).

  Multiple regressions predict that a combination of predictor variables will influence the outcome on a criterion variable.

  Logical regressions, *hierarchical linear modeling*, and *causal modeling* are regression designs that examine more complex interactions of variables.

Factor analysis explores the meaning of a theoretical construct that is being measured.

Predictor variable (PV) is the name given to the IV in correlations research.

Criterion variable (CV) is the name given to the DV in correlations research.

And one very important point must always be kept in mind: Correlation does not mean causation!

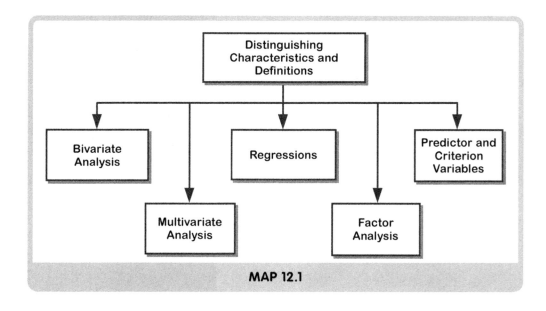

MAP 12.1

KEY ELEMENTS IN A CORRELATIONS RESEARCH ARTICLE   MAP 12.2

Research Review and Theory

As in a nonexperimental group comparison, the researcher provides a comprehensive research review in order to establish a theory or to develop a framing construct to guide the study.

Sample and Sampling

Ideally, samples in correlations research are randomly selected from a target population and described in detail. This enables the researcher to generalize results. In addition, the sample should be of adequate size to enable the researcher to apply the appropriate statistics. In fact, the larger the sample, the better. Larger samples add to representativeness and also help to reduce error.

Data Collection

The most commonly used measures for data collection are survey questionnaires and test scores. These allow researchers to investigate relationships between or among variables for one group. The data may be archived or may be collected for the purpose of the study. Measures with strong construct validity are preferred.

Data Analysis

All analysis begins with bivariate analyses and the generation of a value that describes the direction and strength of a simple correlation. Depending on the nature of the dependent variable, the researcher will use one of the correlation statistics from Table 12.1.

As noted in Chapter Seven, most researchers use the following (based on Cohen, 1988, and Salkind, 2004) as a guide for evaluating the strength of a correlation.

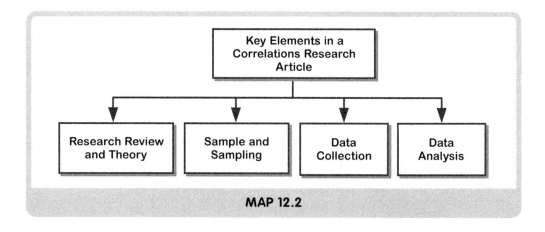

MAP 12.2

TABLE 12.1. Correlation Statistics	
Type of DV	**Statistic**
Continuous	Coefficient of correlation (r)
Ordinal (ranked)	Spearman's rho (ρ)
Categorical	Phi coefficient (ϕ) Cramer's V (V)

Weak correlations: ±.24 or less

Moderate correlations: ±.25 to .49

Moderately strong correlations: ±.50 to .74

Strong correlations: ±.75 to .99

DESIGNS IN CORRELATIONS RESEARCH   MAP 12.3

Simple and Multiple Regressions   MAP 12.4

Simple and multiple regressions depend on the calculation of a *coefficient of determination.*

> A *coefficient of determination* provides an estimate of the degree to which the change (or *variance*) in the PV will predict (or explain) the change (or variance) in the CV.
>
> > r^2 is the coefficient of determination for a simple regression; it is the square of a simple correlation (r).
> >
> > R^2 is the coefficient of determination for a multiple regression; it is the square of a multiple correlation (R, or "big R").

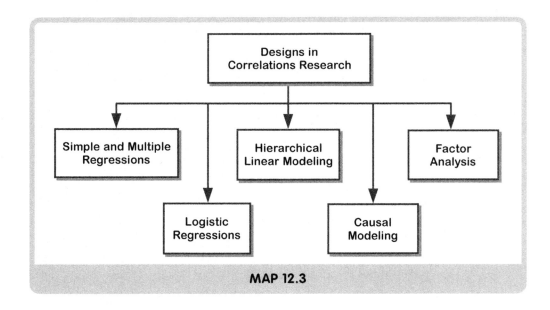

MAP 12.3

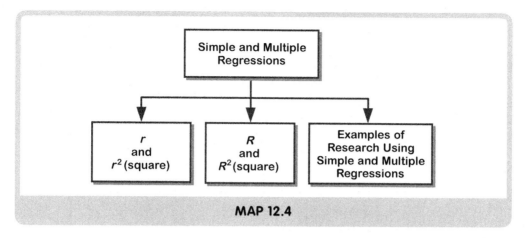

MAP 12.4

For example, consider a study that investigates the relationship between SAT Critical Reading scores and freshman GPA in college:

PV = SAT Critical Reading score   PV = GPA
$r = .47$ $r^2 = .22$

These data indicate that (1) there is a moderate correlation between SAT Critical Reading scores and freshman GPA and (2) SAT Critical Reading scores predict (or explain) 22% of the variance in freshman GPA. That leaves 78% of the difference unaccounted for.

Now consider what happens when a researcher investigates the combination of three variables and their relationship to the CV:

CV = freshman college GPA

PV 1 = SAT Critical Reading score

PV 2 = SAT Mathematics score

PV 3 = high school GPA

Multiple-regression analysis requires a three-step process.

1. The first step is to calculate three simple correlations; that is, to do a bivariate analysis of each of the three predictor PVs against the CV and arrive at an r for each PV. Figure 12.1 shows these calculations.

2. The second step involves a *multivariate analysis* that yields R, or "big R."

$$R = .60$$

3. The final step is to square the R.

$$R^2 = .36$$

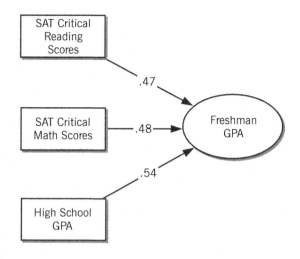

FIGURE 12.1. Bivariate analysis of SAT scores and freshman GPA.

This is the total variance that is explained by the three variables. That is, taken together, the three variables account for (or explain) 36% of the variance in freshman GPA. This leaves 64% of the difference in freshman GPA unaccounted for. It also leaves admissions officers grasping at other information to help them in their deliberations.

Examples of Research Using Simple and Multiple Regressions

1. Fernald, J. (2002). *Preliminary findings on the relationship between SAT scores, high school GPA, socioeconomic status, and UCSC freshman GPA.* Santa Cruz: University of California, Santa Cruz.

Most selective colleges use the SAT as a filter for admitting students. The assumption is that the SAT is a good predictor of success in college. The Senate of the University of California at Santa Cruz (UCSC) conducted a study of the relationship of SAT to freshman success, which they operationalized as the GPA at the end of the freshman year at the university (UCSC freshman GPA) (see Figure 12.2). The results showed a weak positive correlation ($r = .290$) that was statistically significant ($p = .0000$).

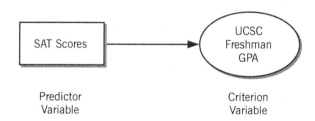

FIGURE 12.2. SAT as PV, and UCSC freshman GPA as CV, in the Fernald (2002) study.

The conclusion of this study might be presented as follows: "There is a significant positive correlation between SAT scores and success in college." Although true in fact, this statement overlooks an important consideration: A weak, statistically significant correlation is still a weak correlation. In effect, this correlation is not substantial enough to be important or useful; nor does it account for much in the way of differences in UCSC freshman GPA, as evidenced by the simple regression analysis that followed. The researcher calculated the variance (change) in UCSC freshman GPA (the CV) that could be accounted for by the SAT I (the PV). This required squaring the r (r^2 = .084). This means that the SAT I predicted 8.4% of the variance (or change) in UCSC freshman GPA, leaving 93.6% of the variance unaccounted for.

To investigate further the predictors of college success, the researchers added two more PVs (SAT II scores and high school GPA, or HS GPA) and conducted a multiple-regression analysis (see Figure 12.3).

The first step in the analysis was to calculate the correlation of each PV to the CR. The correlation matrix in Table 12.2 shows these correlations. To read the matrix, look across each row or look down each column. You will see that there is a perfect correlation of UCSC GPA to itself, a weak correlation to SAT II (r = .029), a somewhat stronger correlation to SAT II (r = .306), and the strongest correlation to HS GPA (r = .345). Note that all of these correlations are also statistically significant (p = .0000).

The next step was to calculate the multiple correlation (R = .425). To calculate the combined variance for the three PVs, the R was squared (R^2 = .181). This means that, together, the three variables accounted for 18.1% of the variance in UCSC freshman GPA. This is better than any one criterion taken separately, but it still leaves 81.9% of the difference in UCSC freshman GPA unaccounted for.

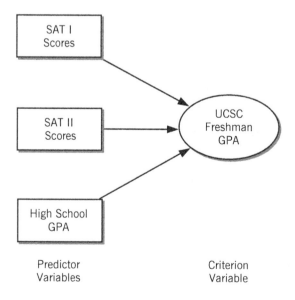

FIGURE 12.3. PVs in the Fernald (2002) study = SAT I, SAT II, HS GPA; CV = UCSC freshman GPA.

TABLE 12.2. Correlation Matrix for UCSC Freshman GPA, SAT I, SAT II, and HS GPA

	UCSC GPA	SAT I	SAT II	HS GPA
UCSC GPA				
Pearson r	1.000	.290	.306	.345
Significance		.000	.000	.000
SAT I				
Pearson r	.290	1.000	.816	.150
Significance	.000		.000	.000
SAT II				
Pearson r	.306	.816	1.000	.220
Significance	.000	.000		.000
HS GPA				
Pearson r	.345	.159	.220	1.000
Significance	.000	.000	.000	

Note. Data from Fernald (2002).

The researcher presents the following conclusions for UCSC freshmen: (1) The single best predictor of UCSC freshman GPA was HS GPA, which accounted for 11.9% of the variance; (2) the next best predictor was SAT II scores, which accounted for 9.4% of the variance; (3) SAT I scores were the lowest predictor and accounted for 8.4% of the variance; and (4) the combination of all three PVs explained more of the variance in UCSC freshman GPA than any of these variables taken alone. Together, they accounted for 18.1% of the UCSC freshman GPA.

2. Adams, E. (1999). Vocational teacher stress and internal characteristics. *Journal of Vocational and Technical Education, 16*(1), 7–22.

Adams (1999) conducted a more complex multiple-regression study with six PVs. Drawing the sample from vocational teachers in one state, the researcher examined to what degree the variables could predict teacher stress. Adams selected these PVs after conducting an extensive review of prior research.

> PVs = role preparation, job satisfaction, life satisfaction, illness symptoms, locus of control, and self-esteem
>
> CV = teacher stress

In the first step of the analysis, the researcher correlated each of the PVs to the CV. Figure 12.4 represents those correlations. As this figure shows, each PV had a moderate to moderately high correlation with teacher stress. One variable, locus of control (feeling in control of oneself), had a negative correlation ($r = -.375$) with teacher stress. In other words, as locus of control went up, teacher stress went down—or "the less control vocational teachers believe they have over the events that occur in their lives, the more intense is their stress" (Adams, 1999, p. 9).

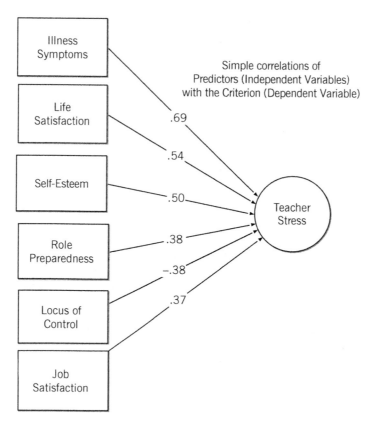

FIGURE 12.4. Simple correlations of PVs to CV in the Adams (1999) teacher stress study.

In the next two steps, the researcher calculated the R (the combination of all PVs) and then squared the R.

$$R = 74.6659226153$$
$$R^2 = .5575$$

This means that almost 56% of the variance in stress was accounted for by the combination of variables.

The final step involved a process to identify which of the six predictors had the most impact. This required an examination of the probability level for each variable. Table 12.3 provides this information.

To explain how this works, we like to make an analogy to the TV program *Survivor.* In the program, a large group of contestants begin on the island, but there is progressive elimination of contestants. With multiple regressions, the same process occurs. The researcher can "kick some variables off the island" by looking at the p-values to see which are significant correlations. The last column on the right in Table 12.3 shows the p-values for each predictor.

TABLE 12.3. Teacher Internal Characteristics—Multiple-Regression Results of Internal-Related Variables on Vocational Teacher Stress

Variable	Metric regression coefficient (beta)	Standard error	Standardized regression coefficient (beta-weight)	t-test	Probability
Role preparedness	.382202	.1468	.1344	2.60	.0092
Job satisfaction	.009817	.0098	.0056	0.10	.9125
Life satisfaction	.135020	.0995	.0673	0.99	.3229
Illness symptoms	.833539	.0869	.5180	9.58	.0000
Locus of control	.044400	.0271	−.0813	1.64	.1018
Self-esteem	.379038	.1360	.1586	2.69	.0053

Note. R^2 = .5575. Adapted from Adams (1999) under a Creative Commons agreement.

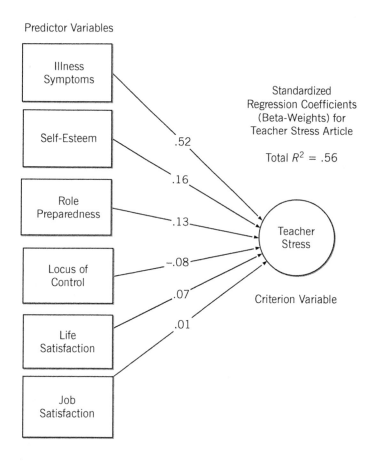

FIGURE 12.5. Standardized regression coefficients (beta–weights) in the Adams (1999) study.

- The three predictors with $p > .05$ "leave the island" and are not included in the calculation of R and R^2. These are job satisfaction ($p =. 9125$), life satisfaction ($p =.3229$), and locus of control ($p = .1018$).

- The three predictors with $p < .05$ get to stay. These are illness symptoms ($p = .0000$), role preparedness ($p =. 0092$), and self-esteem ($p = .0053$).

These are the three variables that are included in the calculation of R and R^2. What R^2 tells us, then, is this: Taken together, illness symptoms, role preparedness, and self-esteem account for 55.75% of the variance in teacher stress.

Table 12.3 also lists the *standardized regression coefficient* or *beta-weight* for each PV. These appear in the fourth column from the left in this table and are also shown in Figure 12.5. These are special correlations that indicate how much of the change in the CV can be attributed to each PV. The three highest beta-weights are as follows:

Beta-weight for illness symptoms = .518

Beta-weight for role preparedness = .134

Beta-weight for self-esteem = .158

This means that for every 1–unit change in the measure of illness symptoms, there is a .518–unit change in the measure of teacher stress; for every 1–unit change in role preparedness, there is a .134–unit change in stress; and for each 1–unit of change in self-esteem, there is a .158–unit change in teacher stress. The size of the beta-weights is another indication of the preeminence of some predictor PVs over others.

This is a rather complicated study and requires careful attention to detail. It is important to remember that a researcher can eliminate some variables by looking at their p-values and beta-weights.

Other Correlational Designs

Logistic Regressions, Hierarchical Linear Modeling, and Causal Modeling

MAP 12.5

In addition to the approaches described above, you may encounter more regressions that use more complex statistics. The aim of these approaches is to more closely approximate causation. The most commonly used are *logical regression, hierarchical linear modeling*, and *causal modeling*.

Logistic regressions predict the variance in one categorical CV that can be explained by more than one continuous or categorical PV. The *odds ratio* is the statistic used to calculate the odds (probability) that the CV will increase due to the influence of the PVs. For example, Gofin and Avitzour (2012) used a logistic regression to analyze the likelihood of boys versus girls as bullies. Both the PVs and CV were categorical variables. The researchers found a higher odds ratio (a significant difference) for boys as traditional bullies.

Hierarchical linear modeling is an approach to analysis of hierarchical or nested data. It is used to estimate the influence of PVs at different levels. For example, Ming

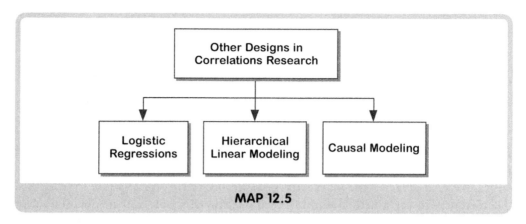

MAP 12.5

(2007) examined the interrelationships of the effects of students' countries and families on students' science achievement. The study was based on data from the 2002 Program for International Student Assessment (PISA) study of 15 countries.

PVs = gross domestic product (GNP) of country

equality of household incomes (GINI) of country

CVs = student achievement (Level 1)

school achievement (Level 2)

country achievement (Level 3)

Causal modeling designs predict outcomes of multiple PVs on one CV, calculate the interactions/indirect effects of PVs on one CV, and calculate interactions/indirect effects of PVs on other PVs. Causal modeling is based on correlations with the purpose of examining complex interactions of variables. For example, Phan (2010) combined two separate theoretical orientations (achievement goals and study processing strategies) into one overall causal model. Over a 2-year period, these theoretical constructs were measured with a variety of self-reported inventories, and academic performance was measured by overall course marks and final examination scores. The results showed relationships between two sets of predictors: (1) performance-approach goals, mastery goals, effort, and academic performance and (2) performance-approach goals, deep processing, mastery goals, effort, and academic performance.

Factor Analysis   MAP 12.6

Factor analysis is a special application of correlations research. It is used to explore and develop the meaning of a theoretical construct that is being measured.

Krathwohl (2004, p. 430) has defined factor analysis as "a statistical procedure that, by examining interrelationships among items or tests, help to identify the dimensions underlying a measure and hence what it is measuring." Because research

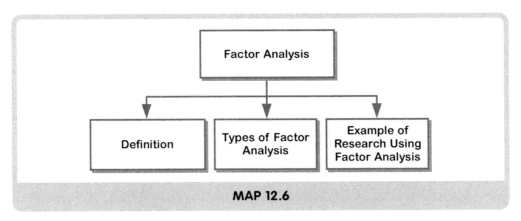

MAP 12.6

concerns itself with understanding theoretical constructs, like achievement, stress, and motivation, it is important to develop a measure or instrument that quantifies each construct, which is also known as a *factor*. Factor analysis is used to examine and identify connections and patterns in lengthy surveys and tests, and to identify the general construct that is being measured. In standardized tests that measure achievement or evaluate a clinical condition, all of the items on the test relate to one factor. That is, they all measure different aspects of the same construct and their supporting ideas. For example, tests are labeled with the general construct they measure (e.g., general intelligence), and they have subscales or subtests that measure aspects of the construct (e.g., spatial, quantitative, and verbal intelligence).

Factor analysis sounds more complicated than it really is. It all comes back to understanding the coefficient of correlation, with values ranging from +1.0 to −1.0. A factor analysis quantifies the interrelationships among ideas; as such, it is an empirical, quantitative reasoning process. The results are interpreted similarly to correlations, and in this case, the bigger the correlations (called *factor scores or factor loadings*), the better. There are no tests of statistical significance and no *p*-values, so the interpretation is done strictly with the factor scores (factor loadings).

Types of Factor Analysis

There are two types of factor analysis: *exploratory* and *confirmatory*.

Exploratory factor analysis seeks to discover the patterns of interrelationships among factors.

Confirmatory factor analysis is a follow-up procedure to determine whether the predicted interrelationships are found.

Both types examine the complex interrelationships of general constructs and their unique, underlying factors; both types yield quantitative results that represent the size of the empirical relationships between and among these factors and constructs.

Example of Research Using Factor Analysis

Cheng, E. (2011). The role of self-regulated learning in enhancing learning performance. *International Journal of Research and Review, 6*(1), 1–16.

Cheng completed a factor analysis of a survey instrument that explored the relationship between self-regulated learning and learning performance. The abstract reads as follows:

> The paper aims to explore the relationship between students' self-regulation ability and their learning performance. In this study, self-regulation ability is conceptualized by four dimensions: learning motivation, goal setting, action control and learning strategies. [A total of] 6,524 students from 20 aided secondary schools in Hong Kong participated in the questionnaire survey. Factor analysis and reliability test[ing] were used to confirm the constructed validity and the reliability of the survey instrument.

Figure 12.6 is a visual representation of the four factors constituting the construct of learning performance in this article.

Since there was no way to observe all of these processes directly, the survey approach was used to elicit responses to these correlated processes. The researcher developed a survey questionnaire based on prior research models to measure relevant variables, and used factor analysis to detect whether specific items in the questionnaire corresponded to the theoretical constructs of self-regulated learning. Through

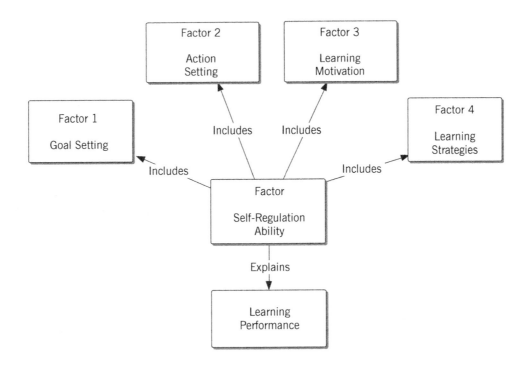

FIGURE 12.6. Theoretical construct and factors for the Cheng (2011) study.

factor analysis, the author concluded that the variables were in fact measured in the questionnaire, and that the questionnaire was valid and reliable, with all Cronbach's alpha coefficients of variables higher than .50. These results showed that there were positive relationships between/among learning strategies, action control, goal setting, learning motivation, and learning performance. The author also conducted multiple-regression analyses to sort out the relative effects of each factor as a predictor of learning performance.

EVALUATING CORRELATIONS RESEARCH   MAP 12.7

As explained in Chapter Eleven with regard to nonexperimental group comparisons, because correlations research involves no treatment and minimal researcher control, the category of *theory and treatment* does not apply here. As in group comparisons, we use the term *theory or framing construct* to describe what guides the study. In some instances, researchers establish a theory to guide the correlations, state a research hypothesis, and conduct hypothesis testing. In other instances, researchers will conduct exploratory studies, develop a framing construct to guide the study, and raise research questions.

Theory or Framing Construct

The primary considerations in evaluating the first category are the quality of the literature review and how well it established a theory or develops a framing construct to guide the research.

1. How well does the research review establish a theory or generate a construct to guide the study? For a theory, does the review support a research hypothesis that can be tested? For a framing concept, does the review link various ideas to develop the framing construct?
2. Are relevant and adequate (10 or more) research studies reviewed?
3. Are the PV and CV clearly identified?

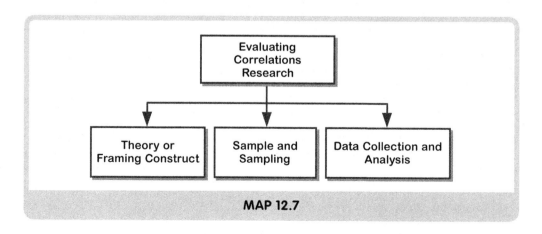

MAP 12.7

Sample and Sampling

The major considerations in evaluating sample and sampling are methods of sample selection and the sample size.

1. Is there a clear description of how the sample was selected? Was it selected randomly or nonrandomly?
2. Are sample characteristics described? What were they?
3. What was the size of the sample? Was it of adequate size?

Data Collection and Analysis

The key elements in evaluating data collection and analysis are the validity and reliability of the measures and the appropriateness of the statistical analysis and of the process of statistical reasoning.

1. How good are the validity and reliability of the measure(s)?
2. How well were the measured data reported and analyzed?
3. Were appropriate statistics applied for continuous and categorical criterion variables (CVs)? What was the alpha level established for statistical significance?
4. Were the results statistically significant?
5. Does the author stay close to the data and not overconclude?

Figure 12.7 is a rubric for evaluating correlations research.

Example: Evaluation of the Teacher Stress Study

Theory or Framing Construct

Because the Adams (1999) study used surveys to measure teacher stress, it is an example of a quantitative, empirical study. The author's aim was to investigate and explore the concept of teacher stress; hence there was no intervention. Numerous studies focusing on stress and related internal characteristics in psychology, sociology, and medicine are cited in the article as the rationale for the study. The author describes the study's purpose as measuring the internal characteristics of stress, such as role preparedness, job satisfaction, life satisfaction, illness symptoms, locus of control, and self-esteem.

There are no specific hypotheses or research questions given in the article, but there are two specific objectives: "(a) identify variables emanating from teacher internal characteristics that explain vocational stress and (b) build and test a model to explain the inter-relationships among inter-related variables and vocational teacher stress" (p. 10). The model for stress was based on the relationship of the internal characteristics of teachers with teacher stress. The theory of the study seems to be well documented and clear.

Criterion	Strong	Moderate	Weak
Theory or framing construct	Clear, current, and sufficient literature review that either establishes a theory or links ideas to develop a framing construct and includes 10 or more references; clear identification of hypothesis or research questions; strong support for the PV and CV.	Literature review may not adequately link ideas to a framing construct or make a clear connection to the research question, or may include fewer than 10 references; hypothesis or research questions implied; adequate support for the PV and CV.	Unclear literature review that fails to link ideas to a framing concept; fewer than five references; no hypothesis or research questions evident; inadequate support for the PV and CV.
Sample and sampling	Clear description of the sample characteristics and the population; clear description of sample; evidence of sufficient size (60 or more); random selection of sample.	Description of sample is present, but lacking in details about characteristics and the population; insufficient sample size; nonrandom sample.	No description of the sample; total lack of details about the population; nonrandom sample.
Data collection and analysis	Clear description of measures selected to collect data on PV and CV, including evidence of validity and reliability (r); correct use of tests for; description of statistical significance (p) and alpha level, as well as of the inferential tests used; researcher stays close to data and does not overconclude; article includes explanatory charts and narratives.	Mention of measurement, but lacking in details about validity and reliability (r); mention of statistical significance (p) without including inferential tests used; researcher avoids overconcluding; article includes explanatory charts and/or narratives.	Minimal or no mention of measurement; no mention of validity or reliability; no mention of significance; researcher may overconclude; article does not include adequate visual or narrative explanations.

FIGURE 12.7. Rubric for evaluating correlations research.

Prior research indicated that there could be an important distinction between the levels of stress in teachers' lives and the perception or experience of stress by teachers. Ultimately the researcher would like to provide more insights into teacher burnout and leaving the teaching profession. While the research provides insights into the relationship, the author does not claim that internal characteristics cause stress.

Purpose and Design

The author clearly indicates that the study was a correlational study, because it examined the relationships among key variables. As mentioned, Adams states no hypotheses, but the study clearly focused on the internal characteristics of stress as reported by a sample of vocational education teachers. The correlational design fit the purpose of the study, because the relationships among variables were being studied. Multiple regression was appropriate, because the researcher wanted to determine the most predictive variables from the six PVs. The teachers being studied were not receiving any treatment for stress; the study was simply a measurement of their stress level during the school year.

Based on the correlations, the researcher used multiple-regression analysis to create a predictive model for teacher stress. The IVs or PVs were the internal characteristics (role preparedness, job satisfaction, life satisfaction, illness symptoms, locus of control, and self-esteem), and the DV or CV was the amount of teacher stress. No other factors (e.g., age or experience) were measured or used in the study.

Sample and Sampling

Although vocational teachers in general were the target group or population being studied, the population from which samples were taken consisted of vocational teachers in Virginia. There were two steps in the sampling process. "All of the vocational teachers teaching in five targeted school systems" (p. 10) were included in the first step, amounting to a sample size of 182 teachers. In the second step, a random sample of vocational teachers was taken from all of the remaining vocational teachers in the state. There was no specific total given, but the researcher ended up with 235 usable surveys from 85 male and 150 female teachers. "The random selection from the remainder of the state was added to increase the number of participants as well as to produce a more inclusive study of vocational teachers in the state" (p. 10). The final sample was larger and more representative of the state's population of vocational teachers than the first one. Because of the nonrandom sampling process, however, the generalizability of the study is reduced.

Data Collection

Several instruments were used to collect the data for this correlational multiple-regression study, as described below. The descriptive statistics for all variables for this sample are shown in Table 12.3.

Four of the IVs/PVs were measured by subscales on the Teacher Stress Measure (TSM), an instrument with 70 items or questions that uses a 6-point Likert scale for measurement. The TSM has good internal consistency estimates using Cronbach's alpha, as well as evidence of reliability, construct validity, and predictive validity.

Two other instruments used to measure IVs/PVs were the Personal Behavior Inventory (PBI) and the Self-Esteem Scale (SES). The PBI contains 46 items or questions that measure locus of control. On a 5-point scale, teachers indicated whether they felt as if they were in control of their lives (a low score) or whether they felt like victims of fate (a high score). Although no specific evidence of reliability or validity for the PBI was provided, the researcher points out studies that have validated the PBI with teachers. The SES has a total of 10 items, uses a 4-point scale, and has a test–retest reliability of .62. This instrument is thus on the margin of acceptable reliability.

The DV or CV was measured by the Tennessee Stress Scale–R (TSS-R), which was developed to measure stress in "selected service-oriented professions" (p. 5). The instrument has 60 items or additive statements with a yes–no forced-choice scale.

The TSS-R was validated with national stress norms. The TSS-R has a test–retest reliability coefficient of .88, making it a reliable measurement tool for this study.

Data collection for the sample consisted of multiple attempts to contact non-respondents by mail and telephone. To check for bias, when nonrespondents were contacted by phone, their responses to one question were compared to the responses of the teachers who completed the survey. There were no significant differences in the responses.

Data Analysis, Interpretation, and Conclusions

There were three steps in the data analysis: (1) descriptive statistics, (2) correlations, and (3) multiple regression. Correlations between the predictors and stress, the CV, ranged from strong for illness symptoms ($r = .69$) to weak for job satisfaction ($r = .37$). There was a negative correlation between locus of control and stress ($r = -.38$).

The total explained variance (R^2) was 56% for all of the PVs on teacher stress, as shown in Table 12.3 and Figure 12.5; this means that 56% of the variation in stress was explained by the variables. The three PVs that were the strongest predictors were illness symptoms, self-esteem, and role preparedness. These variables are identified by the p-values in Table 12.3; for all three, $p < .05$. This means that they were significantly different from zero or no predictive value, and higher in predictive value than the other three PVs (locus of control, life satisfaction, and job satisfaction).

This research has a clear purpose, and the theoretical base is well documented; stress is linked with teachers' wellness and potential burnout. The sample size was adequate, but the sample was nonrandom, and we do not know the characteristics of the state population of vocational teachers (e.g., for gender or age). The measurement was done with established instruments like the PBI, SES, and TSS-R. There is no hypothesis, but the results do show that a large proportion of the total variance of stress could be explained by three out of the six PVs, which may help future researchers to examine these factors in depth. Instrumentation was one of the strong points of the study, but I would rate the study's overall quality as moderate.

CHAPTER SUMMARY   MAP 12.8

✓ Correlations research is a form of nonexperimental research that uses correlation statistics to quantify the relationship or associations between or among variables.

✓ Correlation does not mean causation.

✓ Correlations research may be explanatory or predictive.

✓ Correlational research depends on large, representative samples.

✓ Correlational research depends on surveys and questionnaires as measures.

✓ Data analysis rises in complexity as it moves from explanation to prediction and as the number of variables increases.

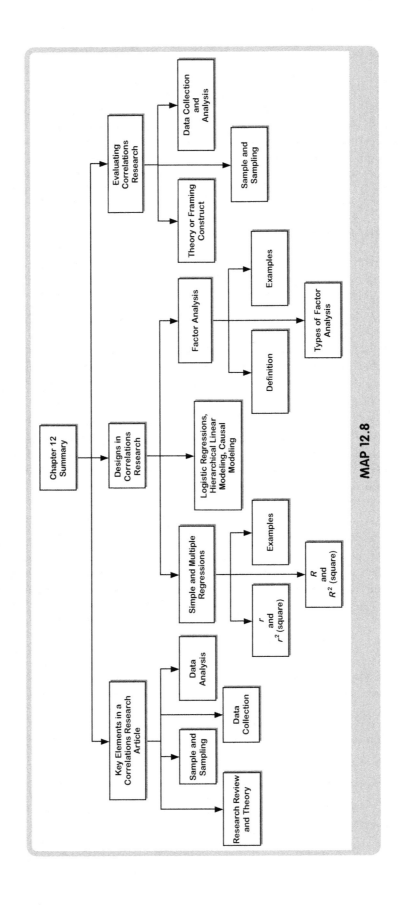

MAP 12.8

236

✓ The basic correlational designs are simple correlations/regressions and multivariate correlations/multiple regressions.

✓ Simple correlations are represented by the correlation coefficient (r); simple regressions are represented by the coefficient of determination (r^2).

✓ Multivariate correlations are represented by the multiple-correlation coefficient (R); multiple regressions are represented by the coefficient of determination (R^2).

✓ Advanced regression analyses include logical regression, hierarchical linear modeling, and causal modeling.

✓ Factor analysis is a special application of correlations research; it is used to explore and develop the meaning of a theoretical construct that is being measured.

✓ The two types of factor analysis are explanatory and confirmatory.

✓ Correlations research is evaluated on the basis of statistical conclusion validity and external validity.

KEY TERMS AND CONCEPTS

beta–weight

bivariate analysis

causal modeling

coefficient of correlation

coefficient of determination

confirmatory factor analysis

correlation research

criterion variable

exploratory factor analysis

factor

factor analysis

hierarchical linear modeling

logistic regression

multiple correlation (R)

multiple regression (R^2)

multivariate analysis

predictor variable

simple correlation (r)

simple regression (r^2)

REVIEW, CONSOLIDATION, AND EXTENSION OF KNOWLEDGE

1. In your own words,

   a. Describe how correlations studies are similar to and different from nonexperimental group comparison studies.

   b. Identify the statistics that explain relationships between or among variables.

   c. Identify the statistics that predict how one variable predicts an outcome on another variable.

   d. Explain how a correlation can be significant but not important.

2. Using an electronic database, search for a regression study on a topic of interest. Follow the Guide to Reading below as you work through the article. Then, with the Guide as a template, write a critique of about 750 words of the study you have selected. See the Appendix for an exemplar.

Guide to Reading

Research Review: What is the purpose of the research review? What is the theory or framing construct of the study?

Purpose and Design: What is the purpose of the study? Are research questions raised? If so, what are they? What are the PVs and CVs?

Sample and Sampling: How was the sample selected, randomly or nonrandomly? Who was in the sample? What were the characteristics of the sample? What was the sample size?

Data Collection: How were data collected: survey, questionnaire, test report? Are there indications of validity and reliability for each measure? What information does the instrument collect? What is the response format of the questions?

Data Analysis, Interpretation, and Conclusions: What statistical tests were used to analyze the data? Were the results (p-values) significant or nonsignificant? What does the researcher conclude about the findings? Does the researcher avoid overconcluding?

Evaluation: How do you rate the overall quality of the study? Strong? Moderate? Weak? How do you rate the categories below, and what is your reason for the ratings in each category?

Theory or framing construct: Strong, moderate, weak

Sample and sampling: Strong, moderate, weak

Data collection and analysis: Strong, moderate, weak

PART VI

Mixing and Creating Methods

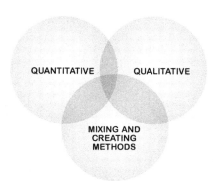

QUANTITATIVE   QUALITATIVE

MIXING AND
CREATING
METHODS

"The real voyage of discovery consists not in seeking
new landscapes, but in having new eyes."

—MARCEL PROUST

Part VI concentrates on approaches to research that challenge the established categories discussed in previous parts. Not all topics for investigation lend themselves to the established categories of research discussed in previous sections. Some benefit from creating a synergy of traditional qualitative and quantitative methods, while others require the development of new approaches to inquiry.

CHAPTER THIRTEEN

Mixed Methods Research

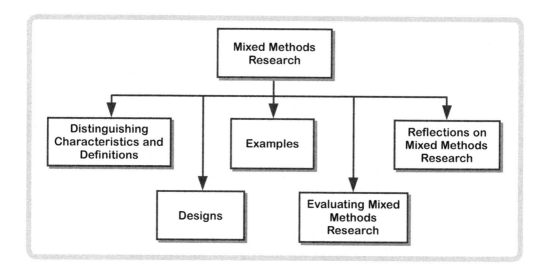

M ixed methods research combines traditional qualitative and quantitative methods to answer questions that neither method can answer on its own.

CHAPTER OBJECTIVES

✓ Understand the purpose and premise underlying mixed methods research.
✓ Understand how mixed methods research combines quantitative and qualitative methods.
✓ Understand the difference between concurrent and sequential mixed methods designs.
✓ Understand triangulation and embedded procedures for concurrent mixed methods research.
✓ Understand explanatory and exploratory procedures for sequential mixed methods research.

DISTINGUISHING CHARACTERISTICS AND DEFINITIONS

MAP 13.1

Mixed methods research combines and integrates quantitative and qualitative methods in a single study.

The purpose of mixed methods research is to investigate a problem fully by drawing on quantitative measures to determine frequencies and relationship of variables, as well as on qualitative tools to provide insight into meaning and understanding. It combines qualitative and quantitative methods in a way that emphasizes the strengths of each method and avoids overlapping weaknesses.

> It involves the recognition that all methods have their limitations as well as their strengths. The fundamental principle is followed for at least three reasons: (a) to obtain convergence or corroboration of findings, (b) to eliminate or minimize key plausible alternative explanations for conclusions drawn from the research data, and (c) to elucidate the divergent aspects of a phenomenon. (Johnson & Turner, 2003, p. 299)

The philosophy that undergirds mixed methods research is *pragmatism*, which is a quintessentially American philosophy advocated by William James, Charles S. Peirce, and John Dewey. Pragmatists propose that the value of an inquiry can best be judged by its practical consequences. Mixed methods research fits the pragmatic idea because it makes practical use of both induction and deduction to achieve understanding and explanation (Johnson & Onwuegbuzie, 2004, p. 14).

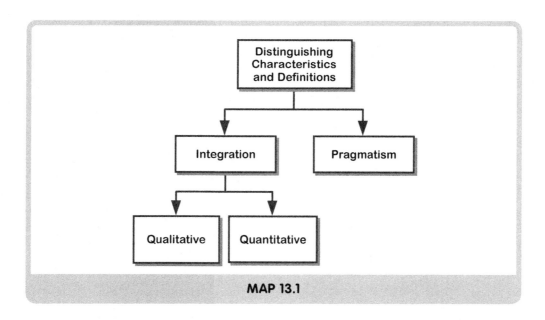

MAP 13.1

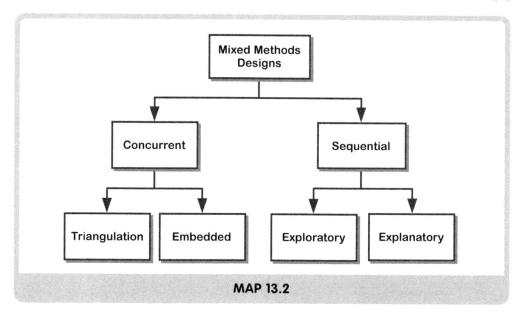

MAP 13.2

MIXED METHODS DESIGNS

MAP 13.2

Some mixed methods studies weight the qualitative and quantitative strands equally, while others weight one strand more heavily than another. It is important to distinguish mixed methods designs from multiple-methods research that uses more than one method of data collection and analysis within the same research tradition. For example, ethnographies and case studies use interviews, observations, and documents/discourses. Similarly, quantitative studies may depend on both surveys and measures of academic achievement. A unique feature of mixed methods research is that qualitative and quantitative data are separately collected and analyzed, and are then brought together in a final interpretation, in what are known as *metainferences* or *integrated mixed inferences* (Tashakkori & Teddlie, 2003a). There are two basic types of mixed methods designs: *concurrent* and *sequential*, each with specific procedures for data collection and analysis.

Concurrent Designs

Concurrent mixed methods designs "are those in which the researcher converges or merges quantitative and qualitative data in order to provide a comprehensive analysis of the research problem" (Creswell, 2009, p. 228). There are two procedures for data collection and analysis in concurrent designs: *triangulation* and *embedded*.

1. In the *concurrent triangulation design*, there is one data collection phase in which the qualitative and quantitative data are collected simultaneously, and there are two separate analyses of the qualitative and quantitative data. In the interpretation phase, either the findings are merged, or they are compared in a discussion section. In this procedure, the qualitative and quantitative strands are usually weighted equally. Figure 13.1 illustrates this design.

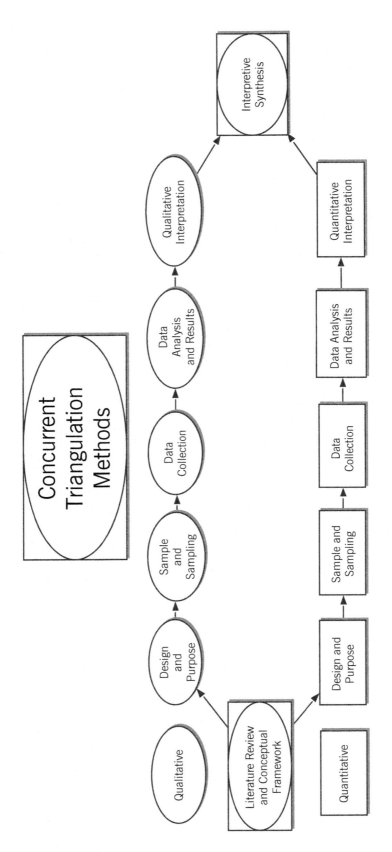

Concurrent Triangulation Methods

Qualitative

Design and Purpose → Sample and Sampling → Data Collection → Data Analysis and Results → Qualitative Interpretation → Interpretive Synthesis

Literature Review and Conceptual Framework

Quantitative

Design and Purpose → Sample and Sampling → Data Collection → Data Analysis and Results → Quantitative Interpretation → Interpretive Synthesis

FIGURE 13.1. Concurrent triangulation procedures.

2. In the *concurrent embedded design*, the procedure for data collection is similar to that in the triangulation design: There is one data collection phase in which qualitative and quantitative data are collected simultaneously. However, during the data analysis phase one strand is nested within another stage, which is more heavily weighted. Figure 13.2 illustrates this design.

Sequential Designs

Sequential mixed methods designs "are those in which the researcher seeks to elaborate on or expand on the findings of one method with another method" (Creswell, 2009, p. 234). Within sequential designs, there are also two procedures for data collection and analysis: *explanatory* and *exploratory*.

1. In the *sequential exploratory design*, the qualitative strand is weighted more heavily. The quantitative strand is used to assist in interpreting the qualitative findings. Figure 13.3 illustrates this design.

2. In the *sequential explanatory design*, the quantitative strand is weighted more heavily and informs procedures in the qualitative strand. The qualitative analysis is used to examine or clarify quantitative findings. Figure 13.4 illustrates this design.

EXAMPLES OF MIXED METHODS DESIGNS

1. Concurrent Embedded Design

Feldon, D., & Kefai, Y. (2008). Mixed methods for mixed reality: Understanding users' avatar activities in Virtual Worlds. *Educational Technology Research and Development,* 56(5–6), 575–593.

This study investigated the use of avatars in a game called Virtual Worlds, and it used several methods of data collection and analysis. There were 595 participants in the game, who created avatars that had to survive and progress in their environment, respond to other avatars, and deal with disease and health risks. Over 33% of participants in the game engaged in avatar activities through computer clicks, hits, and navigations. An avatar-related activity might be a change in physical appearance or the exchange of facial features as a trade or a symbol of friendship. The participants visited over 6.93 million screen locations over the 6-month duration of the study.

The authors used log data, online and offline observations, interviews, and surveys as data sources. The logs represented the raw data of participants' actions—the total count of clicks and hits. A 30-item online survey administered after the game included an outbreak of a smallpox virus, which produced spots on the face of each avatar. All but one of the survey questions were closed-response questions that focused on general use and user preferences. Interviews of 35 participants were conducted at the end of the study and consisted of questions such as "How is your avatar like you and/or not like you?" and "How often do you change your avatar?"

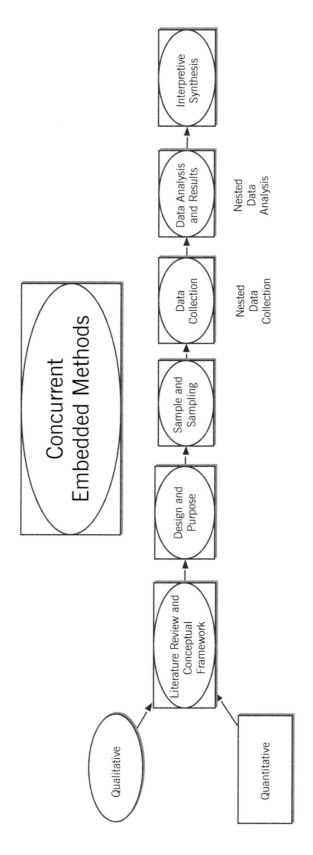

FIGURE 13.2. Concurrent embedded procedures.

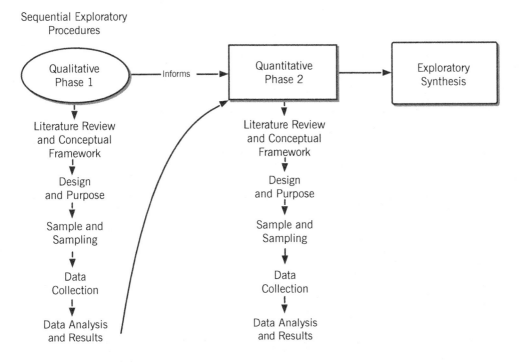

FIGURE 13.3. Sequential exploratory procedures.

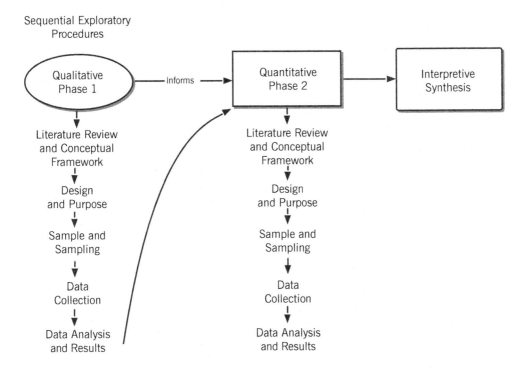

FIGURE 13.4. Sequential explanatory procedures.

(p. 583). A researcher, who was embedded in the game as a reporter, collected the observations in the online environment. The researcher visited virtual locations to observe the movements and interactions of avatars.

Data from the server logs and the surveys were analyzed, and three types of participants/users were identified: casual users, social users, and heavy users. This categorization formed the basis for analyzing differences across the total sample, and it provided a key quantitative comparison for the overall time and effort spent on avatar-related activities. The comparison of the three groups used an ANOVA, which showed that participants from the three groups were very similar in their avatar-related activities.

The combination of methods in this study provided an understanding of the incidence of participants' activities, the details of their motivation and questions, and their concerns about their virtual experiences. The researchers attempted to balance quantitative and qualitative methods and designs. There was a progression of methods, beginning with server logs and quantitative method, and ending with interviews and observations. This study is thus a good example of a concurrent embedded design.

2. Sequential Explanatory Design

Gasiewski, J., Eagan, M., Garcia, G., Hurtado, S., & Chang, M. (2012). From gatekeeping to engagement: A multi-contextual, mixed method study of student academic engagement in introductory STEM courses. *Research in Higher Education*, 53(2), 229–261.

This study "employed a sequential, explanatory mixed method approach to provide a richer understanding of the relationship between student engagement and introductory science instruction" (p. 229). The authors explained, "With this research design, we sought not only to examine the predictive power of specific learning strategies and classroom contexts that relate to STEM students' engagement in introductory courses but also to further support and enrich these findings through students' narrative experiences of being enrolled in these courses" (p. 230). The researchers reviewed research on academic engagement, active learning pedagogies, motivation, and faculty behavior to establish a theoretical framework for the study.

The more heavily quantitative strand was conducted first. The sample was drawn from 73 introductory science, technology, engineering, and mathematics (STEM) courses from 15 colleges and universities. The researchers administered surveys at the beginning and end of the courses; 2,873 students completed both surveys. The DV was academic engagement, which included these eight factors: "frequency with which students asked questions in class, discussed course grades or assignments with the instructor, attended professor's office hours, participated in class discussions, tutored other students in their introductory STEM course, reviewed class material before it was covered, attended review or help sessions to enhance understanding of course content, and studied with students from their introductory STEM course" (p. 237). An extensive multivariate analysis "suggested that 3.1 and 4.1% of the variance in academic engagement was attributable to differences across classrooms and institutions, respectively. In other words, classrooms and institutions appear to have a marginal effect on students' academic engagement, and the vast majority of variance we see in academic engagement can be attributed to differences between students" (p. 239).

The qualitative strand used a purposeful, criterion sample of 8 colleges and universities selected from the original 15, based on survey responses and evidence of innovation in teaching practices. The researchers conducted 41 focus groups with students who had completed the quantitative surveys or who were currently enrolled in an introductory STEM course. A constant comparative strategy was used to code and analyze data. In the final step of analysis and interpretation, the researchers combined findings from the quantitative and qualitative strands. Though the statistical analysis yielded no significant connection between student engagement and teaching practice, it did provide evidence about the relationship between student attributes such as excitement about learning, competitiveness, and career orientation on the one hand, and engagement and success in the courses on the other. Interviews with students supported this connection and provided insights that furthered understanding.

The researchers integrated the quantitative and qualitative findings to develop two composite types of STEM instructors: *gatekeeper* and *engaging* professors. Gatekeeper professors "disregard individual learning styles because they are so focused on conveying the abundance of information that must be passed on to students who are worthy of passing through the gates. Their expectation is that students can and should understand the content at a sophisticated level" (p. 252). By contrast, an engaging professor "uses strategies that encourage active learning, cooperation among students, and student–faculty contact. . . . facilitates student excitement in the classroom through humor, enthusiasm, and practical application . . . is highly accessible to students and encourages them to participate in additional learning opportunities offered by the university" (p. 253).

The researchers concluded, "If educators are the key change agents in this dynamic, the findings suggest that introductory STEM course instructors must think just as carefully and thoroughly about how they interact with and come across to students as they do about the course content and how to assess its mastery, especially when it comes to scaling up STEM achievement and increasing student persistence" (p. 256).

EVALUATING MIXED METHODS RESEARCH   MAP 13.3

The evaluation of mixed methods studies builds on the categories and criteria for qualitative and quantitative research, and adds a third consideration: the mixing or interpretation of the methods. Accordingly, there are three steps in evaluating mixed methods studies:

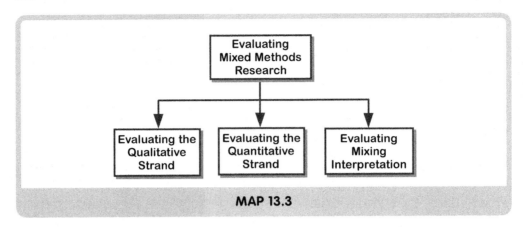

MAP 13.3

1. Evaluating the qualitative strand. The criteria for this strand are trustworthiness and transferability.

2. Evaluating the quantitative strand. The criteria for this strand are theory or framing construct, sample and sampling, and data collection and analysis.

3. Evaluating mixing/interpretation: Is there a clear description of how the data were mixed in the study? Were they mixed at the sampling, data collection, and/or data analysis (interpretation) stage? This step involves an evaluation of two elements:

   • Timing: What was the timeline of the study in terms of the sampling, data collection, and data analysis? Does the article include a timeline that visually depicts the timing of each step?

   • Weight: What was the emphasis on each strand? Did the study emphasize qualitative and quantitative methods equally? Or was there a clearly communicated emphasis on one strand or the other?

The rubric in Figure 13.5 provides the criteria for evaluating mixed methods studies.

Example: Evaluation of the Virtual Worlds Study

Qualitative Strand

   • **Trustworthiness:** The Virtual Worlds study (Feldon & Kefai, 2008) merits a moderate to strong rating for trustworthiness. There is a thorough literature review, together with lengthy descriptions of the researchers' involvement in the study and of the online and offline environments. The study included triangulation of sources of data as well as a team of researchers to check for accuracy. A variety of qualitative data were collected and analyzed, both online and offline, so that users' perspectives were represented well. The article includes little or no discussion of coding and development of themes.

Qualitative strand	Strong	Moderate	Weak
Trustworthiness	Thick description and quotes provided; purposive or theoretical sampling described; explicit triangulation; checks for accuracy; clear procedures for coding and development of themes; sufficient engagement to earn trust.	Some thick description and quotes provided; sampling discussed; triangulation implied; limited checks for accuracy; partial description of procedures for coding and development of themes; sufficient engagement to earn trust.	Limited or no thick description and quotes provided; scant mention of sampling; triangulation not in evidence; no reported checks for accuracy; limited (if any) description of procedures for coding and development of themes; insufficient engagement.
Transferability	Detailed description of context and actors' actions, thoughts, verbatim language from interviews and documents.	Partial description of context and actors' actions, thoughts, verbatim language from interviews and documents.	Limited description of context and actors' actions, thoughts, verbatim language from interviews and documents.

Quantitative strand	Strong	Moderate	Weak
Theory or framing construct	Well-developed literature review that establishes either a theory or a framing construct and includes 10 or more references; strong support for the IV and DV; clear identification of hypothesis or research questions and the DV.	Literature review may not adequately develop a theory or framing construct, or includes fewer than 10 references; research questions implied; adequate support for the IV and DV.	Unclear literature review that does not develop a theory or framing construct; fewer than five references; no research questions evident; inadequate support for the IV and DV.
Sample and sampling	Clear description of the sample characteristics and the population; clear description of sample; evidence of sufficient size (60 or more); random selection of sample or sample matching.	Description of sample is present, but lacking details about characteristics and the population; scant detail about variability of sample; insufficient sample size.	No description of the sample; total lack of details about the population; sample neither randomly selected nor matched.
Data collection and analysis	Clear description of measures selected to collect data on DV and evidence of validity and reliability (r); correct use of tests for DV clear; description of statistical significance (p) and alpha level, as well as of the inferential tests used; researcher stays close to data and does not overconclude; article includes explanatory charts and narratives.	Mention of measurement, but lacking in details about validity and reliability (r); mention of statistical significance (p) without including inferential tests used; researcher avoids overconcluding; article includes explanatory charts and/or narratives.	Minimal or no mention of measurement; no mention of validity or reliability; no mention of significance; researcher may overconclude; article does not include adequate visual or narrative explanations.

(continued)

FIGURE 13.5. Rubric for evaluating mixed methods studies.

Mixing/ Interpretation	Strong	Moderate	Weak
Timing	Clear and well-developed rationale for mixing data; article identifies organization of the design as concurrent or sequential; clear visual representation of the timeline–methods mix (timeline could stand on its own).	Mention of strategies for mixing data, but incomplete description; article may be unclear whether design is concurrent or sequential; unclear or missing visual representation of timeline–methods mix.	No mention of strategies for mixing data; no mention of concurrent or sequential design; missing visual representation of timeline–methods mix.
Weight	Clear and well-organized discussion about the purpose of the study and how it affects the weighting of the data.	Mention of the purpose of the study, but insufficient explanation of how it affects the weighting of the data.	No mention of the purpose or how the purpose affects the weighting of the data.
Overall rating	Strong	Moderate	Weak

FIGURE 13.5. *(continued)*

- **Transferability:** The study's transferability is strong. There are detailed descriptions of the context, both the online and offline environments. Specific quotes from field notes, videotaped interviews, and observations depict the actors' action and thoughts. In addition, the article includes photographs of avatars and the gaming "dashboard" to engage the readers.

Quantitative Strand

- **Theory or Framing Construct:** The Virtual Worlds study merits a moderate rating for theory or framing construct. The study examined online avatar-related activities, but the article provides little discussion about the value of online environments for learning or leisure. Rather, the study appeared to focus more on the use of mixed methods and an effort to address the shortcomings of a quantitative study based on the use of surveys and server data.

- **Sample and Sampling:** The study's sample and sampling are strong. The sample was large enough for a nonexperimental design based on correlations, with 595 children responding to the survey, and a subset of 88 students responding to additional survey questions. Approximately 70 million lines of server log data were analyzed as well.

- **Data Collection and Analysis:** The study's data collection and analysis also merit a strong rating. As mentioned earlier, there was a nonexperimental group comparison analysis of casual, social, and heavy users with server log data, including time spent on activities in a variety of online gaming locations. The 30-item online surveys used for pre- and postactivity analysis are described in detail, and the overall Cronbach's alpha reliability coefficient was .72.

Mixing/Interpretation

- **Timing:** The study earns a moderate rating for timing. The researchers used a framework for the mixing and analysis of data: expansion, triangulation, complementarity, initiation, and development. However, the article includes no explicit timeline or visual representation of the mixed methods.

- **Weight:** The study also earns a moderate rating for weight. From the authors' description of the study, it seems that their intent was to have an equal weighting of qualitative and quantitative data. The purpose of collecting the qualitative data was to provide the researchers with understanding of the gaming culture and the motives of users and their avatars, but it is not made clear how this was enacted.

Example: Evaluation of the STEM Course Study

Qualitative Strand

- **Trustworthiness:** The Gasiewski et al. (2012) study merits a strong rating for trustworthiness. The literature review of approximately 100 references establishes a very good rationale for the study of STEM courses in higher education. The study used a sequential explanatory design with a purposeful sampling strategy. The large volume of focus groups, with 2–10 students per group, provided triangulated data and increased the likelihood of data saturation. The researchers' categories are illustrated by numerous quotes and descriptions; intercoder reliability was established through multiple steps to strengthen the integrity of data.

- **Transferability:** The study's transferability is also strong. Based on the interviews, the authors created composite representations of the professors and students that were not identifiable. The representations were developed with numerous quotes and observations and in-depth descriptions of college classrooms and campuses.

Quantitative Strand

- **Theory or Framing Construct:** The study merits a strong rating for theory or framing construct. The literature review is current and includes approximately 100 references, discussing both the questions about engagement in STEM learning and the use of mixed methods research designs for investigations. The DV was student engagement (including persistence and academic performance in STEM courses); the IVs of interest were quality of teaching and the learning environment (in particular, the items on the behavioral academic inventory). The research questions are clearly stated and match the study's purposes.

- **Sample and Sampling:** The study's sample and sampling are also strong. The sample was large enough for a nonexperimental correlations design, with 15 higher education institutions and 73 classrooms. Although the sample was nonrandom, a total of 3,205 students filled out the surveys; of those, 2,873 students were included in the data analysis.

• **Data Collection and Analysis:** The study likewise earns a strong rating for data collection and analysis. Survey data were collected from both students and college professors. The behavioral academic inventory was developed from an earlier survey on the development of scientific dispositions and collegiate habits of mind. Factor analysis of this survey helped to ensure construct validity, with the identification of multiple factors used as both IVs and DVs. Reliability for survey was established by using Cronbach's alpha; for example, the factor for academic engagement had a Cronbach's alpha of .75. Extensive techniques were used to weight the data and to account for missing data in the hierarchical linear model statistical analysis.

Mixing/Interpretation

• **Timing:** The study earns a strong rating for timing. The design of the study was identified as a sequential explanatory design. The rationale for timing and mixing qualitative and quantitative methods is made very clear in the article and is presented in a visual model (a flow chart of the mixed methods design procedures).

• **Weight:** The study merits a moderate to strong rating for weight. The purpose of the study was to use the qualitative data to explain the quantitative findings, thus separating the study into two major phases. The article makes no mention of the precise weighting of the data, however.

REFLECTIONS ON MIXED METHODS RESEARCH

Mixed methods research is not without its critics. Methodological purists hold that research is either qualitative or quantitative, and that nothing can exist in between. Despite these reservations, most researchers acknowledge mixed methods research as a promising development. The publication of the *Handbook of Mixed Methods in Social and Behavioral Research* (Tashakkori & Teddlie, 2003b) added to its legitimacy, as did the founding of the *Journal of Mixed Methods Research*. Further evidence of its entry into the mainstream is establishment of a special interest group within the American Education Research Association that has the following as its goal: "To support, encourage, and increase dialogue and idea exchange among educational researchers utilizing mixed methods and those interested in integrating qualitative and quantitative research approaches" (see *www.aera.net/SIG158/MixedMethodsResearchSIG158/tabid/12201/Default.aspx*).

However, there are some lingering concerns about mixed methods approaches. They take longer to implement, entail more resources, require separate inductive and deductive analyses, and add a step to articulating qualitative and quantitative results. After interviewing 20 social scientists who had conducted mixed methods studies, Bryman (2007a) concluded that "insufficient attention has been paid to the writing up of mixed methods findings, and in particular to the ways such findings can be integrated. Indeed, it could be argued that there is still considerable uncertainty concerning what it means to integrate findings in mixed methods research" (p. 22).

CHAPTER SUMMARY

MAP 13.4

✓ Mixed methods research combines qualitative and quantitative methods of data collection and analysis.

✓ The two mixed methods designs are concurrent and sequential.

✓ Concurrent mixed methods designs combine or merge quantitative and qualitative data.

✓ Sequential designs expand on the findings of one method with another method.

✓ Mixed methods researchers combine findings in a final interpretation, called *metainferences/integrated mixed inferences*.

✓ Mixed methods research is evaluated according to the criteria for qualitative and quantitative studies and also according to two criteria for mixing/interpretation (i.e., timing and weight).

KEY TERMS AND CONCEPTS

concurrent embedded methods

concurrent designs

concurrent triangulation methods

metainferences/integrated mixed inferences

mixed methods research

multiple-methods research

pragmatism

sequential designs

sequential explanatory methods

sequential exploratory methods

REVIEW, CONSOLIDATION, AND EXTENSION OF KNOWLEDGE

1. Using an electronic database or a search engine, locate a mixed methods study on a topic of interest. Read the article, and then answer the questions below.

   a. What research is reviewed? Does it provide a rationale for the study? Does it provide a rationale for using mixed methods?

   b. What was the purpose of the study?

   c. What design was employed? Concurrent (triangulation or embedded) or sequential (explanatory or exploratory)?

   d. How were the strands weighted?

   e. What were the results of the analysis of each strand?

   f. How were the two analyses integrated? What is the researcher's interpretation?

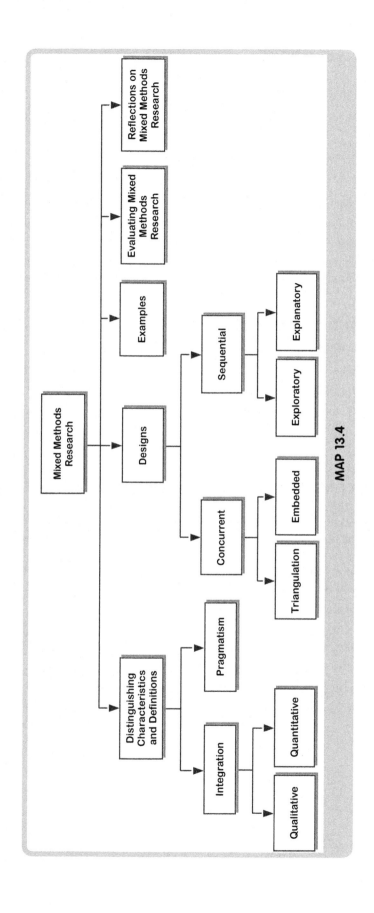

MAP 13.4

256

CHAPTER FOURTEEN

Program Evaluation and Teacher Evaluation

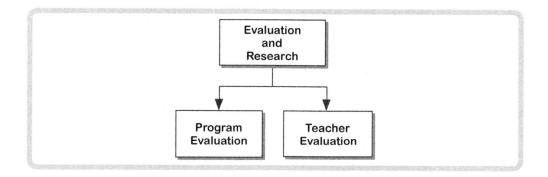

This chapter brings the fields of research and evaluation together. It discusses the commonalities and differences between these two fields, and provides examples of program evaluation and teacher evaluation.

CHAPTER OBJECTIVES

✓ Understand how program evaluation differs from research in the social sciences.

✓ Understand the difference between formative and summative evaluation.

✓ Understand the established standards for program evaluation research.

✓ Understand the policy and purpose of teacher evaluation.

✓ Understand the application of research methods to teacher evaluation.

PROGRAM EVALUATION   MAP 14.1

Distinguishing Characteristics and Definitions   MAP 14.2

Program evaluation, as the term is used in education, gathers evidence in order to monitor the progress or judge the merits of a program or curriculum. It is related to but not the same as *accreditation,* which is a peer assessment of organizations and institutions according to established standards; nor is it the same as a personnel evaluation. Because program evaluation is used in diverse fields and disciplines, it has been characterized as a *transdiscipline* (Scriven, 1991). It has also been labeled *applied research.*

Formative and Summative Evaluation

Formative evaluation (also known as *implementation evaluation* or *process evaluation*) provides evidence about how to improve a program as it is developing.

Summative evaluation (also known as *impact evaluation* or *outcome evaluation*) provides evidence about whether to continue or discontinue a program after it has been in place for a sufficient time to produce results.

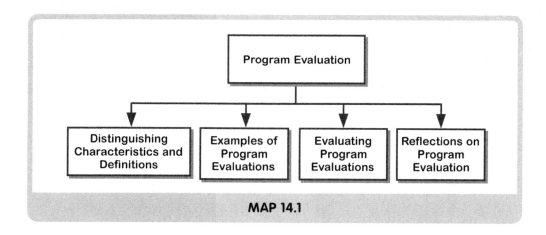

MAP 14.1

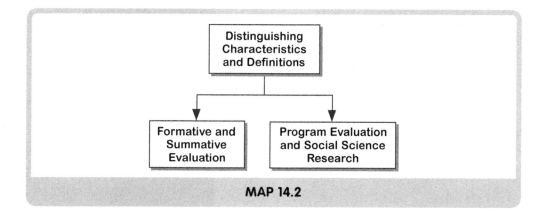

MAP 14.2

In other words, formative evaluation seeks to maximize feedback as a basis for making changes and improvements. It asks questions such as these (Frechtling & Sharp, 1997, pp. 1–2):

- To what extent do the activities and strategies match those described in the plan? If they do not match, are the changes in the activities justified and described?
- To what extent were the activities conducted according to the proposed timeline? By the appropriate personnel?
- To what extent are the actual costs of project implementation in line with initial budget expectations?
- To what extent are the participants moving toward the anticipated goals of the project?
- Which of the activities or strategies are aiding the participants to move toward the goals?
- What barriers were encountered? How and to what extent were they overcome?

On the other hand, summative evaluation measures the effects of a program as objectively as possible and provides information that allows stakeholders to judge program success or failure. Summative evaluations raise questions such as these (Frechtling & Sharp, 1997, pp. 2–3):

- To what extent did the project meet its overall goals?
- Was the project equally effective for all participants?
- What components were the most effective?
- What significant unintended impacts did the project have?
- Is the project replicable and transportable?

Program Evaluation and Social Science Research

Although program evaluation uses the same tools and methods of basic qualitative, quantitative, and mixed methods approaches, it has a very different purpose. It aims to acquire knowledge that can guide decision making and improve practice. It also has a different audience: It is directed to practitioners, stakeholders, and decision makers who use findings to decide on how to improve programs and whether to continue or terminate them. In distinguishing between evaluation and research, Mathison (2008, p. 188) quotes Michael Scriven, a pioneer in the evaluation field, who made the following statement in an interview:

> Evaluation determines the merit, worth, or value of things. The evaluation process identifies relevant values or standards that apply to what is being evaluated, performs empirical investigation using techniques from the social sciences, and then integrates conclusions with the standards into an overall evaluation or set of evaluations.
>
> Social science research, by contrast, does not aim for or achieve evaluative conclusions. It is restricted to empirical (rather than evaluative) research, and bases its conclusions only on factual results—that is, observed, measured, or calculated data. Social science research does not establish standards or values and then integrate them with factual results to reach evaluative conclusions. In fact, the dominant social science doctrine for many decades prided itself on being value free.

However, in deference to social science research, it must be stressed again that without using social science methods, little evaluation can be done. One cannot say, however, that evaluation is the application of social science methods to solve social science problems. It is much more than that.

Examples of Program Evaluation

1. Formative Evaluation

Friday Institute for Educational Innovation. (2009). *Formative evaluation report: North Carolina Virtual Public School.* Raleigh: North Carolina State University.

This evaluation examined the second year of implementation of the North Carolina Virtual Public School (NCVPS). The report states: "The primary purpose of this formative evaluation is to provide data to NCVPS administration to improve their existing courses and services, to design new services where needs warrant, and to promote the school with indicators of success" (p. 9). The Friday Institute's team of evaluators used a survey that combined quantitative and qualitative methods. The quantitative data were in the form of responses to a Likert scale; the qualitative data were in the form of responses to open-ended questions about barriers to implementation and recommendations for improvement. The surveys were administered online to students, teachers, distance learning advisors, and high school principals. The researchers compared the quantitative responses with those on same surveys that had been administered the previous year. Using ANOVA, the researchers found significant improvements in the teachers' reports of student learning; the teachers' own use of digital media; the usefulness of resources to support teaching diverse learners; the rigor of course assignments; and the teachers' use of resources to further their professional development in teaching the 21st-century skills of career and life planning, innovation, and technological literacy. Students also reported significant improvements in the use of 21st-century skills; both teachers' and students' responses showed significant decreases in technical problems. Qualitative responses indicated that teachers and distance learning instructors saw barriers in students' lack of direction and motivation, while students listed barriers that had to do with personal issues and teachers' responsiveness and quality. The report concluded with a series of recommendations about modifying teaching and curriculum (especially in math and world languages), adding to professional development, increasing administrative support, and improving the design of a virtual school.

2. Summative Evaluation

Vahey, P., & Crawford, V. (2002) *PALM Education Pioneers Program: Final evaluation report.* Menlo Park, CA: SRI International.

The PALM Education Pioneers (PEP) study evaluated a project in which teachers used PALM technology as instructional tools in their classrooms. The explicit purpose of the evaluation was to provide an empirical base of information for assisting educators, researchers, and other users of handheld computers in making decisions about choice of technology and implementation. The researchers used a single quantitative method: They administered survey questionnaires to 102 teachers who had been awarded grants to implement PALM technology in their classrooms. After analyzing the survey data, the researchers concluded that teachers across grade levels were positive about using PALM devices, that elementary teachers were more positive than middle and high school teachers, and that teachers deemed the PALM devices most useful in science and writing activities. Teachers also reported that it was important to have peripheral software available to support the program; that personal use of the PALM technology was more effective than shared use; and that benefits to students included increased motivation, collaboration, and communication. Drawbacks included inappropriate student use and equipment dysfunctions. Final recommendations to decision makers included the need to provide appropriate time and training for teachers to learn how to integrate the PALM, purchase additional software, develop appropriate use policies, and put in place logistics for equipment maintenance and efficient use.

Program Evaluation Standards   MAP 14.3

Because evaluation is applied research, it is evaluated for quality according to a different set of criteria. These are based on a set of professional, rather than purely academic, standards. Several organizations (the American Psychological Association, the American Educational Research Association, the National Council on Measurement in Education, and others) have come together as the Joint Committee on Standards for Educational Evaluation to develop a set of professional standards for program evaluation. The first version of these standards was published in 1981; they are now in their third edition (Yarbrough, Shulha, Hopson, & Caruthers, 2011). In the current version, there are a total of 30 standards organized under the categories of utility, feasibility, propriety, accuracy, and accountability.

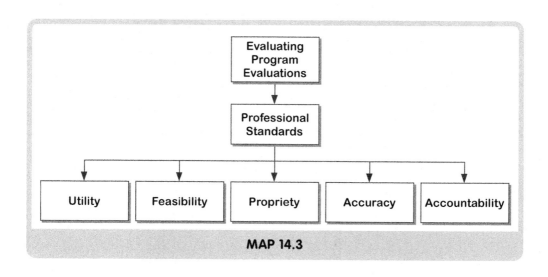

MAP 14.3

Utility Standards

1. Evaluations should be conducted by qualified people who establish and maintain credibility in the evaluation context.
2. Evaluations should devote attention to the full range of individuals and groups invested in the program and affected by its evaluation.
3. Evaluation purposes should be identified and continually negotiated based on the needs of stakeholders.
4. Evaluations should clarify and specify the individual and cultural values underpinning purposes, processes, and judgments.
5. Evaluation information should serve the identified and emergent needs of stakeholders.
6. Evaluations should construct activities, descriptions, and judgments in ways that encourage participants to rediscover, reinterpret, or revise their understandings and behaviors.
7. Evaluations should attend to the continuing information needs of their multiple audiences.
8. Evaluations should promote responsible and adaptive use while guarding against unintended negative consequences and misuse.

Feasibility Standards

1. Evaluations should use effective project management strategies.
2. Evaluation procedures should be practical and responsive to the way the program operates.
3. Evaluations should recognize, monitor, and balance the cultural and political interests and needs of individuals and groups.
4. Evaluations should use resources effectively and efficiently.

Propriety Standards

1. Evaluations should be responsive to stakeholders and their communities.
2. Evaluation agreements should be negotiated to make obligations explicit and take into account the needs, expectations, and cultural contexts of clients and other stakeholders.
3. Evaluations should be designed and conducted to protect human and legal rights and maintain the dignity of participants and other stakeholders.
4. Evaluations should be understandable and fair in addressing stakeholder needs and purposes.
5. Evaluations should provide complete descriptions of findings, limitations, and conclusions to all stakeholders, unless doing so would violate legal and propriety obligations.
6. Evaluations should openly and honestly identify and address real or perceived conflicts of interests that may compromise the evaluation.
7. Evaluations should account for all expended resources and comply with sound fiscal procedures and processes.

Accuracy Standards

1. Evaluation conclusions and decisions should be explicitly justified in the cultures and contexts where they have consequences.
2. Evaluation information should serve the intended purposes and support valid interpretations.
3. Evaluation procedures should yield sufficiently dependable and consistent information for the intended uses.
4. Evaluations should document programs and their contexts with appropriate detail and scope for the evaluation purposes.
5. Evaluations should employ systematic information collection, review, verification, and storage methods.
6. Evaluations should employ technically adequate designs and analyses that are appropriate for the evaluation purposes.
7. Evaluation reasoning leading from information and analyses to findings, interpretations, conclusions, and judgments should be clearly and completely documented.
8. Evaluation communications should have adequate scope and guard against misconceptions, biases, distortions, and errors.

Accountability Standards

1. Evaluations should fully document their negotiated purposes and implemented designs, procedures, data, and outcomes.
2. Evaluators should use these and other applicable standards to examine the accountability of the evaluation design, procedures employed, information collected, and outcomes.
3. Program evaluation sponsors, clients, evaluators, and other stakeholders should encourage the conduct of external metaevaluations using these and other applicable standards.

Reflections on Program Evaluation

There is still debate about whether and to what degree evaluation research qualifies as research. Is evaluation a "profession," as implied above? Or is it better understood as "applied research" because of its usage in the real world of policy and practice? Michael Scriven (2010) has argued that these distinctions are becoming blurred, as more and more social science research is oriented toward solving social problems. He advocates for a shift in evaluation from being viewed as either a "profession" or "applied research" to becoming seen as a discipline.

> While evaluation has been practiced for many years, it is only now developing into a discipline. In this way evaluation resembles technology, which existed for thousands of years before there was any substantive discussion of its nature, its logic, its fundamental differences from science, and the details of its distinctive methods and thought. In recent years we have begun to see more discussions within the field about evaluation-specific methodology. We are moving toward the general acceptance of evaluation as a discipline, but there is still a long way to go. (p. 110)

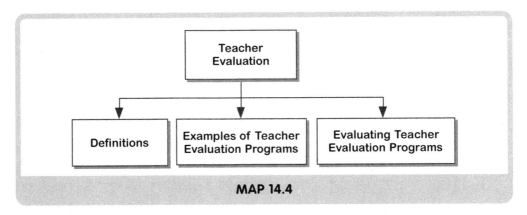

MAP 14.4

TEACHER EVALUATION

MAP 14.4

In the United States, the emphasis on accountability in public education has prompted new policies in the evaluation of both student and teacher performance. Although research on teacher evaluation goes back to the 1980s, since 2011 teacher evaluation has been at the center of policy making for school improvement (Darling-Hammond, 2013; Popham, 2013). Each U.S. state has its own unique policy regarding teacher evaluation, but all of these policies focus on the connections between teachers' classroom practices and student growth. Each state education agency has developed its own model (as in Tennessee or Washington), or has reviewed and approved commercially developed models by Charlotte Danielson, Kim Marshall, or Robert Marzano (as in Maine and New York). Teacher evaluation is part of a general plan for educator evaluation, in which the mandates for teacher evaluation are accompanied by requirements to evaluate principals and superintendents. This chapter presents teacher evaluation in the context of research literacy and alongside program evaluation because it is a practical and complex application of research methods.

Definitions

Teacher evaluation: The process of research design, data collection, and data analysis that includes evidence of student growth, and that results in formative and summative evaluations of teachers' performance.

Administrator evaluation: The process of research design, data collection, and data analysis that includes evidence of teachers' performance, student growth, and community involvement, and that results in formative and summative evaluations of administrators' performance.

Student growth: Changes in student performance based on a variety of data sources and methods of data collection and analysis; the data come primarily from classroom assessments and large-scale standardized assessments.

Teacher evaluation model: A framework or design to organize the timeline, data sources, and decisions for teacher evaluation; it is designed either by a state's department of education or by a professional consultant like Danielson, Marzano, or Marshall.

Examples of Teacher Evaluation Programs

This section presents summaries of two teacher evaluation programs, one from Arizona and the other from Maine. The Arizona program is called Teacher/Principal Evaluation, and the name of the Maine program is Educator Effectiveness. The ultimate purpose of teacher evaluation is the improvement of classroom practice and the growth in student learning. Both the Arizona and Maine programs rely on multiple measures, and individual school districts or local education agencies are responsible for the implementation of the programs and must make the choices for precise levels of each method of data collection to fit their design.

In Maine, the Educator Effectiveness program is spelled out in the Performance Evaluation and Professional Growth (PEPG) systems (Maine Department of Education, n.d.; see *http://maine.gov/doe/effectiveness/index.html*). The key components of the PEPG systems are (1) standards of professional practice; (2) multiple measures, including professional practice and student growth data; (3) a 4-point rating scale of educator effectiveness, with professional development opportunities and employment consequences for each level; and (4) a process for using this information to make decisions. The primary sources of data are classroom observations, surveys of students and parents, evidence of student work in classroom assessment, school/district common assessments, and state standardized assessments. In Maine, student growth may account for up to 20% of the total rating score for teacher effectiveness. The largest proportion of data comes from the evaluation of professional practice, and in Maine school districts may select from a variety of professional/commercial teacher effectiveness models: (1) the model of the National Board for Professional Teaching Standards, (2) Danielson's Framework for Teaching, (3) Marzano's Teacher Evaluation Model, or (4) Marshall's Teacher Evaluation Rubrics.

The Teacher/Principal Evaluation program in Arizona uses the following data sources: (1) student growth on classroom assessments (33–50%), (2) surveys of parents or students (17%), and (3) teaching performance and professional practice measures (50%) (Arizona Department of Education, 2014; see *www.azed.gov/teacherprincipal-evaluation*). Student growth is to be measured by a mix of classroom assessments, school/district common assessments, and state standardized tests. In Arizona, student growth is to be measured by standardized tests using a value-added measurement approach to account for at least 20% of the student growth. A timeline for data collection, and a rubric for judging and interpreting data, are laid out in specific terms.

Evaluating Teacher Evaluation Programs   MAP 14.5

The examples of teacher evaluation programs given above use mixed methods research designs, since they contain a mix of qualitative and quantitative data. The teacher evaluation programs must contain evidence of teacher practice as documented

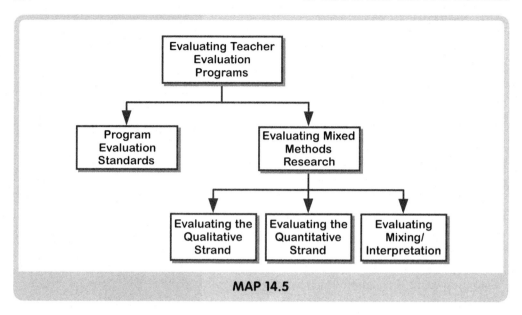

MAP 14.5

by classroom observation and teacher reflection, as well as student growth data, test scores or other assessments, and surveys of students' and parents' dispositions.

As we've noted, program evaluation has an established set of standards for evaluating quality: (1) utility, (2) feasibility, (3) accuracy, (4) propriety, and (5) accountability. In addition to these standards, evaluations of teacher evaluation programs should include the criteria for evaluating mixed methods research, as discussed in Chapter Thirteen. To review briefly, the criteria for evaluating specific mixed methods studies include the following:

1. Qualitative strand
   a. Trustworthiness
   b. Transferability
2. Quantitative strand
   a. Theory or framing construct
   b. Sample and sampling
   c. Data collection and analysis
3. Mixing/interpretation
   a. Weight
   b. Timing

A full discussion of evaluating teacher evaluation programs is beyond the scope of this book, but here are some suggestions based on our comparison of the program evaluation standards with our criteria for evaluating mixed methods studies. There is good alignment with accuracy (clear approaches to data collection, analysis, and storage); propriety (responsive, transparent, and ethical evaluation processes); and accountability (full documentation of and critical reflection on the process and products). The purpose of the present textbook is to educate researchers, which also addresses utility (available resources and qualified, trained evaluators).

CHAPTER SUMMARY

MAP 14.6

✓ Program evaluation gathers evidence in order to report on the progress or merits of a program to improve or make judgments about program or curriculum success.

✓ There are two types of program evaluation: formative and summative.

✓ Formative evaluation provides feedback on implementation.

✓ Summative evaluation makes judgments about value.

✓ Program evaluation is evaluated for quality according to professional standards of utility, feasibility, propriety, accuracy, and accountability.

✓ Teacher evaluation represents a policy in the United States adopted by individual states to improve teaching practice and student learning.

✓ Educator evaluation is the broad policy that includes teacher evaluation and administrator evaluation.

✓ Teacher evaluation is a specific example of program evaluation prescribed by most states to include multiple methods of evaluation—classroom observations, surveys of perceptions, and student growth scores (both classroom scores and standardized test scores).

✓ Teacher evaluation designs are mixed methods designs.

✓ The criteria for evaluating mixed methods designs inform teacher evaluation.

✓ The criteria for evaluating mixed methods designs align with the program evaluation standards, which can be used to provide more specificity.

KEY TERMS AND CONCEPTS

accountability standards

accreditation

accuracy standards

feasibility standards

formative evaluation

program evaluation

propriety standards

summative evaluation

teacher evaluation

utility standards

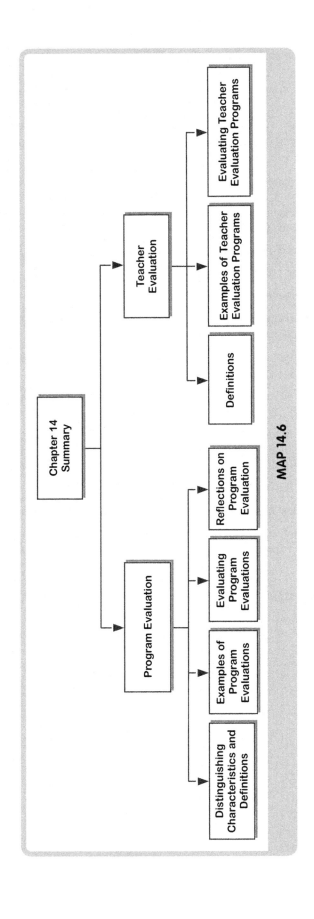

MAP 14.6

REVIEW, CONSOLIDATION, AND EXTENSION OF KNOWLEDGE

1. Using an electronic database or a search engine, locate a program evaluation study on a topic of interest. Read the article and answer the questions below.

    a. What is the purpose of the evaluation?

    b. What kind of evaluation is it: formative or summative?

    c. Who commissioned the evaluation? Who conducted the evaluation?

    d. What methods of data collection were used?

    e. How were data analyzed?

    f. How would you rate the evaluation (strong, moderate, weak) in relation to the standards?

    > Utility:
    >
    > Feasibility:
    >
    > Propriety:
    >
    > Accuracy:
    >
    > Accountability:

2. What are the similarities between program evaluation and teacher evaluation?

3. What are the similarities and differences between the program evaluation standards and the criteria for evaluating the quality of mixed methods studies?

CHAPTER FIFTEEN

Practitioner Research

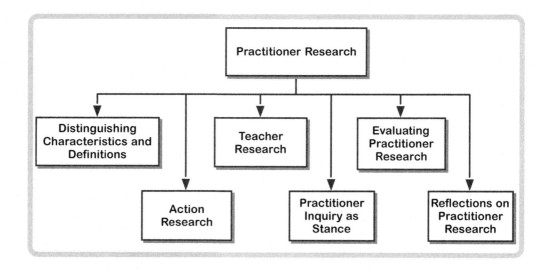

Practitioner research has gained respect as an approach that is geared to both describing and improving practice.

CHAPTER OBJECTIVES

✓ Understand how practitioner research differs from professional academic research.

✓ Understand the roots of practitioner research and current iterations.

✓ Understand the three types of practitioner research.

✓ Understand the steps in the action research spiral.

✓ Understand how teacher research was defined by Cochran-Smith and Lytle.

✓ Understand the Cochran-Smith and Lytle typology of teacher research.

✓ Understand how inquiry as stance is different from teacher research.

✓ Understand the meaning of inquiry as stance and its goals.

DISTINGUISHING CHARACTERISTICS AND DEFINITIONS   MAP 15.1

Research Perspective

Practitioner research focuses on issues that arise in professional practice and is designed and implemented by the people who are most likely to use knowledge for the benefits of their students.

Practitioner research traces its roots to the work of Kurt Lewin (1946), a psychologist and social reformer who stated, "Research that produces nothing but books will not suffice" (p. 35). Many researchers have adapted Lewin's central idea under a variety of descriptors, such as *action science* (Argyris, Putnam, & Smith, 1985), *participatory research* (Freire, 1970), and *collaborative practitioner research* (Heron, 1996). Since its introduction, the idea of practitioner research has gained recognition and legitimacy. It is published nationally and internationally and has generated its own peer-reviewed journals, such as *Action Research, Educational Action Research, Journal of Invitational Theory and Practice*, and *Networks: An On-line Journal for Teacher Research*. The nation's premier professional education research organization, the American Educational Research Association, has recently established an Action Research Special Interest Group.

Practitioner research invests in practitioners the authority usually reserved for professional researchers to identify a problem or question, to decide on methods of data collection, and to analyze and interpret results. Privileging collaboration over individual authorship and craft knowledge over abstract theory, practitioner research has a twofold purpose: (1) to deepen understandings of practice and (2) to promote actions that lead to change, improvement, and (in some cases) social transformation.

Comparison to Professional Research

Proponents of practitioner research offer it an alternative to professional research, which they view as being externally driven, motivated by institutional and professional interests, and "being in the hands of a 'monopoly' of expert knowledge

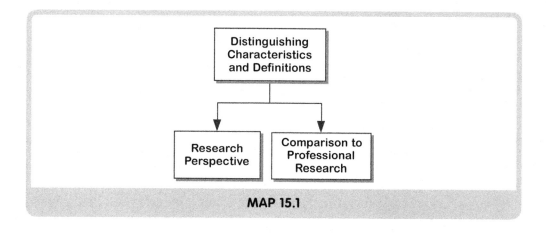

MAP 15.1

TABLE 15.1. Practitioner and Professional Research Compared	
Professional research	**Practitioner research**
Is conducted by professionals who are located in universities and other research centers.	Is conducted by practitioners in their own settings.
Generates research questions from the academic disciplines or the literature in a field.	Generates research questions from the realities of practice.
Views professional researchers as the legitimate producers of knowledge and practitioners as consumers of knowledge.	Views practitioners as legitimate producers as well as consumers of knowledge.
Findings are useful to other professional researchers and policy makers.	Findings are useful to practitioners and may become part of a social movement for school transformation.
Depends on traditional data collection and rules of evidence.	Depends on both traditional and innovative data collection and rules of evidence.

producers, who exercise power over others through their expertise" (Gaventa & Cornwall, 2006, p. 123). Table 15.1 highlights some of the differences between professional and practitioner research.

In order to navigate the wide landscape of practitioner research, this chapter focuses on three current approaches: *action research*, *teacher research*, and *inquiry as practice*.

ACTION RESEARCH   MAP 15.2

Premises and Purposes

> *Action research* is "comparative research on the conditions and effects of various forms of social action and research leading to social action" (Lewin, 1946, p. 35).

Kurt Lewin's definition of action research continues to serve as the prototype of a genre of practitioner research that is oriented toward problem solving and improvement. It utilizes a six-step process called the *action research spiral*, which is represented in Figure 15.1 and described next.

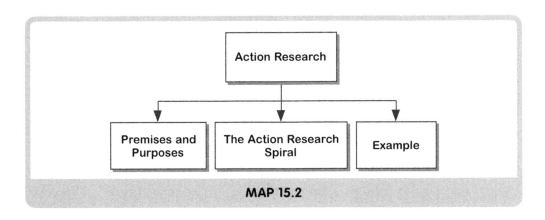

MAP 15.2

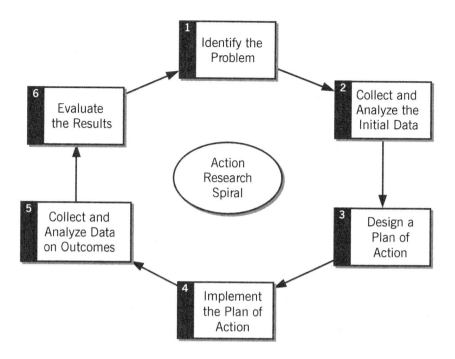

FIGURE 15.1. The action research spiral.

1. *Identify the problem.* The first step is for the action researcher to identify a problem that is important personally and professionally, is of interest to other practitioners, and needs to be solved in order to improve practice and educational outcomes.

2. *Collect initial data.* The next task is to collect and analyze baseline data that are directly related to the problem and that can be compared to data collected after the intervention or action (see Step 5, below). Data may be qualitative, in the form of interviews, documents, or observations; or data may be quantitative in the form of surveys and tests; or data may represent a combination of the two methods.

3. *Design a plan of action.* In designing a plan of action, the researcher has to choose an intervention that has some likelihood of solving the problem. There are basically two sources for this information: research reviews of promising practices and consultation with colleagues. In action research, both sources are considered legitimate and of value. This is in keeping with the view expressed by Corey (1953) that "the consequences of our own teaching is more likely to change and improve our practices than is reading about what someone else has discovered of his teaching" (p. 70).

4. *Implement the plan of action.* The researcher carefully implements the action or intervention and documents the process.

5. *Collect and analyze data on outcomes.* The researcher collects and analyzes the data on outcomes of the implemented action. In analyzing qualitative data, the

researcher codes the data and develops themes that are grounded in the data. For quantitative data, the researcher calculates and displays data in visual form.

6. *Evaluate the results.* The last stage of the research process involves the researcher in reflecting on the project and evaluating whether it has met its goals. This sometimes involves sharing the results with others.

Example of Action Research

Don Chouinard, an English teacher in a rural high school, conducted an action research project that focused on changing the reading achievement and attitudes of the male students in his classes (Chouinard, 2011). He defined the problem as "How can I improve the reading attitudes achievement of my ninth-grade male students?" (p. 1) and conducted his project in four of his ninth-grade classes. In reviewing achievement data from the early fall, he found that males scored lower than females on all standardized tests of reading. Results of a Google survey about attitudes toward reading for pleasure indicated that 88% of females reported they "loved or liked" to read, as opposed to only 18% of males. In devising an intervention and an action plan, Chouinard reviewed literature to help clarify his intentions. He decided on this course of action: (1) developing a reading loft, a comfortable reading space stocked entirely with donations from community members; (2) compiling a "Guy List" of approximately 200 male-friendly novels; and (3) providing alternative assessments on book tests to those students who failed the first assessment.

The plan was implemented in January, when the reading loft was open for use. Furnished with a carpeted floor, three recliners, a rocking chair, a beanbag chair, a sofa, and several large throw pillows, it ultimately housed over 500 donated high-interest books. The "Guy List" was compiled and consisted of over 200 male-friendly novels. Alternative assessments, which included students' writing "novel responses" and having oral conferences with Chouinard about the books they read, were also put in place. Data collection and analysis depended on a Yin mixed methods case study of three purposefully selected male students. Chouinard used qualitative interview and observation methods, and gathered quantitative data from achievement tests administered periodically (Northwest Evaluation Association assessments). His analysis showed that while standardized test scores remained unchanged for two of the three students, the student who was weakest in reading showed progress. Book test scores and observed engagement in reading improved for all three students. Most important for Chouinard, there was a noted improvement in attitudes toward reading. Students attributed the change in attitudes to the "Guy List" and the reading loft.

Chouinard (2011) concluded that the actions he took produced the results he had desired. He noted, "Although the loft has taken longer to create than I anticipated, once operating, it was a much more effective tool in promoting literacy and positive attitudes toward reading than I had originally imagined" (p. 12). As a result of sharing his project with colleagues, the reading loft, the "Guy List," and alternative forms of assessment were regularized as features of language arts instruction in the school.

TEACHER RESEARCH

MAP 15.3

Premises and Purposes

Teacher research is "systematic and intentional inquiry carried out by teachers" (Cochran-Smith & Lytle, 1993, p. 7) that leads to deeper knowledge of teaching and learning.

Since 1987, Marilyn Cochran-Smith and Susan Lytle have been the major voices for teacher research. As they explained,

> Neither interpretive nor process–product classroom research has foregrounded the teacher's role in the generation of knowledge about teaching. What is missing from the knowledge base for teaching, therefore, are the voices of the teachers themselves, the questions teachers ask, the ways teachers use writing and intentional talk in their work lives, and the interpretive frames teachers use to understand and improve their own classroom practices. (1990, p. 2)

Like Lewin, Cochran-Smith and Lytle challenged the long-held views of what research entails and who should be doing it, and they provided guidelines for doing the work. They also proposed a typology of teacher research, which is presented in Table 15.2.

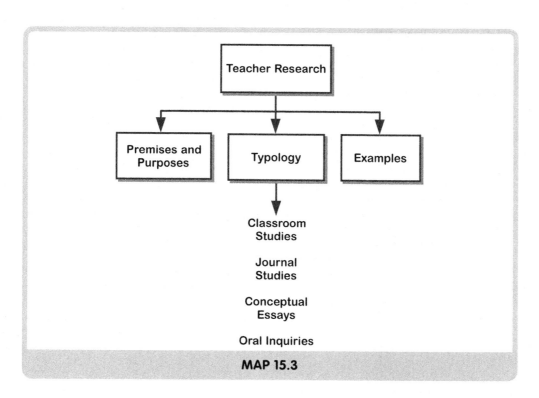

MAP 15.3

TABLE 15.2. The Cochran-Smith and Lytle Typology of Teacher Research

Type	Purpose	Method
Classroom/school studies	To study one's own practice and share understandings with colleagues.	Established qualitative and quantitative methods of data collection and analysis.
Journal studies	To illuminate one's practice, examine and reconstruct understandings, clarify questions, and seek answers.	Written records that capture personal experiences and reflections as they occur.
Conceptual essays	To explore big issues or answer broad questions and reach a wide audience.	Reflective essays intended for dissemination to an audience of teacher researchers.
Oral inquiries	To explore issues of teaching and learning through structured and protocol-based dialogue with colleagues.	Reflective conversations, descriptions of children's work, staff reviews of children.

Examples of Teacher Research

These three examples of teacher research are drawn from contributions to Cochran-Smith and Lytle's (1993) book.

1. Penny Starr, a teacher of deaf students, conducted a classroom study. She wanted to understand how deaf children transfer what they compose in the visual language of American Sign Language to the language of written English. She focused on one student in her classroom and observed his development as a writer over 2 years, making notes on his adaptations and changes. She came to view the process of writing for deaf children as being a form of second-language acquisition; the result of her inquiry was a firmer understanding of how "valuing a native language in all its aspects encourages deaf learners to take risks in acquiring a second language"(Starr, 1993, p. 193).

2. Lynne Yermanock Strieb, an elementary teacher in an urban school, engaged in a journal study and identified two audiences for her inquiry. She saw herself as her first audience; she used her journals to help with her teaching and to provide a way to record and reflect on how she planned, how she looked at students, how she thought about her curriculum, and how she might think and act differently. Her journals were spaces in which she could raise questions and seek answers, identify problems, and seek solutions (Strieb, 1993). Her second audience was the group of teachers who participated with her in the Philadelphia Writing Project, a long-established teacher research community. There Strieb joined with Deborah Jumpp to develop a collaborative research project about journaling. Both Jumpp and Strieb had been using individual journals in their classes when they decided to join forces. Their collaboration led to seeing their own practices differently, raising new questions to explore, and uncovering new ways to share perceptions. They also discovered how they used the journals as curriculum, "to help students learn about their own learning and to help them learn about journals as a versatile genre" (Jumpp & Strieb, 1993, p. 146).

Finally, they found that they used their journals as tools for assessing student interests and progress.

3. Robert Fecho, a high school English teacher, and Samona Joe, a sixth-grade teacher of math and science, published conceptual research essays. Both were active members of the Philadelphia Writing Project, the local teacher research and writing community mentioned in regard to Strieb's study. Fecho (1993) wrote a conceptual piece about what it means to read as a teacher. He argued that "teachers constitute a distinctive interpretive community—particularly as it related to the reading of educational research and theory—that has clear values and standards that dominate the ways teachers ultimately interpret readings" (p. 266). Joe's (1993) essay raised questions about how issues of gender, race, and class played out in her teaching and her students' learning.

PRACTITIONER INQUIRY AS STANCE   MAP 15.4

Premises and Purposes

> *Inquiry as stance* is "a continual process of making current arrangements problematic; questioning the ways knowledge and practice are constructed, evaluated, and used; and assuming that part of the work of practitioners individually and collectively is to participate in educational and social change" (Cochran-Smith & Lytle, 2009, p. 121).

Sixteen years after the publication of their 1993 book, Cochran–Smith and Lytle (2009) revisited their ideas in a book whose title, *Inquiry as Stance: Practitioner Research for the Next Generation*, signaled two important shifts in their thinking. In selecting the term *practitioner research*, they extended their original method to a broader community of educators to include administrators, university teachers, parents, community-based educators, and social activists, as well as preschool and kindergarten teachers. They described this new approach as "a continual process of making current arrangements problematic: questioning the ways knowledge and practice are constructed are constructed, evaluated, and used" (p. 121). Their intention was

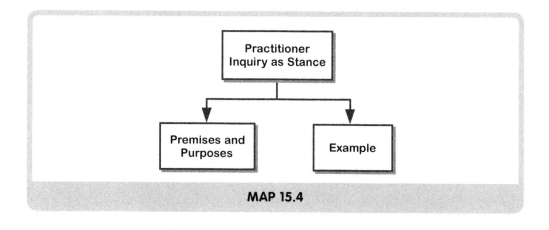

MAP 15.4

to respond to what they saw as the "trying times" (p. 5) that educators were facing on both national and local stages—times in which generic, "expert" knowledge was valued, and the contextualized and craft knowledge of practitioners was devalued. And they issued "a call for practitioner researchers in local settings across the country and the world to ally their work with others as part of larger social and intellectual movements for social change" (p. viii).

The process of inquiry as stance thus both embraces and expands upon the goals of action and teacher research. Like teacher research, it seeks to examine practice with the aim of increasing knowledge and insight. Like action research, it is problem oriented and explicitly promotes an agenda of social improvement. It expands on these other forms by looking to critical theories of race, gender, and class as organizing concepts in developing strategies for transforming educational arrangements toward norms of democratic practice and social justice.

Example of Inquiry as Stance

Gary McPhail (2009), a teacher in the primary grades, focused his inquiry on the interplay of gender and writing. Having used the Writer's Workshop approach for over 10 years as a teacher of first graders, he came to the reluctant conclusion that

> this writing instructional model biases certain literary interests over others. Many of the genres and styles to which many boys gravitate (e.g., comic books, adventure stories, silly fictitious stories, sports pages) are considered low status by many teachers (and parents) and are not welcome in many classrooms during writing time because they are either "inappropriate" for school or deemed not worthy of instructional time. . . . Thus many boys come to realize that their interests are not worthy of being taught in the classroom and as a result come to view writing as more of a female activity than male. (p. 91)

McPhail decided to create a new Writer's Workshop curriculum that included some units especially appealing to boys and others especially appealing to girls. He titled his inquiry "Teaching the 'Bad Boy' to Write," and focused on the development of David—who, like boys in many primary classrooms, pushed boundaries and sought attention in inappropriate ways, and was also reluctant to write about personal issues.

McPhail quoted extensively from his research journal as he described the changes in David's writing over the course of the school year. As the curriculum shifted from personal narratives to letter writing and units on comic books and fiction that engaged David's interests, his writing became more expressive and less violent. His behavior changed as well; his abandonment of the "bad boy" stance became most evident in the anti-war poem that David wrote at the end of the year. McPhail (2009) noted:

> By writing this happy anti-war poem, David allowed himself to be vulnerable, and showed his classmates that he was kind and that he wanted to change his reputation as resident bad boy. This social transformation took time, but by the end of the year, when our poetry unit took place, David managed to break out of his emotional straight jacket and abandon the boy code.

It is important to note that if the writing curriculum had not been able to connect with David's interest in violence, he would not have been able to write about his interest freely, which contributed to his desire to change his social reputation. By being more inviting, the writing curriculum helped David rebel less against the classroom culture and become more interested in Writer's Workshop. (p. 102)

McPhail concluded his piece by looking at the broader social implications of his inquiry: He urged a rethinking of the writing curriculum for boys by "diffusing the personal from the curriculum" (2009, p. 102) and attending to their tastes and interests.

EVALUATING PRACTITIONER RESEARCH   MAP 15.5

Because practitioner research challenges many of the assumptions of professional academic research, it is not appropriate to apply those criteria in evaluating practitioner inquiries. We recommend that an evaluation of a practitioner study be based on the trustworthiness and usefulness of the work, and on how the following questions are answered.

- Is the issue, problem, or concern clearly defined?
- Is the purpose of the inquiry and its audience made clear?
- Are practitioners the chief researchers?
- How are results used?
- Do the findings make a contribution to practitioner knowledge and practice?

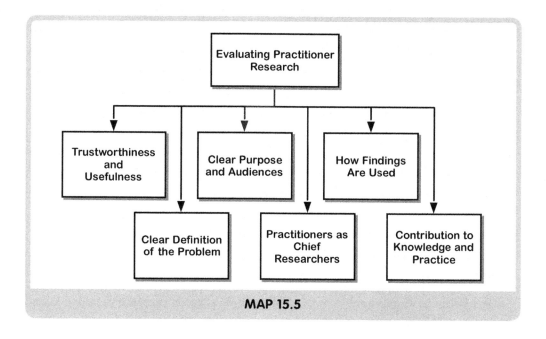

MAP 15.5

REFLECTIONS ON PRACTITIONER RESEARCH

Critics of practitioner research question its validity because it does not meet the established standards or ethics of university-based research in terms of (1) the importance of the research questions, (2) the sufficiency of evidence to draw conclusions, and (3) the ability of researchers to be objective in studying their own practice. At the root of these criticisms are the questions of what, in fact, constitutes knowledge and who is capable of producing it.

There is also apprehension among practitioner researchers themselves about possible misuses of the method. They are concerned that, too often, school administrators who are under pressure to show improvement in student achievement appropriate practitioner research to have teachers collect data for the externally driven agenda of raising test scores. In addition, there are concerns that practitioner research tends to be conflated with professional development and is viewed as yet another staff development strategy.

CHAPTER SUMMARY   MAP 15.6

✓ Practitioner research has its roots in the work of Kurt Lewin and has been adapted and modified by various theorists.

✓ Practitioner research challenges academic research in terms of who has the authority to identify questions and conduct inquiry; the audience for the research and the uses of findings; and methods of data collection and rules of evidence.

✓ Practitioner research may be oriented toward solving problems of practice, developing deeper understanding of teaching and learning, and/or transforming educational arrangements in support of equity and social justice.

✓ Action research solves identifying and solving context-specific problems of practice and uses as a template Lewin's spiral of six steps: (1) problem identification, (2) initial data collection and analysis, (3) designing a plan of action, (4) implementing the plan of action, (5) collecting data on outcomes of the plan, and (6) evaluating results.

✓ Cochran-Smith and Lytle (1993, p. 7) defined teacher research as an approach that develops understanding and insight through "systematic and intentional inquiry carried out by teachers."

✓ Cochran-Smith and Lytle developed a typology of four approaches: classroom and school studies, journal studies, conceptual essays, and oral inquiries.

✓ Cochran-Smith and Lytle (2009) refined their earlier ideas and replaced teacher research with the notion of practitioner inquiry as stance—extending the community of researchers to include all educators, and expanding the purpose of inquiry to include the transformation of education in support of equity and social justice.

✓ Practitioner research is evaluated on criteria of trustworthiness and usefulness, plus clear definition of the problem, clear purpose and audience, practitioners as chief researchers, how results are used, and contribution to knowledge and practice.

✓ Despite its academic critics and internal sources of apprehension, practitioner research has gained legitimacy as a research approach that is acknowledged in peer-reviewed journals and in research organizations and conferences.

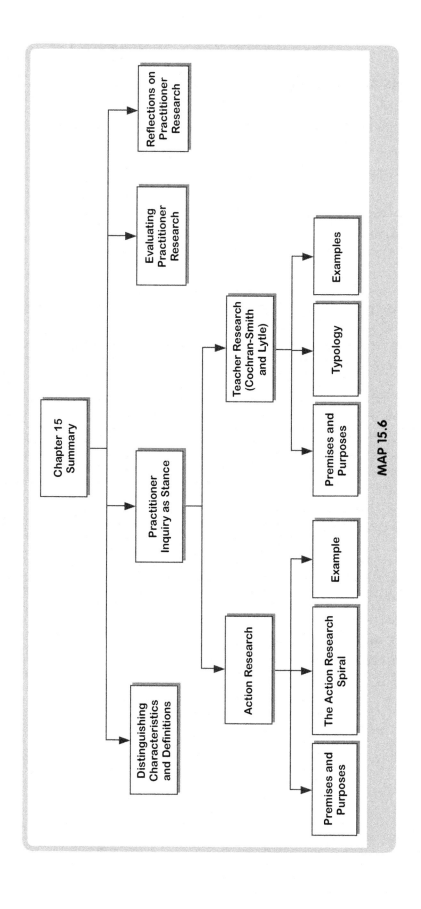

MAP 15.6

Chapter 15 Summary

- Distinguishing Characteristics and Definitions
- Practitioner Inquiry as Stance
  - Action Research
    - Premises and Purposes
    - The Action Research Spiral
    - Example
  - Teacher Research (Cochran-Smith and Lytle)
    - Premises and Purposes
    - Typology
    - Examples
- Evaluating Practitioner Research
- Reflections on Practitioner Research

281

KEY TERMS AND CONCEPTS

action research

action research spiral

classroom and school studies

conceptual research essays

descriptions of children's work

descriptive review of the child

inquiry as stance

journal studies

oral inquiries

orientation toward problem solving

orientation toward transformation

orientation toward understanding

practitioner research

reflective conversations

teacher research

teacher research typology

REVIEW, CONSOLIDATION, AND EXTENSION OF KNOWLEDGE

1. The practitioner research focus for both Chouinard (2011) and McPhail (2009) was the "boy problem" in literacy. They used different methods to conduct their inquiries. Compare the action research approach of Chouinard to the inquiry-as-stance approach of McPhail. What is similar? What is different?

2. Choose a problem of practice that you want to solve in an action research project, and either complete Steps 1–3 of the action research spiral, or complete all six steps.

3. Either independently or in collaboration with a colleague, choose one or more of the approaches from the Cochran-Smith and Lytle (1993) teacher research typology to explore.

4. Using an electronic database, search for a practitioner research (action or teacher research) study on a topic of interest. Read the article and comment on the following:

   • Its purpose.
   • Its methods.
   • Its findings.
   • Its usefulness to you as a practitioner.
   • Is it research or staff development?

PART VII
Research
Reviews

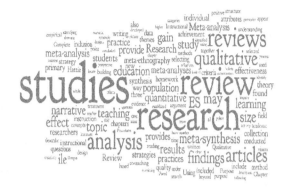

"Knowledge comes by taking things apart: analysis.
But wisdom comes by putting things together."
                    —JOHN A. MORRISON

Part VII demonstrated how researchers move from analysis
to synthesis to gain a wider perspective on a given topic by
reviewing and critiquing research in the area of interest.

CHAPTER SIXTEEN

Professional Research Reviews

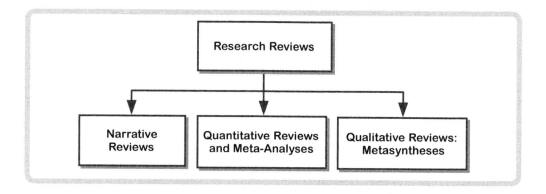

In previous chapters, the focus has been on reading and critiquing individual, primary, empirical studies that appear in peer-reviewed journals. Such studies provide direct access to the evidence-based results of an investigation. However, when taken one at a time, they may become an overwhelming pile of individual bits of information that beg for order and coherence. A research review provides that order and coherence.

A *research review* is a written summary of research on a particular topic or question.

A research review presents the big picture in a field of inquiry, points to promising practices, and provides the rationale for future research. High-quality reviews go far beyond opinion pieces, commentaries, articles, and books that purport to summarize research, but that make little or no reference to the primary research articles on which the summary is based. This chapter provides descriptions and examples of three types of reviews: (1) narrative reviews, (2) quantitative meta-analyses, and (3) qualitative metasyntheses/metaethnographies.

NARRATIVE REVIEWS   MAP 16.1

Purpose and Designs

A *narrative review* "summarizes different primary studies from which conclusions may be drawn into a holistic interpretation contributed by the reviewers' own experience, existing theories and models" (Narrative Review Literature, 2014).

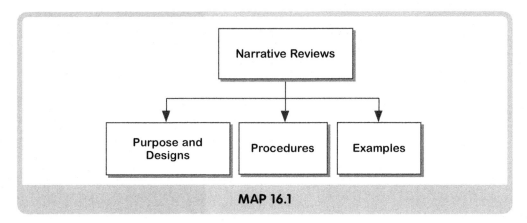

MAP 16.1

A narrative review, which is also referred to as a *traditional review* (Light & Pillemer, 1982), provides an author's written perspective on selected studies in a particular field.

- Short narrative reviews appear in the sections of research articles usually titled "Review of the Literature," where they set the stage for the research that follows and provide the rationale and framework for qualitative studies and the theory to support hypotheses in quantitative studies.

- Long narrative reviews appear as chapters in dissertations and theses and as articles in peer-reviewed journals. For example, the American Educational Research Association regularly publishes books as well as a quarterly journal (the *Review of Educational Research*) devoted to long research reviews. A relatively new European journal, *Educational Research Review,* is another source for high-quality reviews.

Procedures

There are accepted procedures for completing a narrative review. The journal *Educational Research Review* provides the following guidelines to authors, which can also serve as a rubric for readers.

- A clear description of the research problem, the strategy for the review, and the significance of the study.
- An explicit explanation of the criteria and procedures for selecting studies.
- Accessible writing that adheres to a coherent, organized, and logical structure.
- A full research review that includes for each study its aims and theoretical foundations, research question, sample, design, methods of data collection and analysis, and results; this last includes significance values for quantitative studies and a description of how themes were derived for qualitative studies.
- A synthesis that identifies commonalities and themes as well as inconsistencies and tensions across the studies, develops explanatory theories, and makes recommendations for further study.

Examples

- Goldrick-Rab (2010) completed a narrative review of the success of community college students by examining academic and policy research that looked at "the macro-level opportunity structure; institutional practices; and the social, economic, and academic attributes students bring to college" (p. 437).

- Cavagnetto (2010) examined 54 studies having to do with the research on the use of argumentation to improve scientific inquiry, in order "to determine structural patterns of the various argument interventions: (a) the nature of the argument activity, (b) the emphasis of the argument activity and (c) the aspects of science included in the argument activity" (p. 336).

- Andiliou and Murphy (2010) looked at the literature on teacher creativity and developed a framework "for sustained programs of research regarding beliefs about creativity and their role in educational practice," including investigations of teacher beliefs about creativity and intelligence (p. 218).

QUANTITATIVE REVIEWS: META-ANALYSES   MAP 16.2

Purpose and Designs

Quantitative reviews are based on the calculation and manipulation of collective data; these reviews are most often labeled as meta-analyses.

Meta-analysis is "the statistical analysis of a large collection of analysis results for the purpose of integrating the findings" (Glass, 1976, p. 3).

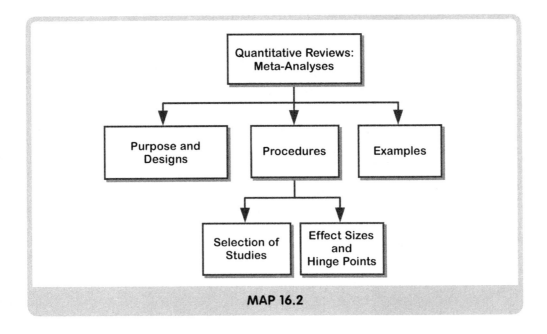

MAP 16.2

Meta-analysis is an efficient way to obtain an estimate of the overall effects of an intervention or treatment strategy (Glass, McGaw, & Smith, 1981) on outcomes. A treatment strategy may be an instructional method, an experimental condition, a curriculum, or a program. Meta-analysis has grown as a method of review research since its inception in the 1970s, as evidenced in the publication of the second edition of *The Handbook of Research Synthesis and Meta-Analysis* (Cooper, Hedges, & Valentine, 2009). Meta-analysis makes important contributions to education research by identifying primary research studies and organizing them so that they can be read and reviewed by outside readers. However, meta-analysis is not a "silver bullet" (Hattie, 2009) that can deliver the answer to everyone's questions about effectiveness. Critics may voice concerns about the diversity of study designs that are included in a meta-analysis and their inconsistencies in quality; the danger of overgeneralizing; and the subjectivity involved in selecting studies for inclusion. Nevertheless, meta-analysis has become a research methodology in its own right and is an important addition to the repertoire of research methodologies.

Procedures

Meta-analysis applies to research summaries the same level of rigor that is used in experiments. Researchers must first identify and define the theory or treatment that drives the analysis. The next step is perhaps the most essential: selecting the studies to include in the analysis. A meta-analysis can only include explanatory studies that have outcome variables, control and treatment groups, and sufficient statistical information (such as means, standard deviations, adequate sample sizes, and t- or F-values). Because the number of published studies that qualify for inclusion may be limited, meta-analysis researchers must often hunt for so-called "grey" or "fugitive" studies (Rothstein & Hopewell, 2009)—that is, studies that have not been published. These may include dissertations and conference papers. Fugitive studies serve to expand the range of articles for inclusion and to ensure that nonsignificant results are included. This last precaution protects against the bias of publications that tend to include only positive findings. Authors of meta-analyses spend considerable time describing their process of searching for articles in detail, so that others can replicate and validate the results. Once a group of qualifying studies, called the *population*, is selected for a meta-analysis, the researchers will use a computer program to calculate results.

Meta-analysis uses the *effect size* statistic, which, as you will remember from Chapter Eight, is a quantitative estimate of the impact of treatments on outcomes. After completing an extensive study of meta-analyses in education, Hattie (2009) concluded that the average effect size for educational innovations was $d = 0.4$. As a result, he recommended that $d = 0.4$ serve as the *hinge point* marking the *zone of desired effects*. (See Figure 16.1.)

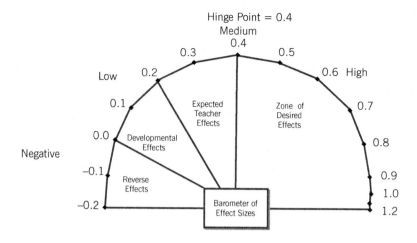

FIGURE 16.1. Hattie's (2009) barometer of effect sizes.

Examples

• Marzano (2003) conducted a series of meta-analyses on the impact of various instructional strategies on student achievement, using locally developed measures. He identified nine strategies with very positive effect sizes and translated these into percentile gains, as indicated in Table 16.1.

• Hattie (2009) also looked at influences on student achievement. He employed a strategy that involved summarizing other effect size estimates. He examined over 800 meta-analyses and found a total of 138 influences for which different effect size estimates could be made. Table 16.2 shows the influences for which effect sizes of 0.4 or more were obtained.

TABLE 16.1. Marzano's Teacher-Level Factors

Instructional strategy	Average effect size	Percentile gain	Number of effect sizes	Standard deviation
Identifying similarities and differences	1.61	45	31	0.31
Summarizing and note taking	1.00	34	179	0.50
Reinforcing effort and providing recognition	0.80	29	21	0.35
Homework and practice	0.77	28	134	0.36
Nonlinguistic representations	0.75	27	246	0.40
Cooperative learning	0.73	27	122	0.40
Setting objectives and providing feedback	0.61	23	408	0.28
Generating and testing hypotheses	0.61	23	63	0.79
Questions, cues, and advance organizers	0.59	22	1,251	0.26

Note. Data from Marzano (2003).

TABLE 16.2. Influences on Student Achievement for Which Effect Sizes of 0.4 or More Were Obtained

Student	Effect size	Teaching	Effect size	Curriculum	Effect size
Self-reported grades	1.44	Providing formative evaluation (and action research)	0.90	Vocabulary programs	0.67
Piagetian programs	1.28	Microteaching (video + reflection)	0.88	Repeated reading programs	0.67
Prior achievement	0.67	Comprehensive interventions for students with disabilities	0.77	Creativity programs	0.65
Preterm birth weight	0.54	Teacher clarity	0.75	Phonics instruction	0.60
Concentration, persistence, engagement	0.48	Reciprocal teaching	0.74	Tactile stimulation programs	0.58
Motivation	0.48	Feedback	0.73	Comprehension programs	0.58
Early intervention	0.47	Teacher–student relationships	0.72	Visual-perception programs	0.56
Preschool programs	0.45	Spaced vs. mass practice	0.71	Outdoor/adventure programs	0.52
Self-concept	0.43	Metacognitive strategies	0.69	Play programs	0.50
Reducing anxiety	0.40	Self-verbalization, self-questioning	0.64	Second-/third-chance programs	0.50
		Professional development	0.62	Mathematics	0.46
		Problem-solving teaching	0.61	Writing programs	0.44
		Not labeling students	0.61	Science	0.40
		Teaching strategies	0.60	Social skills programs	0.40
		Concept mapping	0.60		
		Cooperative vs. individualistic learning	0.59		
		Study skills	0.59		
		Direct instruction	0.59		
		Mastery learning	0.58		
		Worked examples	0.57		
		Goals	0.57		
		Peer tutoring	0.55		
		Cooperative vs. competitive learning	0.54		
		Keller's PIS (programmed instruction sequence)	0.53		
		Interactive video methods	0.52		
		Questioning	0.46		
		Quality of teaching	0.44		
		Teachers' expectations	0.43		
		Behavioral organizers/adjunct questions	0.41		
		Matching style of learning	0.41		
		Cooperative learning	0.41		

Note. Data from Hattie (2009, pp. 297–300).

• Cooper, Robinson, and Patall (2006) examined homework effectiveness studies that had been conducted in the United States since 1987. They grouped the studies into four research designs and found that although all of the studies had design flaws, there was generally consistent evidence for a positive influence of homework on achievement. Studies that reported simple homework–achievement correlations revealed evidence that a stronger correlation existed (a) in grades 7–12 than in K–6 and (b) when students rather than parents reported time on homework. No strong evidence was found for an association between the homework–achievement link and the outcome measure (grades as opposed to standardized tests) or the subject matter (reading as opposed to math).

• Rakes, Valentine, McGatha, and Ronau (2010), in their study of effective instructional strategies for teaching algebra, identified 82 studies that met their criteria. Together, these studies represented a sample of 22,424 students. Analysis yielded five categories of strategies that showed positive results: technology curricula, non-technology curricula, instructional strategies, manipulatives, and technology tools. The researchers also found that "interventions focusing on the development of conceptual understanding produced an average effect size almost double that of interventions focusing on procedural understanding" (p. 372).

QUALITATIVE REVIEWS: METASYNTHESES   MAP 16.3

Purpose, Designs, and Procedures

Qualitative metasynthesis is "the bringing together and breaking down of findings, examining them, discovering essential features, and, in some way, combining phenomena into a transformed whole" (Schreiber, Crooks, & Stern, 1997, p. 314).

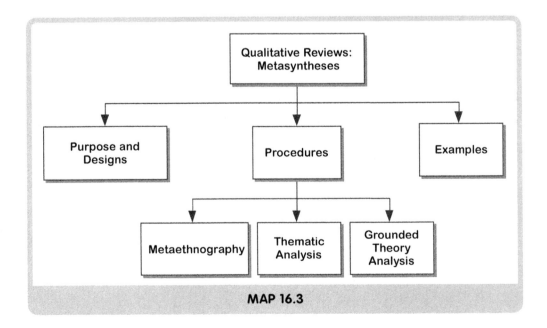

MAP 16.3

Other terms used to describe this approach include *metaethnography, metanarrative, metastudy,* and *metainterpretation* (Ring, Ritchie, Mandava, & Jepson, 2011). Qualitative metasynthesis answers the question of "how to 'put together' written interpretive accounts" (Noblit & Hare, 1988, p. 7) with the goal of producing "a new and integrative interpretation of findings that is more substantive than those resulting from individual investigations and to build theory" (Finfgeld, 2003, p. 894).

It may seem counterintuitive to synthesize qualitative work, and some critics have argued that those who attempt to do so are distorting the research. On the other hand, there is an equal concern (Scruggs, Mastropieri, & McDuffie, 2007) for the durability of qualitative research if researchers fail to collect and synthesize findings in a field. There is a growing belief that qualitative metasyntheses can provide in-depth analyses of questions that are difficult to quantify and that go beyond quantitative effect size, especially in education and in health-related fields.

As in a quantitative meta-analysis, the process of conducting a qualitative metasynthesis includes identifying the topic, establishing inclusion criteria, and selecting the population of studies (which tends to comprise 15 studies or so). The idea of qualitative metasynthesis is quite new, making it difficult to capture what it entails and to develop clear guidelines. However, three promising approaches are emerging, each with a specific goal (Centre for Reviews and Dissemination [CRD], 2009):

> *Metaethnography* seeks to create new interpretations or concepts. It involves reading and rereading studies, listing and comparing key concepts, determining how they are related, translating the studies into one another, and identifying concepts which "go beyond individual accounts and can be used to produce a new interpretation" (CRD, 2009, p. 228).

> *Thematic analysis* seeks to uncover recurrent themes. It involves developing thematic headings from the individual studies and combining these to present a coherent whole.

> *Grounded theory analysis* seeks to build theory by applying the constant comparative method to evidence from individual studies. (See Chapter Three for a fuller discussion of grounded theory.)

As a method of research, qualitative metasynthesis is gaining recognition as a way to codify and preserve qualitative findings. Better established in health and education than in other disciplines, it holds promise for informing decision making, complementing effectiveness reviews, and contributing to the knowledge base about educational practice.

Examples

• Scruggs et al. (2007) conducted a thematic metasynthesis of team teaching in inclusive classrooms. Specifically, they wanted to know the answers to these questions: "How is co-teaching being implemented?" and "What are the benefits perceived to be?" (p. 394). The researchers selected 32 qualitative studies of co-teaching in inclusive classrooms and conducted a metasynthesis, employing qualitative research integration techniques. They concluded that although co-teachers generally supported co-teaching, they expressed a number of important needs that were linked to administrative support; these included planning time and professional development. The usual model of co-teaching was found to be "one teach, one assist," with the special education teacher usually playing a subordinate role. Classrooms were characterized by traditional instruction, and instructional techniques that were recommended for special education teachers (such as the use of peer mediation, study skills instruction, self-advocacy skill development, and self-regulation and monitoring) infrequently occurred.

• Savin-Baden, McFarland, and Savin-Baden (2008) completed a metaethnography that focused on thinking, learning, and teaching practices in higher education. They approached the review with three questions:

1. What does the literature indicate about thinking and practices about teaching and learning in higher education?

2. What are the tensions and differences across practices and communities?

3. What is the relationship between theories of teaching and learning and actual practices?

After searching and analyzing articles for inclusion, the researchers divided the articles into three categories of themes: teaching practice, transfer of learning, and communities that supported teaching and learning. Next, they engaged in a process of reading and rereading the studies, using annotations and maps to identify methods, concepts, metaphors and findings. Savin-Baden et al. concluded their final synthesis as follows:

> Whilst this review presents research and practice, disciplinary differences and similarities, it also shows that issues of pedagogical stance, disjunction, learning spaces, agency, notions of improvement, and communities of interest all help to locate overarching themes and hidden subtexts that are strong influences on areas of practice, transfer and community. Nevertheless, these are areas that are sometimes ignored, marginalised or dislocated from the central arguments about teaching and learning thinking and practices in higher education. (2008, p. 225)

• Pielstick (1998) conducted a metaethnography on transformational leadership. He used a software program to assist in coding and analysis, and employed the constant comparative method. Beginning with open coding and progressing to axial coding, Pielstick developed a profile of the transformational leader that included seven elements: (1) creating a shared vision, (2) communicating the vision, (3) building relationships, (4) developing a supporting organizational culture, (5) guiding implementation, (6) exhibiting character, and (7) achieving results. This metaethnography produced a concept of tranformational leadership that Pielstick described as follows:

> A clear picture of goals based on a shared vision provides meaning and purpose beyond the noise and turmoil of conflicting demands. Interactive dialogue promotes understanding and inspires followers to overcome the challenges and to enjoy the thrill of accomplishment. Strong relationships pull a team together to achieve more than can be done by individuals

paddling alone. Guidance through the most challenging whitewater minimizes the chances of overturning the raft. A supporting culture of understanding and trust builds the confidence needed to overcome obstacles. Exhibiting character enhances the confidence and trust of an entire team to achieve its shared vision. (p. 34)

CHAPTER SUMMARY   MAP 16.4

✓ Research reviews consolidate and summarize findings and understandings from a collection of studies within a field of inquiry.

✓ A research review presents the "big picture" about a well-defined topic, points to established and promising practices, and provides the rationale for future research on that topic.

✓ Research reviews provide empirical knowledge that challenges deeply held beliefs, help to validate professional judgment, and assist in decision making and policy formation.

✓ There are three types of research reviews: narrative reviews, quantitative meta-analyses, and qualitative metasyntheses. In each case, researchers must clearly define a topic, identify a theoretical perspective, establish criteria for inclusion, conduct a search for articles and papers, select a population of studies, complete an analysis, and present a synthesis.

✓ A narrative review provides an author's written perspective on selected studies in a particular field. Such reviews may be short reviews at the beginnings of articles or long reviews that appear as chapters in books and dissertations or in journals dedicated to reviews.

✓ Meta-analysis is "the statistical analysis of a large collection of analysis results for the purpose of integrating the findings" (Glass, 1976, p. 3) and uses the effect size statistic to determine effectiveness.

✓ An effect size of 0.4 is the hinge point for determining effectiveness.

✓ Qualitative metasynthesis "is the bringing together and breaking down of findings, examining them, discovering essential features, and, in some way, combining phenomena into a transformed whole" (Schreiber et al., 1997, p. 314).

✓ Types of metasyntheses include metaethnography, metathematic analysis, and metagrounded theory analysis.

KEY TERMS AND CONCEPTS

effect size hinge point   narrative/traditional review

fugitive study   population of studies

metaethnography   qualitative metasynthesis

metagrounded theory analysis   quantitative meta-analysis

metathematic analysis   research review

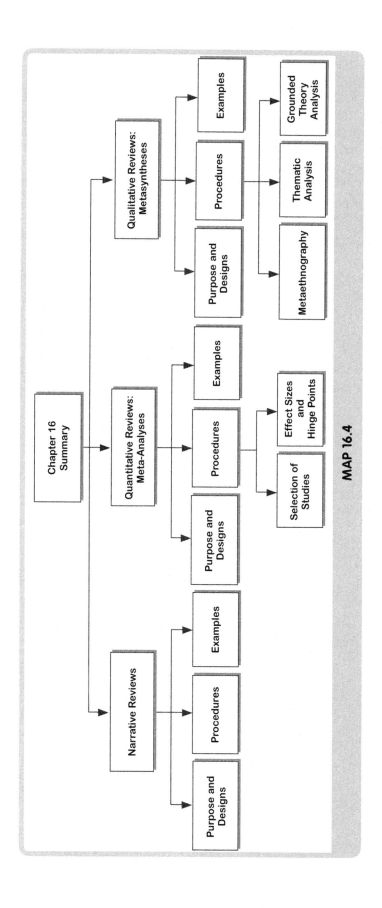

MAP 16.4

REVIEW, CONSOLIDATION, AND EXTENSION OF KNOWLEDGE

1. Using an academic or commercial database, locate a meta-analysis on the topic of
    your choice and describe the following:

    a. Criteria for selecting the population.
    b. The size of the population.
    c. The effect size of findings.
    d. Conclusions about effectiveness.

2. Using an academic or commercial database, locate a metasynthesis on the topic of
    your choice and describe the following:

    a. Criteria for selecting the population.
    b. The size of the population.
    c. The design and procedures.
    d. Conclusions and implications of the synthesis.

CHAPTER SEVENTEEN

Writing a Student Review Essay

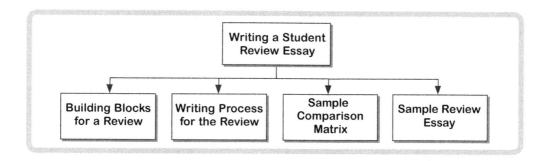

BUILDING BLOCKS FOR A REVIEW

This chapter brings together the material covered in the previous chapters by guiding you through the process of writing a student review essay—an essay that demonstrates your mastery of the methods of research described in this text, as well as your ability to communicate your knowledge both verbally and visually. The building blocks for writing a review essay include knowing how to do the following:

- Search for primary, empirical, peer-reviewed articles that use different methods of research.
- Read and analyze articles that use different research methodologies and conventions.
- Write critiques of qualitative, quantitative, mixed methods, and applied research articles.
- Use APA guidelines for within-text citations and full references.

WRITING PROCESS FOR THE REVIEW (SEE MAP 17.1)

MAP 17.1

Follow these steps in the process of writing your review essay:

1. Decide on a broad topic of interest.

2. Use the databases and search strategies described in Chapter Two to identify

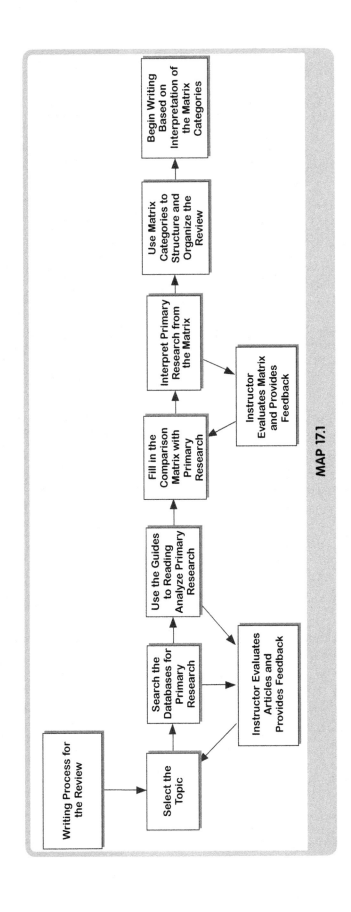

MAP 17.1

six primary, empirical, peer-reviewed articles on your chosen topic for the review. It is best to limit your search to the basic categories of quantitative, qualitative, and mixed methods. You may have identified a good number of articles if you have completed the various end-of-chapter activities. Once you have selected your six articles, ask your instructor to provide feedback on your choices.

3. Use the Guides to Reading for the types of research you have selected as you go through each article. (These Guides are provided in the end-of-chapter activities for Chapters Four, Eight, Nine, Ten, Eleven, and Twelve. Informal guidance is also provided in the end-of-chapter exercises for Chapters Thirteen through Fifteen.) You may want to answer the questions on the Guides in bulleted list format, or you may decide to write a separate critique for each article. Again, you may already have written critiques for some of the articles if you have completed the various end-of-chapter activities. **MAP 17.2**

4. Before you begin to write, fill in the comparison matrix provided in Figure 17.1. This matrix will help you organize your review. Fill in the basic information for each article. Figures 17.2–17.5 describe the information that should be provided in each cell for each type of research. Once you have filled in the matrix, and your instructor has evaluated it and provided feedback, use it to interpret your primary research.

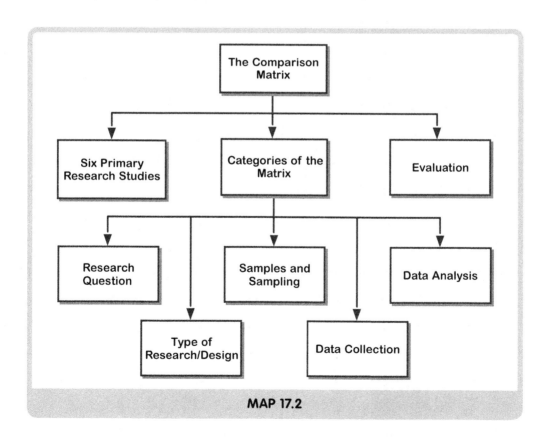

MAP 17.2

Author (date)	Research question	Type/design	Sampling	Data collection	Data analysis	Evaluation
Article 1:						
Article 2:						
Article 3:						
Article 4:						
Article 5:						
Article 6:						

FIGURE 17.1. The comparison matrix.

Author (date)	Research question	Type/design	Sampling	Data collection	Data analysis	Evaluation
Author (date)	What is the research question?	Qualitative: Ethnography Case study Phenomenological study Narrative study Qualitative document analysis Critical discourse analysis	Purposeful or theoretical Characteristics	Multiple sources or single source Observations, interviews, documents/ discourses	Coding Data reduction	Rate each as strong, moderate, weak: Overall quality Trustworthiness Transferability

FIGURE 17.2. Matrix descriptors for qualitative studies.

Author (date)	Research question	Type/design	Sampling	Data collection	Data analysis	Evaluation
Author (date)	What is the research question or the hypothesis (if there is one)?	Quantitative: True experiment Quasi-experiment Factorial design (between-group or repeated-measures) Single-subject	Size of sample Selection (random or nonrandom) Group assignment (random or nonrandom; type of assignment) Characteristics	Measures Validity and reliability IV and DV Response format	Test of significance: t-test (t-value); ANOVA, ANCOVA, MANOVA, or MANCOVA (F-value) p-value Effect size Visual examination	Rate each as strong, moderate, weak: Overall quality Theory/ treatment Sample/ sampling Data collection and analysis

FIGURE 17.3. Matrix descriptors for experimental studies.

Author (date)	Research question	Type/design	Sampling	Data collection	Data analysis	Evaluation
Author (date)	What is the research question or the hypothesis?	Quantitative: Group comparison Correlations	Size of sample Selection (random or nonrandom) Characteristics	Measures Validity and reliability IV/PV and DV/CV Response format	Test of significance: t-test, ANOVA, MANOVA, ANCOVA, MANCOVA chi-square r, r^2, R, R^2 p-value	Rate each as strong, moderate, weak: Overall quality Theory/framing construct Sample/ sampling Data collection and analysis

FIGURE 17.4. Matrix descriptors for quantitative nonexperimental studies.

Author (date)	Research question	Type/design	Sampling	Data collection	Data analysis	Evaluation
Author (date)	What is the research question?	Mixed methods: Sequential (exploratory or explanatory) Concurrent (triangulation or embedded) Quantitative strand: See Figures 17.3 and 17.4 Qualitative strand: See Figure 17.2	Quantitative strand: See Figures 17.3 and 17. 4 Qualitative strand: See Figure 17.2	Quantitative strand: See Figures 17.3 and 17.4 Qualitative strand: See Figure 17.2	Quantitative strand: See Figures 17.3 and 17.4 Qualitative strand: See Figure 17.2	Rate the following as strong, moderate, weak: Overall quality Quantitative strand Qualitative strand Mixing/ interpretation (timing and weight)

FIGURE 17.5. Matrix descriptors for mixed methods studies.

5. Decide on a structure and an organization for the review. You may choose to work across the matrix and summarize each article in terms of methods or to move down the matrix and write a summary of each category of research methods separately.

6. Begin writing. The essay should be about 12 to 15 pages long and should include the following sections: **MAP 17.3**

- A brief introduction that describes the topic for review, the reasons why it is relevant, your search strategy, and a brief overview of each study.
- A narrative summarizing each study you are reviewing in each research category, with headings to guide the reader.
  - An evaluation of each article according to the criteria established in this text.
  - *Qualitative research*: Trustworthiness and transferability.
  - *Quantitative research:* Theory and treatment, or theory or framing construct; sample and sampling; data collection and analysis.
  - *Mixed methods research*: Qualitative and quantitative criteria appropriate for each strand and mixing/interpretation for the entire article.
- A concluding paragraph, covering what you have learned about research methods and about your chosen topic. You may want to develop a chart that summarizes what you have found in your review.
- A full reference list in APA format.

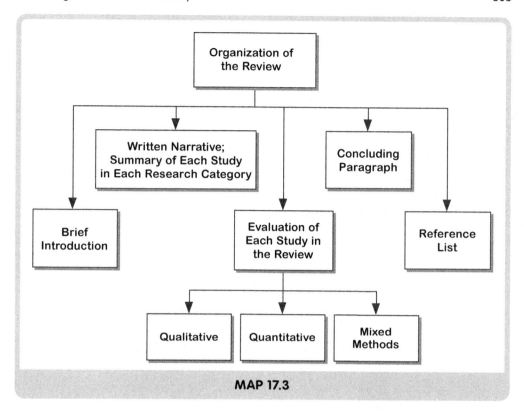

MAP 17.3

SAMPLE COMPARISON MATRIX

Some sample responses to the end-of-chapter exercises in earlier chapters (see the Appendix) have demonstrated how a school social worker with an interest in animal-assisted therapy (AAT) would approach these exercises with an eye toward writing the final review essay. Figure 17.6 is an example of the comparison matrix that would guide the writing of an essay to review articles related to the topic of AAT. Note the inclusion of six articles that are either referenced or critiqued in the Appendix (see the sample responses in the Appendix for Chapters Two, Three, Four, Five, Six, Eight, Nine, and Thirteen).

The following section presents a sample review essay based on this comparison matrix.

Author (date)	Research question	Type/design	Sampling	Data collection	Data analysis	Evaluation
Article 1: Turner (2007)	How do prison inmates experience a therapy dog-training program?	Qualitative: Phenomenological study	Purposeful; 6 inmates in a canine assistance program in one prison	In-depth, audiotaped interviews	Code-and-retrieve method; peer debriefing; six themes related to personal lives and to prison environment	Overall = Strong Trustworthiness = Strong Transferability = Strong
Article 2: Burgon (2011)	How do seven "at-risk" youths experience a therapeutic horsemanship program?	Qualitative: Ethnography	Purposeful; 7 youths in foster care, 11–15 years old	Participant observation: Field notes and interviews	Open coding; four categories of youths	Overall = Strong Trustworthiness = Strong Transferability = Strong
Article 3: Minatrea & Wesley (2008)	How does AAT affect therapeutic alliances?	Quantitative: True experiment	Convenience; 24 adults with substance addiction/abuse; random assignment to treatment and control groups	HAQ-II (valid and reliable)	ANOVA: Significant difference between AAT and non-AAT groups, $F(1, 229) = 25.4, p < .001$	Overall = Moderate Theory/treatment = Moderate to strong Sample/sampling = Moderate to strong Data collection and analysis = Moderate
Article 4: Prothmann, Bienert, & Ettrich (2006)	What effects do AAT have on states of mind of adolescents with psychiatric disorders?	Quantitative: Quasi-experiment and group comparison	Nonrandom; 100 psychiatric patients, 11–20 years old; nonrandomly assigned to groups	BBS (valid and reliable)	Paired t-tests: Significant difference with dog therapy ($t = 4.59, p < .05$); ES = 0.38 ANOVA: No difference by diagnosis ($F = 0.0611, p = .691$)	Overall = Strong Theory/treatment = Strong Sample/sampling = Moderate to strong Data collection and analysis = Strong

Article	Research Question	Design	Sample	Instrument/Measures	Results	Evaluation
Article 5: Somervill, Kruglikova, Robertson, Hanson, & MacLin (2008)	Are there physiological differences when holding a dog or a cat?	Quantitative: Repeated-measures	Nonrandom; 62 college students: 28 males, 34 females, ages 18–29; mostly European American	Health-o-Meter Model 7631 (valid and reliable) Pulse readings	ANOVA for holding/not holding pet = n.s.; t-tests for sequences of holding pets = n.s.	Overall = Strong; Theory/treatment = Strong; Sample/sampling = Moderate to strong; Data collection and analysis = Strong
Article 6: Ewing, MacDonald, Taylor, & Bowers (2007)	What is the effect of equine therapy on youths with severe ED?	Mixed methods: Sequential explanatory; Quantitative strand: Quasi-experiment; Qualitative strand: Case study	Quantitative strand: Convenience; 28 students with ED; nonrandom group assignment; Qualitative strand: Purposeful; 4 students from sample	Quantitative strand: Paired t-tests; no significant differences in five areas measured; Qualitative strand: Method of analysis not stated; observed improvements in specific areas		Overall = Moderate; Quantitative strand = Strong; Qualitative strand = Weak; Mixing/interpretation = Weak

FIGURE 17.6. Sample Comparison Matrix for the Sample Review Essay on AAT.

SAMPLE REVIEW ESSAY

As a school social worker, I have long been interested in therapies that are used with the kinds of students who are referred to me by teachers, guidance counselors, and parents. Animal-assisted therapy (AAT) attracted my interest as a possible treatment option—both because of my love for animals, and because of my strongly held belief that something special in animal–human interactions can unleash untapped potential in students who have not met success with traditional thera-peutic approaches. After searching for articles on the Academic Search Complete database, I was able to settle on six articles that approached the topic from different research perspectives. For this review essay, I have chosen two qualitative studies, three quantitative studies (one true experiment, one quasi-experiment, and one repeated-measures study), and one mixed methods study.

THE QUALITATIVE STUDIES

The two qualitative studies investigated the experiences of actors who were involved in AAT in different settings and with different types of animals. Turner (2007) used a phenomenological approach, while Burgon (2011) conducted a full ethnography.

1. Turner (2007) investigated the experiences of offenders partici-pating in a prison program that trained therapy dogs for children. In this phenomenological study, Turner conducted intensive interviews with a purposeful sample. The sample consisted of six inmates with addiction disorders who volunteered to participate in the dog-training program, which had been introduced as a therapeutic intervention. The research question posed was this: What are the experiences of the prison inmates participating in a service dog-training program? Through a review of the literature on AAT, with a special focus on canine-assisted therapy and its prior use in prison settings, the author has established a clear rationale for the study: "Although dog training programs exist within prisons throughout the United States, there is very little academic research to actually document the ben-efits that these programs have for the offenders" (p. 39). The study drew on the resources of the Indiana Canine Assistant and Adolescent Network (ICAAN).

The researcher relied on unstructured interviews as the method of data collection, beginning each interview with three guiding ques-tions that focused on (a) the experience for the offenders partici-pating in the program, (b) the benefits that the offenders believed they had derived from the program, and (c) how the offenders thought the program had affected them. The interviews were conducted sepa-rately with each participant and were audio-recorded and transcribed. The researcher provided verbatim accounts from the participants and triangulated data. Using a code-and-retrieve method, she established the following themes: patience, parenting skills, helping others, self-esteem social skills, and a calming of the prison environment. Turner also made use of an external peer reviewer for the analysis.

2. Burgon (2011) sought "to explore the experiences of seven 'at-risk' young people who participated in a therapeutic horsemanship program" (p. 165). In a brief research review at the beginning of the article, Burgon focuses on the therapeutic value of interactions between horses and humans, and sets the stage for describing the study. Other relevant reviews occur throughout the article, in order to add insight and to enhance the findings through the lens of the risk-and-resilience literature. The author describes this study as a "qualitative, participative, and reflexive ethnography within a psycho-social approach . . . utilizing a near-practice approach" (p. 169). By this, she means that she acknowledged her presence as a researcher and also paid attention to her own "needs and interests" (p. 169). The author used a purposeful sample of seven young people ages 11–16, who participated in a program providing additional assistance for youth in foster care. The actors were referred by various social service agencies because they had risk factors associated with poor life outcomes. They attended the program over a 2-year period. Of the seven actors, five were female and two were male. The author noted that several of them had attention-deficit/hyperactivity disorder (ADHD) or were on the autism spectrum.

The researcher is a social worker who had prior experience with some of the actors in her study. She noted that her previous engagement with the actors "posed challenges for me during the entire research process; the blurring of lines between practice and research sometimes seemed muddy" (p. 169). The author collected data as a participant observer; she recorded detailed observational field notes and conducted semistructured as well as conversational unstructured interviews. While no evidence of the collection of official or personal documents is provided, the author mentions that the psychological and school records of the actors were examined. The article is replete with thick description and full quotations.

In analyzing the data, the author transcribed all of her field notes and interviews, and used "an open coding process to look for themes and patterns" (p. 170). She was able to reduce the data to the two major themes of social well-being and psychological processes. In line with her stated participatory processes, she shared results with the actors, only three of whom were still available. The researcher identified four main categories that were expressed in the words of the actors. The first was "queen of the world," which connoted growing confidence and self-esteem; the second was "I can't believe I'm doing this!", which connoted an increased sense of master and self-efficacy; the third was "I feel like I can give him love," which connoted the development of empathy through the horses; and the fourth was "I didn't know you could do that," which connoted an openness to new opportunities.

THE QUANTITATIVE STUDIES

Of the three quantitative studies, one was a true experiment (Minatrea & Wesley, 2008); one was a quasi-experimental control–treatment group design (Prothmann, Bienert, & Ettrich, 2006); and one used a repeated-measures design (Somervill, Kruglikova, Robertson, Hanson, & MacLin, 2008).

1. Minatrea and Wesley (2008) investigated whether there would be significant differences in the therapeutic alliances that developed between the therapist and subjects being treated for substance abuse when AAT was added to choice theory/reality therapy (CT/RT) in counseling sessions. The research review examines literature in three areas: CT/RT, AAT, and therapeutic alliances involving both the general population and people addicted to or abusing substances. The review is very comprehensive and includes well over 50 references to research spanning a quarter of a century, with a sufficient number of recent publications.

Based on the review, the authors have stated the research question thus: "Does AAT make a difference in the therapeutic alliance when treating individuals abusing or addicted to substances in a group counselling modality using CT or RT as the counselling theory?" (p. 72). The research adds to the body of literature supporting the thesis that AAT has a positive effect on the therapeutic relationship with persons who abuse substances. The independent variable was CT/RT with AAT. The dependent variable was the therapeutic alliance. This was designed as a posttest-only/control group study, with a sample of 24 individuals who resided in a treatment facility and who met criteria for substance addiction/abuse. Characteristics of the sample in terms of age or gender are not described in any detail. Members of the sample had been previously screened and were assessed on the Pet Attitude Scale. The random assignment of subjects to the control and treatment groups qualified this as a true experiment. The same therapist treated both groups. She used CT/RT approaches with both groups and added AAT with the treatment group, using a 7-year-old beagle mix as a therapy dog.

Data were collected with the Helping Alliance Questionnaire (HAQ-II), which measured the therapeutic alliance. The researchers also administered the Session Rating Scale (SRS) and note that they monitored blood pressure, but they do not report the results of these data. No information is provided about the validity and reliability of the HAQ-II, although it seems to have been used extensively in this line of research. The authors used a series of one-way analyses of variance (ANOVAs) and found significant differences ($F = 25.4$, $p < .001$) in the clients' perceptions of the therapeutic relationship; this implied that the hypothesis was confirmed. The authors state, "A review of effect sizes computed for each variable suggests [that] the addition of

AAT contributed most of the differences observed for the HAQ-II ratings" (p. 72). However, no specific effect sizes were reported.

2. Prothmann et al. (2006) investigated the effects of AAT with a dog on the states of mind of adolescents with psychiatric disorders who were being treated in an inpatient clinic. They also investigated whether there would be any significant differences connected to different diagnoses; this required doing a nonexperimental group comparison as well. The authors used a pre- and posttest/control group design.

The research review focuses on empirical studies of the long- and short-term effects of AAT, and the authors make the case that there was little in the way of previous research on its use with adolescents in psychiatric inpatient clinics. The convenience sample consisted of 100 children and adolescents ages 11–20. The sample was assigned to control and treatment groups. The treatment group consisted of 61 youths who participated in a maximum of five separate therapeutic sessions with a dog; the control group consisted of 39 children and adolescents who were placed on a waiting list. The authors reported that random assignment to groups was not possible, making this a quasi-experiment. The two groups were not significantly different in gender or type of disorder.

Since there were no available measures of states of mind for children, the authors used an instrument designed for adults: the Basler Befindlichkeits-Skala (BBS), a self-rating questionnaire for measuring states of mind over time. The BBS has four subscales that measure vitality, emotional balance, social extroversion, and alertness. The measure was only administered to subjects who were at least 11 years old and had met a reading comprehension requirement; scores on the BBS were measured as the dependent variable before and after each treatment session. The treatment group was video-recorded for five AAT sessions and was tested before and after each session. The control group attended one session without AAT and was measured before and after the session. The researchers compared the means of all pretests with the means of all posttests for the treatment group, and compared these scores with the scores on the pre- and posttests for the control group. There was no significant difference in the pretest scores between the control and treatment groups ($t = 1.66$, $p = .10$), while the difference in means for the posttest scores were significant ($t = 3.5$, $p = .001$). The authors also conducted paired t-tests for each member of the two groups, using the pre- and posttest scores; they found significant differences on all of the subtests for the treatment groups, but no such differences for the control group. In addition, the researchers calculated the effect size of differences and found a medium effect size of 0.38. ANOVA was used to test for significant differences in groups according to diagnosis. No significant differences were found ($F = 0.0611$, $p = .691$).

3. Somervill et al. (2008) sought "(a) to assess the effects of limited exposure to an unfamiliar dog versus an unfamiliar cat on blood pressure and pulse rate on college students, and (b) to increase physical interaction with the animals by having participants hold each animal in their lap for a five minute period" (p. 521). The research review establishes a strong theoretical foundation for the study, and it led the authors to the development of two research questions: (1) Would blood pressure and pulse significantly differ in reactions to a dog or cat? (2) Would the sequence of the presentation of the dog and cat significantly affect blood pressure and pulse? The authors state, "It was tentatively hypothesized that participants would show a reduction in blood pressure while handling both a dog and a cat" (p. 519).

The convenience sample of 62 subjects included 28 males and 34 females. The males ranged in age from 18 to 29, with a mean age of 20.04 and a median age of 19. Of the males, 22 were European Americans and 4 were African Americans. The females ranged in age from 18 to 24, with a mean age of 19.21 and a median age of 19. Of the females, 32 were European Americans, 1 was an African American, and 1 was of unspecified race/ethnicity. The two dependent variables were blood pressure and pulse readings. Blood pressure was measured by the Health-o-Meter Model 7631, which was assumed to be valid and reliable; pulse was measured by readings done by trained research assistants. A total of 10 blood measurements were taken at 5-minute intervals. The measurements taken before and after the first, fifth, and ninth 5-minute intervals—when no animals were present—served as baselines. During the third and seventh 5-minute intervals, each participant held either a dog or cat in his or her lap in alternating orders. A second person was always present to ensure that the animal remained in the participant's lap during the third and seventh 5-minute time periods.

The authors used ANOVAs to analyze the differences between measures at baseline and measures when subjects held a pet. There were no significant differences for systolic blood pressure ($F = 0.671$, $p \leq .613$) or for pulse ($F = 2.373$, $p \leq .053$). To analyze differences in the sequence of holding a dog or cat, the authors used independent t-tests. They found no significant differences for systolic blood pressure ($t = 0.78$, n.s.), for diastolic blood pressure ($t = -1.05$, n.s.), or for pulse ($t = 0.750$, n.s.). The authors also looked for differences in the covariates of (a) liking or disliking cats or dogs and (b) dog ownership (these data were derived from a survey) and found no significant differences.

THE MIXED METHODS STUDY

Ewing, MacDonald, Taylor, and Bowers (2007) investigated the effects of equine-facilitated learning on young adolescents with severe emotional disorders (ED). The research review focuses on the literature on animals as co-therapists and the effects of equine-facilitated psychotherapy in different settings. The authors do not provide a clear rationale for using a mixed methods approach or for their choice of a sequential explanatory design (in which the quantitative/quasi-experimental component preceded the qualitative component and was weighted more heavily).

The Quantitative Component

Based on the review, the authors generated five research hypotheses for the quantitative portion of the study:

1. After participating in equine-facilitated learning, subjects would demonstrate an increase in feelings of self-esteem.

2. After participating in equine-facilitated learning, subjects would demonstrate an increase in feelings of interpersonal empathy.

3. After participating in equine-facilitated learning, subjects would demonstrate an increase in their sense of internal locus of control.

4. After participating in equine-facilitated learning, subjects would demonstrate a decrease in feelings of depression.

5. After participating in equine-facilitated learning, subjects would demonstrate a decrease in feelings of loneliness.

The convenience sample consisted of 28 young adolescents between the ages of 11 and 13 who were enrolled in an alternative day school for students with moderate to severe ED or learning disorders. The mean IQ scores for subjects were as follows: Verbal IQ = 89, Performance IQ = 85, and Full IQ = 86. All of the students received the 9-week treatment, but not at the same time. The subjects who were in the first group to experience the equine therapy served as the first treatment group; their pre- and posttest scores were compared with the scores of the subjects on the waiting list, who served as the first control group. As each new group participated in the therapy, its members served as their own control and treatment groups. Their original posttest scores served as pretest scores when they entered the therapy; posttests were administered to each new group when they completed the equine-facilitated treatment. There was no indication of how the groups were assigned to different waves of treatment.

The measures selected for the study were reported as valid and reliable and included the following: (1) for self-esteem, the Harter Self-Perception Profile for Children; (2) for interpersonal empathy, the Empathy Concern subscale of the Empathy Questionnaire; (3) for internal locus of control, the Nowicki–Strickland Internal–External Control Scale for Children; (4) for feelings of depression, the Children's Depression Scale; and (5) for feelings of loneliness, the

Children's Loneliness Questionnaire. The authors used paired t-tests to analyze results. They found no significant differences between the pre- and posttest scores, with p-values ranging from >.84 to <.22 on the various measures.

The Qualitative Component

The qualitative component involved case studies of four of the members of the quantitative sample who had shown positive results on the quantitative measures. The authors applied the following labels to the four participants in this purposeful sample: (1) "the victim," a 10-year-old who suffered from posttraumatic stress disorder (PTSD) but learned to talk about her fears; (2) "the feral child," an 11-year-old girl with multiple diagnoses who initially could not function in a regular classroom, but who gained reentry into a mainstream class; (3) "the runaway," a 13-year-old boy with ADHD who typically panicked and ran away, but who learned to build trust, and (4) "the boost needed," a 10-year-old boy with a behavior disorder who became more successful in school.

The authors describe the data sources for the qualitative component as "interviews and observations by the special education teachers, therapeutic riding instructor, and volunteers" (p. 67). There is no indication of how the interviews and observations were conducted, recorded, or analyzed. Rather, the authors describe positive outcomes that were reported by the informants; they conclude that these descriptions illuminate the findings of the quantitative component and provide reason for optimism about equine-facilitated therapy.

EVALUATION OF THE QUALITATIVE STUDIES

In evaluating the two qualitative studies, I have applied the criteria of trustworthiness and transferability. I rate the Turner (2007) phenomenological study of participants in a prison therapeutic dog-training program as strong in both categories. Although there is scant detail about the researcher's stance, there is much in the way of thick description. The author provides only a passing reference to how data were coded and reduced, but clearly elaborates on the themes that emerged. The appropriateness of purposeful sampling, the use of thick descriptions, and triangulation make the data credible. The detailed description of data analysis procedures and use of a peer reviewer both add to trustworthiness. And the thick descriptions of context and actors make me think that the results of this study can be transferred to similar settings and actors. It is important to note that the use of a small, purposeful sample is intrinsic to qualitative research; while it does not lend the results to generalizability, it in no way detracts from the quality of the study or its usefulness. Finally, as a reader, I found the thick descriptions (especially the use of verbatim accounts) to be very effective in creating a response of resonance and deeper understanding.

I also rate the Burgon (2011) ethnography of an AAT program for children in foster care as strong in both categories. The author clearly describes her stance as both a researcher and a practitioner and is open about the dilemmas and challenges this dual stance presented. She provides a description of how she transformed data and developed four themes that used the actual words of the actors as organizers. She also provides thick descriptions of the setting and the actors, reproduces the actors' language verbatim, and fully describes what she observed during the program. She connects the experience of the seven actors through a process of triangulation that is implied but not made explicit. She invited the actors to participate fully in the research and to review the findings. The thick description that the author provides, as well as the sample she chose, make it likely that a reader with an interest in improving life outcomes for at-risk youths would resonate with the study and find the findings transferable to another context.

EVALUATION OF THE QUANTITATIVE STUDIES

In evaluating the three quantitative experiments, I have applied the criteria of theory and treatment, sample and sampling, and data collection and analysis.

I give the Minatrea and Wesley study (2008) of the effects on therapeutic alliance of an AAT program for persons being treated for drug abuse an overall rating of moderate. I rate the theory as strong, and the treatment as moderate. The research review establishes the case for AAT. The treatment was appropriate for the theory. However, the authors do not provide adequate information about when, for how long, and under what conditions the treatment was administered, other than the fact that the same therapist treated each group. The sample and sampling are rated as moderate to strong. Although the sample size was a bit limited for an experiment, the rating for sampling is strengthened by the random assignment of subjects to groups. However, the rating for sample is compromised because of the lack of information about subject characteristics. I rate the collection and analysis of data as moderate. The HAQ-II seems to have been an appropriate measure; however, the authors provide no details about the instrument or any specific indications of its reliability and validity. The use of one-way ANOVA was appropriate for data analysis, and results are reported in terms of critical F- and p-values. The authors note that effect size estimates were computed, but they have neglected to provide specifics and are somewhat vague.

I give a stronger rating to the Prothmann et al. (2006) study on the effects of AAT on adolescent psychiatric patients. The theory merits a strong rating; it was well developed in the research review, and the questions for research followed clearly from the literature reviewed. Although the authors used a convenience sample and nonrandomized assignment to groups, their use of pretest and demographic data to demonstrate no significant differences at the beginning of the experiment did control for variability in the groups. The sample size (n = 100) was adequate for an experiment. The methods of data collection and analysis are also rated as strong. The BBS is described in detail and seems an appropriate measure of states of mind. The authors also made certain that the subjects had the language ability to understand this adult measure. The disproportionate number of therapy sessions for treatment and control groups was unavoidable under the circumstances. The analysis of data, from both the experiment and the group comparison was complete and is well presented. The inclusion of the effect size estimate is an added strength. The authors do not overconclude and stay close to the data.

I rate the repeated-measures study by Somervill et al. (2008) as strong. The theory merits a strong rating; the research review led to the generation of clearly stated research questions and a tentative hypothesis. The sample and sampling are rated as moderate to strong; the sample was of adequate size and, as in many repeated-measures designs, was nonrandomly selected. Repeated measurements under several control and treatment conditions were taken for blood pressure and pulse. A reliable and valid instrument was used for the blood pressure measurements, and training was provided to ensure accurate pulse readings. The data analysis is strong. The researchers clearly demonstrated results for main effects through use of ANOVAs and t-tests.

EVALUATION OF THE MIXED METHODS STUDY

In evaluating the mixed methods study, I have applied the qualitative and quantitative criteria to the appropriate components and the criterion of mixing/interpretation (including timing and weight) for the integration of methods. I rate the study as a whole as moderate. I rate the quantitative component as strong, but the qualitative component and the mixing/interpretation as weak.

For the quantitative component, the theory merits a strong rating. The review established credible hypotheses, which are clearly stated by the authors. The selection of the measures is also rated as strong; they were shown to be reliable and valid instruments for assessing the five hypotheses. The convenience sample was appropriate for the study, and the group assignments, while not explicitly defined, were an effective way to measure treatment and control conditions for all of the subjects. The analysis is likewise rated as strong and used appropriate statistical methods. The fact that there were no significant differences due to the treatment does not detract from the quality of the analysis.

The qualitative component, by contrast, seems to have been an afterthought and was not well planned or executed. The authors present no research or theory that grounded the study. The purposeful sample for the case study was chosen from students whose scores on the quantitative measures showed beneficial outcomes. However, these subjects were not included in qualitative data collection. Instead, the researchers used anecdotal comments by adults who participated in the program. This violated the qualitative ideal of seeing the world through the lens of actors. I also rate mixing/interpretation as weak. The findings of the two components were not mixed, adding to the impression that the qualitative component was not planned in advance and was added when the quantitative findings yielded no significant effects of the equine-facilitated therapy.

CONCLUDING REMARKS

As someone who is always looking for new ways to offer therapeutic support to my students with behavioral disabilities, I have found preparing for and writing this review to be very useful. First, it has had the effect of motivating me to find out more about AAT and how I can use it in my practice. As a dog owner, I may be able to do this with some training.

Second, I have learned a great deal about doing research. When I started this project, I was very wary of my ability to understand research, especially the quantitative variety. I think that I have gained the ability to read, understand, and evaluate different kinds of research, and I feel much more confident in dealing with statistics. I have also realized how complex qualitative research is, and have learned that it consists of much more than interesting anecdotes.

REFERENCES

Burgon, H. L. (2011). 'Queen of the world': Experiences of 'at-risk' young people participating in equine-assisted learning/therapy. *Journal of Social Work Practice, 25*(2), 165–183.

Ewing, C. A., MacDonald, P. M., Taylor, M., & Bowers, M. J. (2007). Equine-facilitated learning for youths with severe emotional disorders: A quantitative and qualitative study. *Child Youth Care Forum, 36,* 59–72.

Minatrea, N. B., & Wesley, M. C. (2008). Reality therapy goes to the dogs. *International Journal of Reality Therapy, 28*(1), 69–77.

Prothmann, A., Bienert, M., & Ettrich, C. (2006). Dogs in child psychotherapy: Effects on state of mind. *Anthrozoös, 19*(3), 265–277.

Somervill, J. W., Kruglikova, Y. A., Robertson, R. L., Hanson, L. M., & MacLin, M. H. (2008). Physiological responses by college students to a dog and a cat: Implications for pet therapy. *North American Journal of Psychology, 10,* 519–528.

Turner, W. G. (2007). Experiences of offenders in a prison canine program. *Federal Probation, 71*(1), 38–43.

CHAPTER SUMMARY   `MAP 17.4`

✓ The purpose of the review essay is to demonstrate your mastery of the methods of research described in this text and your ability to communicate your knowledge both verbally and visually.

✓ Previous chapters provided these building blocks for writing a student review essay: searching for (six recommended) primary, empirical, peer-reviewed articles; reading and analyzing articles that use different research methodologies and conventions; writing critiques of qualitative, quantitative, mixed methods, and applied research articles; and using APA guidelines for within-text citations and full references.

✓ In writing a review, the following steps are required: (1) deciding on a topic, (2) searching databases for resources, (3) using the Reading Guides provided, (4) completing the comparison matrix, (5) deciding on an organizational structure, and (6) sitting down to write.

✓ The final essay should be 13 to 15 pages and include an introduction, subheadings to guide the reader, narrative summaries, evaluations of each article, and a concluding paragraph.

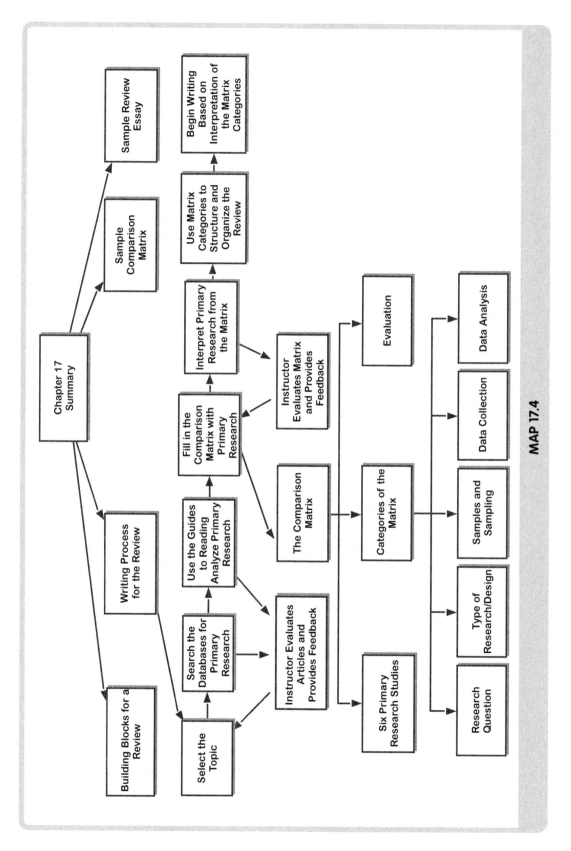

MAP 17.4

317

Sample Answers to Review Questions

CHAPTER ONE

1. **Penning, S. L., Bhagwanjee, A., & Govender, K. (2010). Bullying boys: The traumatic effects of bullying in male adolescent learners.** *Journal of Child and Adolescent Mental Health, 22*(2), 131–143.

    1. The purpose of the study was to investigate the nature and extent of the relationship between bullying and trauma among male adolescent learners.

    2. This study is best characterized as a quantitative, correlational study.

    3. The sample for the study consisted of 486 male adolescent learners between the ages of 12 and 17.

    4. The sample was drawn from a South African male-only high school.

    5. Two objective, quantitative measures were used in this study. These were the Olweus Bullying/Victimisation Scale and the Trauma Symptom Checklist for children, which together measured posttraumatic stress, anxiety, depression, dissociation, and anger.

    6. The two methods of statistical analysis used in the study were a correlations analysis and multivariate analysis of variance (MANOVA).

    7. In general, the findings showed that repetitive stressful events like bullying are related to symptoms of ongoing trauma. More specifically, the study found that the relationship between bullying and trauma was strongest for the victim role and depended on the frequency of bullying. The highest correlation was found between the victim role and depression; next was posttraumatic stress. The study also found that over one-fifth of the students could be diagnosed with posttraumatic stress or dissociation.

2. **Cranham, J., & Carroll, A. (2003). Dynamics within the bully/victim paradigm: A qualitative analysis.** *Educational Psychology in Practice, 19*(2), 113–133.

    1. The purpose of the study was to examine whether high school students within one school could ethically justify bullying behavior.

    2. This study is best characterized as a qualitative interview study.

    3. The purposeful sample consisted of 10 students from one high school.

    4. The 10 students were included in the sample because they assumed specific roles in bullying situations.

    5. Data were collected through semistructured interviews.

6. Data were analyzed through the constant comparative method.

7. Results indicated that there were intricate social structures with the school that students followed when they assumed their roles, and that students who did not comply with these rules risked isolation and exclusion.

3. **Peters, R. D., Bradshaw, A. J., Petrunka, K., Nelson, G., Herry, Y., Craig, W. M., . . . Rossiter, M. D. (2010). The Better Beginnings, Better Futures Project: Findings from grade 3 to grade 9.** *Monographs of the Society for Research in Child Development,* **75(3), 1–174.**

1. The purpose of the study was to investigate the medium- and long-term effects of the Better Beginnings, Better Futures (BBBF) project, an early childhood prevention project for primary school children and families.

2. The study is best characterized as a program evaluation that used a longitudinal experimental design.

3. The sample consisted of 601 children and their families who participated in BBBF programs when the children were between 4 and 8 years old and 358 children and their families from similar communities who did not attend the programs.

4. The sample of children and families all lived in economically disadvantaged neighborhoods.

5. The data were collected through measures of family and school functioning and economic indicators. The abstract does not provide information about the specific measures used.

6. The abstract does not discuss how data were analyzed.

7. Results indicated positive long-term effects on family and school functioning for those students in the program.

4. **Guerra, N. G., Williams, K. R., & Sadek, S. (2011). Understanding bullying and victimization during childhood and adolescence: A mixed methods study.** *Child Development,* **82(1), 295–310.**

1. The purpose of the study was to examine predictors of bullying and victimization and to determine how these varied by age and gender.

2. The study is best characterized as a mixed methods study since it used both quantitative and qualitative approaches.

3. The quantitative sample consisted of 2,678 elementary, middle, and high school students from 59 schools. The qualitative sample consisted of an additional 115 students.

4. The qualitative sample involved students who did not complete the survey.

5. Quantitative data were collected through two "waves" of surveys. Qualitative data were collected through 14 focus group interviews.

6. The abstract does not report on how both kinds of data were analyzed.

7. Results from the surveys indicated that low self-esteem and school climate issues were good predictors of behaviors of both bullies and victims across age and gender lines. In addition, it was found that shared beliefs were predictive of bullying behaviors. The qualitative results indicated that sexuality and identity issues seemed to be connected to bullying behaviors.

5. **DiBasilio, A. (2008).** *Reducing bullying in middle school students through the use of student-leaders.* **Retrieved from ERIC database. (ED501251)**

1. The purpose of the study was to understand the problem of bullying and to figure out how to minimize it through the use of student-leaders.

2. The study is best characterized as action research, conducted by one teacher in a school.

3. The sample consisted of a total of 54 participants (28 eighth graders, two counselors, and 24 teachers from the school). The abstract does not specify how many of the students were school leaders.

4. The abstract does not provide additional information about the sample.

5. Data were collected through three surveys, each designed for a specific role group (counselors, teachers, students).

6. Data were analyzed in terms of the percentages of responses on specific items of the surveys.

7. Results indicated that 71% of the student-leaders had been victims of verbal bullying, and that 26% of students observed social and verbal bullying at least once a week. In addition, the teacher survey showed that 67% of teachers and all of the counselors believed that bullying was an average problem the previous spring.

CHAPTER TWO

1. As a school social worker, I am interested in alternative therapeutic approaches I might use with students who have behavioral and other issues. I have settled on the topic of animal-assisted therapy for investigation. For this topic, I think the best high-quality database is Academic Search Complete.

2. I located the following publications through the following types of searches:

    a. Library website search:

        (1) Qualitative article: Turner, W. G. (2007). Experiences of offenders in a prison canine program. *Federal Probation, 71*(1), 38–43.

        (2) Quantitative article: Prothmann, A., Bienert, M., & Ettrich, C. (2006). Dogs in child psychotherapy: Effects on state of mind. *Anthrozoös, 19*(3), 265–277.

        (3) Mixing and creating methods: Ewing, C. A., MacDonald, P. M., Taylor, M., & Bowers, M. J. (2007). Equine-facilitated learning for youths with severe emotional disorders: A quantitative and qualitative study. *Child and Youth Care Forum, 36*(1), 59–72.

b. Interlibrary loan request:

USM ILLiad

* Logoff jbeaudry
* Main Menu
* New Request
  » Article
  » Book
  » Book Chapter
  » Audio/Video
  » Music Score
  » Conference Paper
  » Report
  » Thesis
* Scan & Deliver from
  USM's Print Collection
  » Article/Book Chapter
* View
  » Outstanding Requests
  » Electronically Received
    Articles
  » Checked Out Items
  » Cancelled Requests
  » History Requests
  » All Requests
  » Notifications
* Tools
  » Change User
    Information

Photocopy/Journal Article Request

*indicates required field

Enter information below and press the Submit Information button to send.
The Interlibrary Loan Office makes every effort to process requests within 24 hours but reserves the right to limit requests handled to 5 per day per patron during peak times.

Describe the Item you want

*Title (Journal, Conference Proceedings, Anthology) Please do not abbreviate unless your citation is abbreviated	Oxford Review of Education
*Volume	38
*Issue Number or Designation	3
Month	
*Year	2012
*Inclusive Pages	323-342
ISSN/ISBN (International Standard Serial/Book Number) If given will speed request processing	
OCLC or Docline UI Number	
*Article Author	Torrance, Harry
*Article Title	Formative Assessment at the Crossroads

c. Library of Congress request: I went to the Main Reading Room and did an advanced search. I came up with the following:

Main title Animal-assisted therapy: therapeutic interventions / authors, Judy Gammonley . . . [et al].

Published/Created Renton, WA : Delta Society, c1997.

Where to Request

Description
1 v. (various pagings): ill. ; 28 cm.
ISBN
1889785032
LC classification (full)
RM931.A65 A55 1997
LC classification (partial)
RM931.A65
Related names
Gammonley, Judy.
Subjects
Animal-assisted therapy.
Human-animal relationships.
Notes
Includes bibliographical references.
LCCN
00502223
Dewey class no.
615.8/515
Type of material
Book
Where to Request

CALL NUMBER	RM931.A65 A55 1997
	Copy 1
Request in	Jefferson or Adams Building Reading Rooms
Status	Not Charged

d. DMOZ:

Therapy Dogs—Links to therapy dogs, animal-assisted therapy, and animal-assisted services, from Dog-Play.-*http://www.dogplay.com/Activities/Therapy/therapyl.html Recreation: Pets: Animal Assisted Therapy (64)*

e. Blog, wiki, YouTube:

Blog URL: *www.servicedogblog.com*

Wiki URL: *https://en.wikipedia.org/wiki/Therapy_dog*

YouTube URL: *www.youtube.com/watch?v=AVum5P3DzYk*

3. Ratings

Source	Resources	Usefulness Rating
Library	Turner, W. G. (2007) Prothmann, A., Bienert, M., & Ettrich, C. (2006) Ewing, C. A., MacDonald, P. M., Taylor, M., & Bowers, M. J. (2007)	High: Ease of access, trustworthy High: Ease of access, trustworthy High : Ease of access, trustworthy
Interlibrary Loan		High: Ease of access, trustworthy
Library of Congress Alcove9	**CALL NUMBER** RM931.A65 A55	Low: Difficulty of access, insufficient information
DMOZ	*http://www.dogplay.com/Activities/Therapy/therapyl.html Recreation: Pets: Animal Assisted Therapy (64*	Medium: A good reference but requires hunting for it; trustworthy
Blog	*www.servicedogblog.com*	Low: Though easy to access, not trustworthy or relevant
Wiki	*https://en.wikipedia.org/wiki/Therapy_dog*	Medium: easy access, questionable trustworthiness, good references and links
YouTube	*www.youtube.com/watch?v=AVum5P3Dzk*	High: easy access, good information on therapy dog visit, trustworthy

CHAPTER THREE

1. Example of placing an X next to terms that need review:

a priori code

axial code **X**

CAQDAS

case study

complete observer

constant comparative method

covert observation

critical race theory **X**

critical theory

discourse **X**

emic and etic perspectives **X**

ethnography

feminism

full participant

generative code **X**
grounded theory
life story interview
Marxism/neo-Marxism
narrative inquiry **X**
observer-as-participant
official documents
open code
overt observation
participant-as-observer
Patton and Spradley questions
personal documents
phenomenological study
phenomenology **X**

purposive sampling **X**
qualitative research
queer theory **X**
selective code **X**
semistructured interview
standardized interview
structured interview
symbolic interaction
text analysis
theoretical sampling **X**
transferability **X**
trustworthiness **X**
verstehen **X**

2. The qualitative article I found in the Academic Search Complete database is this:

> Turner, W. G. (2007). Experiences of offenders in a prison canine program. *Federal Probation, 71*(1), 38–43.

   a. This study used interviews with six inmates as its data source and qualitative coding to uncover themes.

   b. This study used a phenomenological study design.

   c. The findings indicate that the six inmates experienced increased self-esteem and improved social skills.

3. Indicate the appropriate study design for each research purpose from these choices:

   a. ethnography

   b. case study

   c. phenomenological study

   d. text analysis

   e. narrative study

c. This study investigates the way special education teachers in an urban school district think about their working relationship with regular education teachers in the building.

a. This study seeks to understand the culture of special education, from the inside out, within a middle-sized suburban school district.

b. This study investigates how the decision was made to refuse playground privileges to a child with Asperger's syndrome in a rural elementary school.

e. This study aims to understand how one veteran special education teacher has made sense of and given order to her professional and personal life over the past two decades.

d. This study investigates how definitions of qualifying disabilities differ in documents in a K–12 district and a local university.

CHAPTER FOUR

1. Example of placing an X next to terms to review:

actors/informants
Carspecken steps of critical method
Chicago school
critical ethnography **X**
descriptive field notes
ethnography
field notes
grounded ethnography

grounded theory
labeling **X**
reflective field notes
reflexivity **X**
symbolic interaction
theoretical sampling
thick description **X**

2. The ethnography I selected for review is this:

Burgon, H. L. (2011). 'Queen of the world': Experiences of 'at-risk' young people participating in equine-assisted learning therapy. *Journal of Social Work Practice, 25*(2), 165–183.

Research Review

There are two purposes and several locations associated with the research reviews. A brief review is located at the beginning of the article. Its purpose is to set the stage for the study and its focus on the therapeutic value of interactions between horses and humans. Other reviews occur throughout the article; their purpose is to add insight to and enhance the findings through the lens of the risk-and-resilience literature, as risk and resilience are themes that emerge from data collection and analysis. All of the research reviewed is recent and relevant.

Purpose and Design

The purpose of this ethnography was "to explore the experiences of seven 'at-risk' young people who participated in a therapeutic horsemanship program" (p. 165). The author describes this study as a "qualitative, participative, and reflexive ethnography within a psycho-social approach . . . utilizing a near-practice approach" (p. 169). By this, she means that she acknowledged her presence as a researcher to the actors and also paid attention to her own "needs and interests" (p. 169). No specific research questions were raised, though it is implied that the researcher was interested in the question of how this approach might help troubled youths develop resilience.

Sampling

This researcher used a purposeful sample of seven young people between the ages of 11 and 16, who participated in a program she had devised to provide additional assistance for youth in foster care. The actors were referred by various social service agencies because they had risk factors associated with poor life outcomes. They attended the program over a 2-year period. Of the seven actors, five were female and two were male. The author noted that several had attention-deficit/hyperactivity disorder (ADHD) or were on the autism spectrum.

Data Collection

The researcher is a social worker who had prior experience with some of the actors in her study. She noted that the dilemmas of her two roles "posed challenges for me during the entire research process; the blurring of lines between practice and research sometimes seemed muddy" (p. 169). The researcher collected data as a participant observer and recorded detailed observational field notes, conducted "semi-structured, conversational interviews and, laterally, more unstructured, open 'field' interviews" (p. 170). No evidence of the collection of official or personal documents is provided, though the author mentions that the psychological and school records of the actors were examined. The article text is replete with thick description and full quotations.

Data Analysis, Interpretation, and Conclusions

The author transcribed all of her field notes and interviews and used "an open coding process to look for themes and patterns" (p. 170). She was able to reduce the data to the two major themes of social well-being and psychological processes. In line with participatory processes, she shared her results with the actors (only three of whom were still available, due to new foster placements for the others). The researcher identified four main categories and expressed each with a quotation from one of the participants. The first was "queen of the world," which connoted growing confidence and self-esteem; the second was "I can't believe I'm doing this!", which connoted an increased sense of mastery and self-efficacy; the third was "I feel like I can give him love," which connoted the development of empathy through the horses; and the fourth was "I didn't know you could do that," which connoted an openness to new opportunities.

Evaluation

This participative ethnography merits an overall rating of strong. First, it demonstrates strong trustworthiness. The author is clear in describing her position as both a researcher and a practitioner, and is open about the dilemmas and challenges her dual roles presented. She provides a description of how she transformed data and developed four themes that used the actual words of the actors as organizers. She also provides thick descriptions of the setting and the actors, reproduces the actors' language verbatim, and fully describes what she observed during the program. She connects the experience of the seven actors through a process of triangulation that is implied, but not made explicit. She invited the actors to participate fully in the research and to review the findings. The thick descriptions that the author provides, as well as the sample she chose, make it likely that a reader with an interest in improving life outcomes for at-risk youths would resonate with the study and find the findings transferable to another context.

CHAPTER FIVE

1. The major difference between an ethnography and a case study has to do with purpose. The purpose of an ethnography is to understand and interpret a culture or cultural group, while the purpose of a case study is to focus on a specific phenomenon or event. Ethnographies and case studies both depend on multiple sources of data (observations, interviews, and documents/ discourses); however, case studies depend more on structured interviews, while ethnographies depend more on observations and informal interviews. Ethnographies and case studies both involve some form of participant observation and researcher presence in the field; however, ethnographies require fuller immersion and prolonged engagement on site.

Although both phenomenological and narrative studies rely on interviews, they have different purposes and research stances. Phenomenological studies investigate lived human experiences and the meanings these experiences hold for actors; they search for the "essences" of a phenomenon from the perspectives of those who experience it. Narrative studies, on the other hand, describe and give meaning to the lived experiences of individuals through a collaborative process of storytelling that brings order and coherence to the complexity of human lives. In a phenomenological study, the researcher assumes a neutral stance; in a narrative study, the researcher and the narrator become partners in constructing the narrator's story.

Qualitative document analysis and critical discourse analysis both examine the meaning of written documents that are not authored by the researchers. They differ in the stance researchers take toward the documents under study and the goals of analysis. Although researchers engaging in both these types of text analysis tend to use the analytic methods associated with grounded theory, researchers doing critical discourse analysis do so with the aim of identifying underlying ideologies and power relationships. It is content analysis with a political purpose.

2.

	Article 1	Article 2
Title in APA format	Turner, W. G. (2007). Experiences of offenders in a prison canine program. *Federal Probation, 71*(1), 38–43.	Pelto-Piri, V., Engström, K., & Engström, I. (2012). The ethical landscape of professional care in everyday practice as perceived by staff: A qualitative content analysis of ethical diaries written by staff in child and adolescent psychiatric in-patient care. *Child and Adolescent Psychiatry and Mental Health, 6*(1), 18.
Type of design	Phenomenological study	Qualitative document analysis
Research questions/ purpose	How do prison inmates experience a therapy dog-training program?	What are the situations and experiences that gave rise to ethical problems and considerations as recorded in staff journals?
Research stance	Researcher as neutral recorder	Researcher as neutral observer
Data source(s)	Interviews with six prison inmates	Diaries of 68 psychiatric ward staff members
Data analysis	Code-and-retrieve method	Development of meaning units, reduced to themes
Guiding question for trustworthiness	Does the study capture the experience of prison inmates involved in the program?	Does the analysis uncover ethical concerns that appear in the diaries?

3. The two articles are examples of nonethnographic qualitative research methods. The Turner article is an example of a phenomenological study, which relied solely on interviews from six inmates. The Pelto-Piri et al. study is a qualitative content analysis, which used as data the written diaries from 68 subjects. It offers the more complete description of the research process: the purpose, the sampling, and the collection and analysis of data. It meets the criteria for high levels of trustworthiness and transferability through its thick description, sampling, and process of data reduction and theme and pattern development. The Turner study does not provide enough information about data analysis and reduction to warrant as high a rating.

CHAPTER SIX

1. *Sampling*: Quantitative researchers select samples that will allow them to generalize findings to similar samples and populations, whereas qualitative researchers select samples that will allow them to understand and interpret a specific setting, group, event, or phenomenon from a specific context. For quantitative researchers, the most desirable way to select a sample and/or assign a sample to groups is through randomization. Because this is often difficult, they will use convenience/volunteer or intact group sampling and try either to match subjects or to correct for differences. Qualitative researchers use purposeful or theoretical sampling strategies; the choice depends on their professional assessment of the situation.

Data collection: Quantitative researchers use measures that are vetted for validity and reliability, usually through calculation of the coefficient of correlation (*r*). These measures usually use response formats that allow for mathematical calculations of central tendency and standard deviation, though they may include open-ended questions that are then quantified. Qualitative researchers are themselves the instruments for data collection, and they collect data through observations, interviews, and documents/discourses.

2. NAEP, TIMSS, and PISA all use very complex random sampling strategies that do a good job in identifying a representative sample. An Internet search garnered the following information:

> [For NAEP] probability samples of schools and students are selected to represent the diverse student population in the United States. The numbers of schools and students vary from cycle to cycle, depending on the number of subjects and items to be assessed. A national sample will have sufficient schools and students to yield data for public schools, each of the four NAEP regions of the country, as well as sex, race, degree of urbanization of school location, parent education, and participation in the National School Lunch Program. . . . Typically, 30 students per grade per subject are selected randomly in each school. Some of the students who are randomly selected may be classified as students with disabilities (SD) or as English language learners (ELL). NAEP's goal is to assess all students in the sample. (*http://nces.ed.gov/nationsreportcard/about/nathow.asp*)

> TIMSS . . . employ[s] [a] two-stage random sample design, with a sample of schools drawn as a first stage and one or more intact classes of students selected from each of the sampled schools as a second stage. Intact classes of students are sampled rather than individuals from across the grade level or of a certain age because TIMSS . . . pay[s] particular attention to students' curricular and instructional experiences, and these typically are organized on a classroom basis. Sampling intact classes also has the operational advantage of less disruption to the school's day to day business than individual student sampling. (*http://timssandpirls.bc.edu/methods/pdf/TP_Sampling_Design.pdf*)

PISA uses a six-step sampling process, according to one website (*http://nces.ed.gov/surveys/pisa/faq.asp#4*):

> *Step 1:* . . . PISA selects a sample of students that represents the full population of 15-year-old students in each participating country or education system. This population is defined internationally as 15-year-olds (15 years and 3 months to 16 years and 2 months at the beginning of the testing period) attending both public and private schools in grades 7–12. Each country or education system submits a sampling frame to the consortium of organizations responsible for the implementation of PISA 2015 internationally. Westat, a survey research firm in Rockville, Maryland, contracted by the OECD [Organization for Economic Co-operation and Development], then validates each country or education system's frame.

> *Step 2:* Once a sampling frame is validated, Westat draws a scientific random sample of a minimum of 150 schools from each frame with two replacement schools for each original school, unless there are less than 150 schools, in which case all schools would be sampled. A minimum of 50 schools were sampled for benchmarking participants (e.g., U.S. states that opt to participate in 2015). The list of selected schools, both original and replacement, is delivered to each education system's PISA national center. Countries and education systems do not draw their own samples.

> *Step 3:* Each country/education system is responsible for recruiting the sampled schools. They begin with the original sample and only use the replacement schools if an original school refuses to participate. In accordance with PISA guidelines, replacement schools are identified by assigning the two schools neighboring the sampled school in the frame as substitutes to be used in instances where an original sampled school refuses to participate. Replacement schools are required to be in the same implicit stratum (i.e., have similar demographic characteristics) as the sampled school. A minimum participation rate of 65 percent of schools from the original sample of schools is required for a country or education system's data to be included in the international database.

Step 4: After schools are sampled and agree to participate, students are sampled. Each country/education system submits student listing forms containing all age-eligible students for each of their schools using Key Quest, the internationally provided software.

Step 5: Westat carefully reviews the student lists and uses sophisticated software to perform data validity checks to compare each list against what is known of the schools (e.g., expected enrollment, gender distribution) and PISA eligibility requirements (e.g., grade and birthday ranges). The selected student samples are then sent back to each national center. Unlike school sampling, students are not sampled with replacement.

Step 6: Schools inform students of their selection to participate on assessment day. Student participation must be at least 80 percent for a country's/education system's data to be reported by the OECD.

3. The ACT technical manual (*www.act.org/aap/pdf/ACT_Technical_Manual.pdf*) provides the following information for the ACT:

   a. *Sample size and strategy*: Sample size: 2,981 college-bound seniors (1995).

      Strategy: Stratified random sample, weighted by gender, race/ethnic origin, school affiliation, and geographic region.

   b. *Response formats*: Multiple-choice questions (English, math, reading, and science) and an optional extended essay-writing sample.

   c. *Reliability and validity*: Equivalent forms reliability on subtests (r = .74 to .97).

      Content validity based on test specifications.

A report from the College Board (*http://research.collegeboard.org/sites/default/files/publications/2012/7/researchnote-2005-24-reliability-skills-measured-sat.pdf*) provides the following information for the SAT:

   a. *Sample size and strategy*: The SAT was renormed in 1995. Using as its reference group the over 1 million students who took the test in 1995, the test developers applied a complex algorithm to realign the scores in accordance with new demographics. The original norms were set with a random sample of 10,000 students in 1943.

   b. *Response format*: A majority of multiple-choice questions, with a few open-response questions plus an extended essay for a writing sample.

   c. *Validity and reliability*: Predictive validity of the SAT to freshman GPA (r = .49 to .53). Internal reliability (r = .69 to .84 for Critical Reading and Mathematics, .40 to .67 for Writing). Equivalent forms reliability (r = −.80 to .91).

4. A section of the PDK/Gallup Poll website (*www.gallup.com/178685/methodology-center.aspx*) provides the following information:

   a. *Sampling*: The typical Gallup/PDK Poll includes a sample of 1,000 adult Americans over the age of 18, who are drawn from a population of over 60,000 members of what is called the Gallup Panel. It is described as follows:

      The Gallup Panel is one of the nation's few research panels that is representative of the entire U.S. adult population. Members can be reached via phone, Web, or mail. The Gallup Panel allows for a quick "pulse" of U.S. adults' opinions on some of the most pressing issues. Gallup started the Panel in 2004, and it is not an opt-in panel. Gallup maintains demographic profiles of all Gallup Panel members, using this information to draw stratified samples or samples of low-incidence populations that are otherwise difficult to reach.

The Gallup Panel is a multimode Panel with approximately 60,000 members, all of whom can be reached via phone. About 50,000 members can be reached by email to complete a Web survey. Panel members that cannot be contacted by email can be reached by mail. Gallup selects potential panel members using random-digit-dialing (RDD) of landline telephones and cellphones or address-based sampling (ABS) to contact U.S. households at random. Gallup purchases samples for this study from Survey Sampling International (SSI) and Marketing Systems Group (MSG). Because Gallup selects respondents at random, and because all U.S. households have an equal and known probability for selection, the Panel is a representative sample of all American households.

> . . . Gallup weights samples to correct for unequal selection probability and nonresponse. Gallup also weights its final samples to match the U.S. population according to gender, age, race, Hispanic ethnicity, education, and region. Demographic weighting targets are based on the most recent Current Population Survey figures for the aged 18 and older U.S. population.

b. *Response formats*: Multiple-choice, rank-ordered, or dichotomous questions are used, as are Likert-type scales. There is one open-response question.

c. *Validity and reliability*: An Internet search provided no information about the validity and reliability of the poll.

5. The article I found was this one:

> Prothmann, A., Bienert, M., & Ettrich, C. (2006). Dogs in child psychotherapy: Effect on state of mind. *Anthrozoös, 19*(3), 265–277.

a. *Sample*: A convenience sample of 100 children and adolescents ages 11–20, who were undergoing inpatient psychiatric treatment. Intact groups were used; 61 participants were in the treatment group, and the other 39 served as the control group.

b. *Measure*: The Basler Befindlichkeits-Skala (BBS) was used. The authors note that the BBS is "a self-rating method to measure changes in state of mind over time" (p. 268), and that it measures general state of mind, vitality, alertness, social extroversion, and intraemotional balance on four subscales. The authors do not provide specific data on reliability and validity indicators.

6. The Woodcock–Johnson IV (2014) is published by Riverside Publishing. It is a norm-referenced assessment battery that is composed of three individual batteries that can be given individually or together. The three batteries are the Woodcock–Johnson IV Tests of Cognitive Abilities (COG), the Woodcock–Johnson IV Tests of Oral Language (OL), and the Woodcock–Johnson IV Tests of Achievement (ACH). The battery is primarily used in special education for diagnostic purposes. The information presented below is summarized from the WJ IV Assessment Service Bulletin Number 2 (LaForte, McGrew, & Schrank, 2014).

Normative data for the WJ IV were gathered from 7, 416 subjects in the following grades: preschool (n = 664), kindergarten to grade 12 (n = 3,891), college/university (n = 775), and adults over 18 who were not in school or college (n = 2,086). The test developers selected a random sample of participants from a larger stratified random sample that represented different census regions, community types, gender, country of birth, races/ethnicities, parents' level of education, and school type.

As noted, the WJ IV has three parts:

1. The Tests of Cognitive Abilities (COG) assess comprehension, fluid reasoning, short-term working memory, processing speed, auditory processing, long-term retrieval, visualization processes, and information knowledge.

2. The Tests of Oral Language (OL) assess language development, listening ability, phonetic coding, naming facility, and speed and ideational fluency.

3. The Tests of Achievement (ACH) assess reading and writing ability, quantitative knowledge, and content knowledge in science, social studies, and humanities.

The batteries were tested extensively for validity. Content validity was established through expert consensus. Concurrent validity was established through studies with 14 measures. The COG was correlated with 5 measures and had evidence of strong validity (median $r = .74$). The OL was correlated with 4 measures and showed the strongest correlation with oral language (median $r = .71$) and the weakest correlation with speed (median $r = .41$). The ACH was correlated with 5 measures and evidenced the strongest correlations (median $r = .85–.93$). The authors conclude "The procedures used to develop and validate the WJ IV have produced a diagnostic system that can be used with confidence in a variety of settings" (p. 37).

Strong reliabilities were also established for the battery. Reliability coefficients were calculated for each test within each of the three batteries. The median reliabilities for the COG was $r = .90–.97$; for the OL: $r = .89–.95$; and for the ACH: $r = .92–.99$.

CHAPTER SEVEN

1. The *mean* is the average of values that is computed by summing the values and dividing by the number of the values. The *median* is the halfway point of the scores when they are in descending or ascending order; in other words, it represents the point that 50% of scores fall below and 50% fall above. The mean is influenced by the number of high and low values; the median is not.

2. Examples of pie charts, bar graphs, and line graphs from the 2012 SAT Report for Maine.

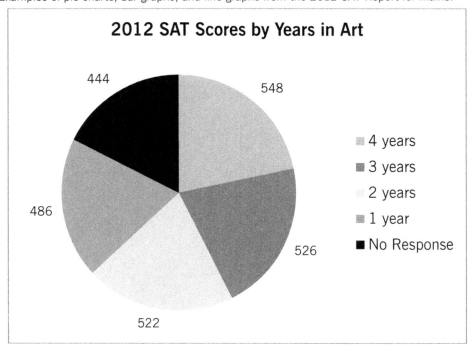

2012 SAT Scores by Years in Art

444
548
4 years
3 years
2 years
1 year
No Response
486
526
522

SAT Score by Family Income

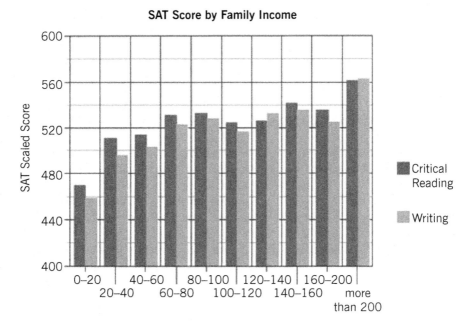

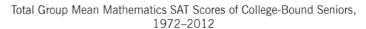

Annual Family Income in Thousands of Dollars

Total Group Mean Mathematics SAT Scores of College-Bound Seniors, 1972–2012

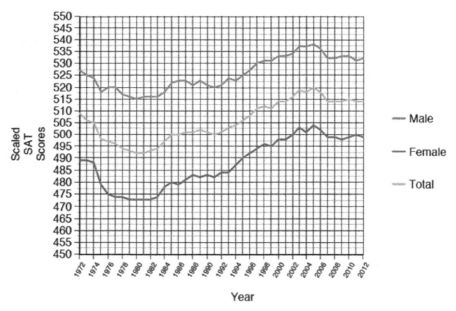

Year

3. Frequency table of test scores on ninth-grade algebra final, all sections:

Score	Frequency	%
90–100	15	15
80–89.9	25	25
70–79.9	40	40
60–69.9	14	14
Below 60	6	6
Total	100	100

4. Stem-and-leaf plot of test scores on ninth-grade algebra final, honors section:

Stem/Leaf
9/8,8,6,6,4,4,2,0
8/8,8,8,6,6,6,4,4,8
7/8,8,6

5. Computation of mean and standard deviation for the scores in honors algebra:

Mean = 88.2 $SD = 6.5827$

CHAPTER EIGHT

1. Terms in Column A matched to answers in Column B:

Column A	Column B
independent variable	the causal variable
true experiment	random assignment to groups
alpha	$p \leq .05$, used in hypothesis testing
null hypothesis	predicts no difference in outcome
effect size	magnitude of difference
Type I error	rejects the null hypothesis when it is true
internal validity	effect is due to the cause
t-test	test for significance

2. The article I found was this one:

Minatrea, N. B., & Wesley, M. C. (2008). Reality therapy goes to the dogs. *International Journal of Reality Therapy, 28*, 69–77.

Research Review

The research review examines literature in two areas: choice theory/reality therapy (CT/RT) and the use of animal-assisted therapy (AAT) in developing therapist–client alliances in mental health counseling. It includes sections on the alliances in counseling involving both the general population and people addicted to or abusing substances. The review is very comprehensive and includes well over 50 references to research spanning a quarter of a century, with a sufficient number of recent publications. Based on the research review, the authors have stated the research question thus: "Does AAT make a difference in the therapeutic alliance when treating individuals abusing or addicted to substances in a group counseling modality using CT or RT as the counseling theory?" (p. 72).

Purpose and Design

The purpose of the study was to see whether there would be significant differences in the therapeutic alliance with patients addicted to/abusing substances when AAT was added to CT/RT in counseling sessions. The IV was CT/RT with AAT. The DV was the therapeutic alliance. This study was designed as a posttest-only true experiment, with a control group and a treatment group.

Sampling

The sample consisted of 24 individuals residing in a treatment facility, all of whom met the criteria for substance addiction/abuse. Members of the sample had been previously screened and were assessed on the Pet Attitude Scale. Subjects were randomly assigned to control and treatment groups, which made this a true experiment, as noted above. The same therapist treated both groups. She used CT/RT approaches with both groups and added ATT with the treatment group. The therapy dog was a 7-year-old beagle mix.

Data Collection

The researchers administered the Helping Alliance Questionnaire–II (HAQ-II) to measure the therapeutic alliance. They also administered the Session Rating Scale (SRS) and monitored blood pressure. All of the measures were administered at the end of the treatments. No information is provided about the validity and reliability of these measures, although they seem to have been used extensively in this line of research.

Data Analysis, Interpretation, and Conclusions

Although several measures are reported as having been administered, the authors only report data on the HAQ-II. They used a series of one-way analyses of variance (ANOVAs) and found significant differences at $p < .001$ in the clients' perceptions of the therapeutic relationship. The authors state, "A review of effect size completed for each variable suggests [that] the addition of AAT contributed most of the differences observed for the HAQ-II ratings" (p. 72). No specific effect sizes are indicated, however.

Evaluation

I give this study an overall rating of moderate. The theory and treatment merit a moderate to strong rating. The research review establishes the case for AAD, and the treatment closely followed the theory and was well controlled, with the use of the same therapist for the control and treatment groups. The sample and sampling are likewise rated moderate to strong. Although the sample size was a bit limited for an experiment, it was strong in appropriateness and in the random assignment of subjects to groups. The collection and analysis of data earn only a moderate rating, however. Validity and reliability tests were applied, but are not made explicit.

Results are only reported on one measure. The authors' conclusions about what the effect sizes "suggested" are somewhat vague and unsubstantiated.

CHAPTER NINE

1. The article I found was this one:

> Somervill, J. W., Kruglikova, Y. A., Robertson, R. L., Hanson, L. M., & MacLin, M. H. (2008). Physiological responses by college students to a dog and a cat: Implications for pet therapy. *North American Journal of Psychology, 10,* 519–528.

Research Review

The review establishes a theoretical foundation for the experiment. The review is current and includes articles that appeared within 5 years of its publication. More than 10 studies are reviewed. There were two research questions: (1) Would blood pressure and pulse significantly differ in reactions to a dog or cat? (2) Would the sequence of the presentation of the dog and cat significantly affect blood pressure and pulse? "It was tentatively hypothesized that participants would show a reduction in blood pressure while handling both a dog and a cat. It was also speculated that male and female participants would react differently to a dog versus a cat" (p. 519).

Purpose and Design

The purpose of the study was "(a) to assess the effects of limited exposure to an unfamiliar dog versus an unfamiliar cat on blood pressure and pulse rate on male and female college students, and (b) to increase physical interaction with the animals by having participants hold each animal in their lap for a five minute period" (p. 521). This was a repeated-measures design with a single group. Each participant held both a dog and a cat for 5 minutes, and the order of presentation was altered.

Sample

The sample size was $n = 62$. Sample characteristics were as follows: For the 28 males, age range = 18–29, mean age = 20.04, median age = 19; 22 of the males were European Americans and 4 were African Americans. For the 34 females, age range = 18–24, mean age = 19.21, median age = 19; 32 of the females were European Americans, 1 was an African American, and 1 was of unspecified race/ethnicity.

Data Collection

There were two DVs. Blood pressure was measured by the Health-o-Meter Model 7631; reliability and validity were implied. Pulse readings were taken by two research assistants; no indication of interrater reliability was provided. There were a total of 10 blood pressure and pulse readings; these readings were taken once at the beginning and once at the end of nine 5-minute intervals.

> During the third and seventh 5-minute interval, each participant held either a dog or cat in their laps for the full 5-minute period. The order of presentation of a dog or cat was alternated. Measurements

taken before and after the first, fifth, and ninth 5-minute interval served as baselines during which no animal was present. Between readings, casual conversation was encouraged. A second person was always in the room to ensure that the animal remained in the participant's lap during the third and seventh 5-minute time period. (p. 522)

Data collection therefore matched the purpose of the study.

Data Analysis, Interpretation, and Conclusions

Data were analyzed by using *t*-tests and ANOVAs.

Main effects: (1) Combined effect for all time periods: Males had slightly higher (but not significantly higher) systolic blood pressure, $F (1, 60) = 4.494$, $p < .038$; females had significantly higher pulse rate, $F (1, 60) = 7.748$, $p < .007$. (2) When animals were held on laps: No significant differences between males and females on systolic blood pressure, $F (1, 60) = 0.226$, $p < .636$, or diastolic blood pressure, $F (1, 60) = 1.491$, $p < .227$; however, females had a significantly higher pulse rate, $F (1, 60) = 6.289$, $p < .015$. (3) Time period immediately following holding an animal: Females had significantly lower systolic blood pressure, $F (1, 60) = 23.64$, $p < .001$, but not diastolic blood pressure, $F (1, 60) = 4.52$, $p < .011$.

Covariates were (1) liking or disliking cats or dogs and (2) dog ownership. Data on these covariates were derived from a survey of participants; no significant differences were found.

The data analysis thus matched the research question and purpose. The interpretation and conclusions stay close to the data; the researchers do not overconclude.

Evaluation

Overall rating = Strong.

Theory and treatment = Strong. Well-developed theory; the treatment fit the theory.

Sample and sampling = Moderate to strong. Convenience sample of adequate size, which is described in detail and was appropriate for the study.

Data collection and analysis = Strong. Reliable and valid measures. Use of *t*-tests and ANOVAs for analyzing the main effects and the covariates was appropriate.

CHAPTER TEN

1. The purpose of single-subject studies is to investigate the effectiveness of a specific intervention on a limited number of subjects, who are individually administered a treatment and measured separately.

2. Using an electronic database, I searched for a single-subject study that was related to the use of animal-assisted therapy as a treatment option for students who were referred to me. Finding none, I changed my search for this task and looked for a single-subject study that focused on the effectiveness of an intervention in reducing aggressive behavior, which is one of the issues that I deal with in my work. This is the article I chose for my critique:

   Gaines, T., & Barry, L. M. (2008). The effect of a self-monitored relaxation breathing exercise on male adolescent aggressive behavior. *Adolescence, 43*(170), 291–302.

Research Review

The research review examines over 30 empirical studies that investigated the effectiveness of successful interventions that reduce aggressive behaviors. The authors note that most of the studies under review examined the combination of two treatments: anger management techniques and relaxed breathing exercises. Through the review of recent and relevant literature, the authors establish the need to examine the efficacy of a single-component treatment in reducing aggressive behavior.

Purpose, Design, and Sample

The purpose of the study was to "assess the effects of an isolated relaxation breathing exercise (RBE) applied to adolescent males in a juvenile justice residential program" (p. 293). The study was "single-subject with multiple baselines across 6 subjects on 2 behavioral measures" (p. 291) and used an ABAB design. The sample consisted of six males between the ages of 15 and 18 who had been recommended as having anger management and impulse control issues, and who had been in residence for more than 1 month. Given the specificity of the research purpose, this is an appropriate sample. The sample size is consistent with the conventions of single-subject research. The target behaviors were the same for all subjects: a reduction in inappropriate behaviors and inappropriate language use. The treatment lasted over 14 days, and there was a withdrawal phase of 2 days.

Data Collection, Analysis, Interpretation, and Conclusions

The direct care staff at the facility were trained to use a daily checklist in which they recorded each subject's behaviors and language. At the end of the day, each subject was given a rating of 0–100. At all times, two staff members were present during observations. In addition, each subject recorded his behaviors after the breathing exercises were introduced. The scores of staff members and subjects were compared for reliability. Maintenance was obtained under the usual conditions at the facility when there were no scheduled interventions. The data were displayed in graphs. Results were mixed: Only one of the subjects showed marked improvement in both behavior and language use over time. The other subjects were less consistent, though none increased the frequency of inappropriate behavior or language use. The researchers are very careful to note the limitations of the study and the possibility of observer effects. They do not overconclude and recommend that further research on single components of dual-treatment interventions be conducted.

Evaluation

Theory and treatment = Strong. The review establishes the empirical evidence supporting a dual-intervention strategy for reducing aggressive behavior and language, and the authors make a case for investigating the efficacy of a single intervention.

Sample and sampling = Strong. The sample size and subject characteristics were very appropriate. The criteria for selection of subjects were also appropriate for a single-subject study.

Data collection and analysis = Moderate. The measurement was weak. The authors note the need for greater reliability measures for the observations, and suggest that future investigations include two independent observers as well as subject self-report. The data analysis was strong, and evidence is presented visually in detailed graphs.

CHAPTER ELEVEN

1a. *Similarities:* Both examine differences in outcomes between groups and apply tests of significance to outcomes.

   Differences: Nonexperimental group comparisons compare differences that already exist between or among existing membership groups; they do not involve an intervention on the part of the researcher; the researcher does not control the IV; the comparisons may demonstrate differences on both continuous and categorical variables; and they do not demonstrate causality.

1b. In analyzing continuous DVs, researchers use the same procedures and tests of significance as they do in analyzing DVs in experiments. That is, they begin by calculating means and standard deviations, and then use one of these tests of significance: t-test, ANOVA, MANOVA, ANCOVA, or MANCOVA. In analyzing categorical DVs, researchers begin by calculating frequencies for each DV in terms of percentages, and then use the chi-square (χ^2) as the test of significance.

2. In my search for a nonexperimental group comparison article, I did not find any articles about animal-assisted therapy that met my criteria. So, instead, I searched for a group comparison article that looked at the quality of life for students with and without behavioral disabilities.

   > Sacks, G., & Kern, L. (2008). A comparison of quality of life variables for students with emotional and behavioral disorders and students without disabilities. *Journal of Behavioral Education, 17*, 111–127.

Research Review

The research review examines 29 articles and scholarly works that dealt with the construct of quality of life (QoL) and its relation to students with diagnosed emotional and behavioral disabilities. The authors define the construct of QoL derived from this review as follows:

> The individual's perceptions of their position in life in the context of the culture and value systems in which they live and in relation to their goals, expectations, standards, and concerns. It is a broad-ranging concept affected in a complex way by the person's physical health, psychological state, level of independence, social relationships, and their relationship to salient features in their environment. (p. 112)

The review does establish a useful construct for the study.

Purpose and Design

The purpose of this nonexperimental group comparison study was to examine differences in QoL assessments between students with and without emotional and behavioral disorders (EBD). The authors examined the following research questions:

1. Does the QoL for middle and high school students with EBD differ from the QoL of their peers without disabilities?
2. What specific QoL domains differ between students with EBD and their peers without disabilities?
3. Does QoL differ between students with EBD in public versus private schools?
4. Does QoL differ between students with EBD in middle versus high school?

5. Does QoL differ for male versus female students with EBD?
6. Do parents' ratings of their adolescents' QoL differ from the adolescents' self-ratings of QoL, and are ratings consistent across dyads including students with and without EBD?

Five group comparisons were studied:

Middle and high school students with EBD/without EBD

Public school students with EBD/private school students with EBD

Middle school students with EBD/high school students with EBD

Male students with EBD/female students with EBD

Parents of students with EBD/parents of students without EBD

Each group comparison served as an IV. The DV was QoL, which was a continuous variable.

Sample and Sampling

The sample consisted of 185 students from a volunteer convenience sample of three public middle schools, two public high schools, and two private schools serving students with EBD.

	EBD	Non-EBD
Gender		
Female	16	59
Male	67	40
Total	86	99
School level		
Middle school		
Public	22	96
Private	27	0
Total	49	96
High school		
Public	12	3
Private	25	0
Total	37	3

In addition, 32 parents of students with EBD and 42 parents of students without EBD volunteered to be in the sample of parent responders.

Data Collection

As stated previously, the IVs were the five comparison groups and the DV was QoL. The DV was measured with the Youth Quality of Life—Revised (YQOL) Perceptual and Contextual surveys. These surveys use Likert scales as the response format and measure the four domains of Self, Relationships, Environments, and General QoL. The Perceptual survey includes 41 statements with responses on a 1–10 scale (from "not at all" to "a great deal"); the Contextual survey includes 15 questions with responses on a 5-point scale (from "never" to "very often"). The parents received a modified version of the survey. The YQOL was vetted for convergent and dominant validity on six instruments, with $r = .94$ to $.96$. Reliability had been established on a predominantly white sample; the authors determined that it did not apply to this sample, which was disproportionately nonwhite.

Data Analysis, Interpretation, and Conclusion

Since the DV was a continuous variable, the authors used ANOVA and MANOVA as the statistical tests of significance. For Question 1, a two-way ANOVA was used; for Questions 2, 3, 4, 5, and 6, a MANOVA was used. The results were as follows:

Question 1: Students with EBD had significantly lower QoL scores ($p < .001$).

Question 2: Students with EBD had significantly lower scores on all four domains ($p = .02$).

Question 3: Private school students with EBD scored significantly higher on the domains of Self ($p < .001$) and Environments ($p = .02$).

Question 4: There were no statistically significant differences between middle and high school students.

Question 5: There were no statistically significant differences between males and females.

Question 6: Parents of students with EBD rated these students significantly lower on the Self ($p < .02$) and Environments ($p = .06$) domains; parents of students without EBD rated these students significantly higher on the General QoL ($p = .01$) and Self ($p = .007$) domains.

The authors conclude that "adolescents with EBD are significantly more dissatisfied with their QoL as well as subareas (Self, Relationships, and Environments) than their non-EBD peers" (p. 123) and state that they did not expect to find that the students with EBD in the special-purpose private schools were more satisfied than their peers in public school. The authors carefully note the limitations of the study, but also state that the results offer "intriguing directions and interesting patterns that merit future follow-up in future research" (p. 123).

Evaluation

I rate this study overall as strong. In regard to a framing construct, it provides a clear definition of QoL and uses this construct to frame the study in a useful way. In terms of sample and sampling, the study earns a rating of moderate. It is limited in that it depended on a volunteer sample and that the sample did not include any students without EBD from private high schools. Data collection and data analysis are both strong. The YQOL is a high-quality measure, with very high validity. The authors wisely decided not to accept the reliability findings because of the inappropriate sample used. The analysis was very strong; correct statistics were applied, and results are clearly reported both verbally and in tables. The authors do not overconclude and clearly state the limitations of the study.

CHAPTER TWELVE

1a. *Similarities:* Both group comparison studies and correlations studies are nonexperimental in nature; there is no intervention by the researcher; the researcher cannot manipulate variables; while these studies cannot demonstrate causality, they can make inferences about the statistical significance of findings; both types of studies are used when it is difficult to maintain the controlled conditions necessary for an experiment.

Differences: (i) Group comparisons investigate whether there are significant existing differences in DVs for existing membership groups; correlations investigate the direction and strength of relationships between and among variables, determine whether those relationships are statistically significant, and make predictions about the extent to which one variable (the PV) can predict the outcome on another variable (the CV). (ii) Group comparisons measure differences on both continuous and categorical DVs; correlations research usually investigates relationships between two continuous variables. (iii) Group comparisons test for statistical significance by consulting a table of critical values for either the t-test, ANOVA, MANOVA, ANCOVA, and MANCOVA, or the chi-square; correlations research establishes significance by consulting a table of critical values for correlations.

1b. The coefficient of correlation (r) describes the relationships between and among variables in terms of strength and direction.

1c. The coefficient of determination for predicting how one variable predicts an outcome on another variable is r^2; the coefficient of determination for determining how multiple variables predict the outcome on other variables is R^2 (or "big R^2").

1d. The statistical significance of a correlation tells the probability that the correlation is true. However, it is possible that a weak correlation can be statistically significant. It is still a weak correlation—and thus not very important, regardless of its statistical significance.

2. The regression study I chose was the following:

> Mathers, M., Canterford, L., Olds, T., Waters, E., & Wake, M. (2010). Pet ownership and adolescent health: Cross-sectional population study. *Journal of Paediatrics and Child Health, 46*, 729–735.

Research Review

The purpose of the review is to establish the need for the study. In the review, the authors cite evidence that pet ownership has positive effects on adults, and they make the case that little is known about its effects on children's health. The theory supporting the study is that pet ownership will increase the health of adolescents.

Purpose and Design

The purpose of the study was to show whether pet ownership would lead to healthy behaviors in adolescents. According to the authors, "It aims to determine whether adolescent health and well-being are associated with (i) having any pet in the household; (ii) having a dog; (iii) having a cat; (iv) having a horse/pony and (v) average daily time devoted to activity caring for the pet." PVs = dogs, cats, or other animals in the household; average daily time caring for pet. CVs = blood pressure, body mass index (BMI), daily activity level, health status, quality of life (p. 730).

Sample and Sampling

A stratified random sample ($n = 960$) was derived from a larger population involved in a longitudinal study from Victoria, Australia. The sample represented students from government, church, and independent private schools.

Data Collection

Data were collected on the DVs/CVs with the following measures:

- *Physical activity:* MARCA, an adolescent self-report software engine that decodes and analyzes daily diaries, was used to determine an overall daily physical activity level (PAL) in METs (Standard Metabolic Equivalent).

- *Blood pressure:* A digital blood pressure monitor (A&D Medical, San Jose, California, Model UA-787) was used by a trained researcher. Three measurements were taken, 1 minute apart. A mean score of the second and third readings was calculated. Systolic and diastolic blood pressure percentiles were calculated according to gender, age, and height.

- *Health status:* The Pediatric Quality of Life Inventory 4.0 (PedsQL 4.0, 13- to 18-year-old self-report and parent-proxy versions, 23 items) was used. Cronbach's alpha = .89 for adolescents, and = .92 for parents. This measure assesses physical, emotional, social, and school functioning, from which Physical and Psychosocial health summary scores were derived. The possible range of scores is 0–100, with 100 representing best possible health.

- *Quality of life:* KIDSCREEN, an adolescent self-report measure (10 items), was used. Cronbach's alpha = .82. This measure assesses the health-related quality of life of healthy and chronically ill children and adolescents ages 8–18 years. Ten domains are measured: physical well-being, psychological well-being, moods and emotions, self-perception, autonomy, parents' relations and home life, peers and social support relations, school environment, bullying, and financial resources. Higher scores indicate higher quality of life.

- BMI status was determined by a trained researcher who used a digital scale to measure weight to the nearest 100 grams and a portable rigid audiometer to measure height to .1 centimeter.

Data Analysis, Interpretation, and Conclusions

The authors used linear regression analysis for the continuous DVs/CVs and proportional odds ordinal logistic regression for the ADD categorical, BMI status outcome. The measurements were carried out separately for each of the IVs/PVs. Go to your library's database and find the interlibrary loan portal. Read the procedures for completing an interlibrary loan request, and complete a request for an article on your topic of interest. The analyses were adjusted for covariates of age and sex. The authors reported *p*-values and effect sizes for each combination of PV and CV. A significant finding was that average daily activity status and BMI were significantly related to health outcomes.

PV	CV
Cat ownership	Increase in blood pressure ($p = .03$)
Horse ownership	Increase in physical activity ($p = .03$)
Time spent in animal care	Decrease in BMI ($p = .001$)

The researchers found that owning a pet predicted few positive or negative outcomes for the adolescents in the study. They conclude:

> The results of this study are incongruent with Banman's and Rew's positive association between pet ownership and health outcomes in young people. . . . Thus, while pets may provide therapeutic benefits for vulnerable adolescent populations they do not seem to afford the same value to healthy adolescents in the community. (pp. 733–734)

They therefore do not overconclude and stay close to the data.

Evaluation

The overall quality of the Mathers et al. (2010) study is strong, as are all of its elements: theory or framing construct, sample and sampling, and data collection and analysis.

CHAPTER THIRTEEN

1. The mixed methods study I chose was the following:

   Ewing, C. A., MacDonald, P. M., Taylor, M., & Bowers, M. J. (2007). Equine-facilitated learning for youths with severe emotional disorders: A quantitative and qualitative study. *Child Youth Care Forum, 36,* 59–72.

   a. The research review focuses on equine-facilitated psychotherapy; in the authors' view, this research provided a strong rationale for investigating this type of therapy with at-risk adolescents. Although the authors have stated no explicit rationale for using a mixed methods approach, they do indicate that the qualitative findings illuminated the quantitative results.

   b. The purpose of the study was to investigate the effectiveness of an equine therapeutic approach on young adolescents with severe emotional disabilities.

   c. The design of this study was sequential explanatory; the quantitative component preceded the qualitative.

   d. The quantitative component of the study was weighted more heavily than the qualitative.

   e. *Quantitative results:* Five hypotheses were investigated: (i) Self-esteem would increase, as measured on a scale from the Harter Self-Perception Profile for Children; (ii) feelings of interpersonal empathy would increase, as measured by the Empathy Concern subscale of the Empathy Questionnaire; (iii) internal locus of control would increase, as measured by the Nowicki–Strickland Internal–External Control Scale for Children; (iv) feelings of depression would decrease, as measured by the Children's Depression Scale; and (v) feelings of loneliness would decrease, as measured by the Children's Loneliness Questionnaire. There were no significant differences between the control and treatment groups on the posttest.

   Qualitative results: Case studies of 4 of the 28 participants showed positive results. These were identified as (i) "the victim," a 10-year-old who suffered from posttraumatic stress disorder (PTSD), but learned to talk about her fears; (ii) "the feral child," an 11-year-old girl with multiple diagnoses who could not function in a regular classroom, but who eventually gained reentry into a mainstream class; (iii) "the runaway," a 13-year-old boy with ADHD who typically panicked and ran away, but who learned to build trust; and (iv) "the boost needed," a 10-year-old boy with a behavior disorder who became more successful in school.

   f. The two analyses were not particularly well integrated. The researchers express surprise in the article that the self-reports did not show significant changes. They attribute this to the severity of the young participants' behavioral problems, their past histories, and their relatively low IQ scores. They also question the validity of the measures with these subjects, many of whom had become overly familiar with self-reported psychological assessments. In effect, the researchers rely more on the qualitative findings, which give reason for optimism for this kind of therapy.

CHAPTER FOURTEEN

1. The program evaluation study I chose was the following:

    > Kemp, K., Signal, T., Botros, B., Taylor, N., & Prentice, K. (2014). Equine facilitated therapy with children and adolescents who have been sexually abused: A program evaluation study. *Journal of Child and Family Studies, 23*, 558–566.

    a. Purpose: To evaluate an equine-facilitated program run by Phoenix House, a sexual assault referral center in Queensland, Australia.

    b. Type of evaluation: Summative.

    c. There is no indication of who commissioned the evaluation. The evaluation was con- ducted by the authors; no institutional affiliations are provided in the article.

    d. Participants were assessed at three points: (1) upon intake and before counseling, (2) prior to beginning the equine-facilitated therapy and after counseling, and (3) upon completion of the equine-facilitated therapy. Measures of trauma symptoms/psycho- pathology for children were the Children's Depression Inventory and the Child Behav- ior Checklist; for adolescents, the measures were the Trauma Symptom Checklist, the Beck Depression Inventory, and the Beck Anxiety Inventory.

    e. Data were analyzed with repeated-measures ANOVA and paired *t*-tests. Differences in scores over time were statistically significant ($p > .001$), with effect sizes of 0.583 to 0.880 for the children and 0.702 to 0.905 for the adolescents.

    f. Ratings of this study in relation to the standards:
    > Utility: Strong
    > Feasibility: Strong
    > Propriety: Strong
    > Accuracy: Strong
    > Accountability: Strong

2. Both program evaluation and teacher evaluation are considered applied research. They are used in real-life situations for formative and summative purposes: to monitor and improve perfor- mance or to assess effectiveness with the aim of continuance or termination. They both gather evidence from a variety of data sources and report findings to specific stakeholders.

3. *Similarities:* Mixed methods research and program evaluation share a concern for accuracy in data collection, for having qualified people do the work, for proper analytic procedure, and for integrating findings when different methods are used.
    Differences: They differ in the audiences to whom they are accountable. Mixed methods research is accountable to an academic audience of peers; program evaluators are accountable to stakeholders. They also differ in purpose. The goal of mixed methods research is to add to a knowledge base in a particular area; the goal of program evaluation is to provide information for improving or terminating a program or activity.

CHAPTER FIFTEEN

1. *Similarities:* Chouinard and McPhail defined the "boy problem" in literacy in the same way— as the reluctance of boys to engage in literacy activities. They both started from the same

assumption: The approaches that their schools required in developing literacy were inappropriate for boys and failed to engage them. Both Chouinard and McPhail decided to develop new approaches. Chouinard developed a reading loft that was stocked with boy-friendly books, and he developed new assessments. McPhail devised a new approach to a Writer's Workshop. Both teachers decided to focus on particular students; Chouinard chose three students, and McPhail chose one.

Differences: The differences had to do with these teacher researchers' approaches to methodology, audience, and intention. Chouinard used a somewhat orthodox mixed methods approach to data collection and analysis, while McPhail kept a journal in which he reflected on what he observed and learned. As a result, two very different products were developed. Chouinard wrote an action research paper that followed the action research cycle, while McPhail wrote a reflective essay. Chouinard wrote for himself and the immediate audience of other teachers in his schools. McPhail wrote and published his findings for a wider audience. Chouinard's purpose was limited to improving his teaching practice with male student readers, while McPhail had a broader social agenda and tied his work to larger social issues.

2. *Step 1, identifying the problem:* The problem I want to address is whether the students who are referred to me as at risk of not graduating would respond to a horsemanship program. *Step 2, collecting and analyzing initial data:* I would want to review the literature on animal-assisted therapy, ideally with a focus on horsemanship programs for at-risk youth. I would also visit the horsemanship program that is 15 miles from my school. *Step 3, designing a plan of action:* I would gain permission from my principal and the school to pursue this study. I would explain my project to parents of at-risk students and seek their consent for their children's participation. I would explore the possibility of having the students earn credit for their participation. I would make sure that all participants knew what to expect.

3. I would like to explore journaling as the research typology to explore. I think that journaling would be very appropriate as I plan and execute my action research project. I think this would help me illuminate my practice and help me understand my students and myself better.

4. Since I could not find any action research projects on my topic, I returned to the topic of the Chouinard and McPhail pieces on developing literacy for this task.

Ziolkowski, J. (1999). "It's friendship, developing friendship": A teacher action research study on reading buddies. *Networks: An On-line Journal for Teacher Research, 2*(1).

Purpose: To better understand what was happening during reading buddies activities in Ziolkowski's middle school class. The author listed the following questions:

1. What is Reading Buddies all about?
2. What will I, as teacher, see taking place during buddies time?
3. Do other types of learning, besides the development of reading skills, take place in a buddies situation?
4. What are the benefits of reading buddies to the younger child?
5. Are there benefits for the older child? If so, what are these?

Methods: Data collection involved transcriptions of four conversations with students and personal journal entries, most of which were written from observations during reading buddy time. These entries included the following, according to the author:

- general and specific observations of student interactions
- what I saw, heard, and felt during reading buddies time

- personal notes and reflections on my research
- comments made by students or buddy teachers
- ideas/suggestions for the course of my research

Data analysis was based on Corsaro's field-note coding system for observations and journal entries, and on identifying matching patterns.

Findings: The focus of the findings was on the development of friendship from the point of view of the teachers and the students. The teachers saw a conflict between the purposes of developing friendship and developing reading skills, while the students saw no such conflict. The older students expressed feelings of gratification at being of assistance, as well as warmth, toward their younger reading buddies.

Usefulness: I think this is very useful to me as a practitioner, especially the way it uncovers the differences in perceptions of students and teachers.

Research or staff development: This study serves both purposes. It is high-quality research, and it also helped a teacher see her practice through new lenses.

CHAPTER SIXTEEN

1. I selected the following meta-analysis for examination:

   Chitic, V., Rusu, A. S., & Szamoskozi, S. (2012). The effects of animal assisted therapy on communication and social skills: A meta-analysis. *Transylvanian Journal of Psychology, 13*(1), 1–17.

   a. *Criteria for selecting articles:* Articles should cover only animal-assisted therapy. Articles should be published in English. Articles should provide data on improvement of social and communication skills. Effect size, descriptive statistics, and statistical significance should be provided.

   b. *Size of sample:* 16,026 potentially relevant studies; 15,994 were excluded due to irrelevance; 32 studies were selected for detailed examination; 28 were eliminated.

   c. *Average effect size of findings:* $d = 0.79$.

   d. *Conclusion:* Animal-assisted therapy has a large-magnitude positive effect on communication and social skills.

2. I selected the following metasynthesis for examination:

   Kramer, J. M., Olsen, S., Mermelstein, M., Balcells, A., & Liljenquist, K. (2012). Youth with disabilities' perspectives of the environment and participation: A qualitative meta-synthesis. *Child: Care, Health and Development, 38*(6), 763–777.

   a. *Criteria for selecting the population:* The authors searched six databases and reviewed 1,287 citations.

      Inclusion criteria [were as follows]: samples with youth ages 3–21 years and diagnosis of autism spectrum disorder, developmental disability (including physical disabilities), deafness or blindness, mental retardation/intellectual disability, and/or chronic illness; research completed in western countries; and studies that addressed participation in the home, school or community and at least one environmental component as defined by the ICF (International Classification of Functioning, Disability, and Health). Exclusion criteria [were as follows]: articles not written in English; not peer reviewed; sample of adults or youth with learning disabilities as primary disability; non-research articles; intervention studies; or other topics not relevant to the research question. (p. 764)

The initial pool was 1,287, of which 15 were selected; this represents the sample size.

b. *Sample size:* 15 qualitative studies.

c. *Design and procedures:* After the 15 studies were identified, the researchers did line-by-line coding and then used the constant comparative method to analyze results.

d. *Conclusions and implications:* The authors concluded, "This meta-synthesis revealed the youth's perspective that the social environment emerged as the factor most likely to influence youth's participation, resonating with findings from quantitative studies exploring barriers to participation" (p. 772).

References

About DMOZ. (2014, March 14). Retrieved from *www.dmoz.org/docs/en/about.html*.

Acklam, P. J. (2015). Random number generator. Retrieved from *http://stattrek.com/statistics/random-number-generator.aspx*.

Adams, E. (1999). Vocational teacher stress and internal characteristics. *Journal of Vocational and Technical Education, 16*(1), 7–22.

Adler, P. A., & Adler, P. (1994). Observational techniques. In N. Denzin & Y. Lincoln (Eds.), *Handbook of qualitative research* (pp. 377–392). Thousand Oaks, CA: Sage.

Agarwal, P. K., Karpicke, J. D., Kang, S. H. K., Roediger, H. L., & McDermott, K. B. (2008). Examining the testing effect with open- and closed-book tests. *Applied Cognitive Psychology, 22*, 861–876.

American Library Association. (2013). Interlibrary loans. Retrieved from *www.ala.org/tools/libfactsheets/alalibraryfactsheet08*.

American Psychological Association (APA). (2010). *Publication manual of the American Psychological Association* (6th ed.). Washington, DC: Author.

Anderson, G. L. (1989). Critical ethnography in education: Origins, current status, and new directions. *Review of Educational Research, 59*(3), 249–270.

Andiliou, A., & Murphy, P. K. (2010). Examining variations among researchers' and teachers' conceptualizations of creativity: A review and synthesis of contemporary research. *Educational Research Review, 5*(3), 201–219.

Argyris, C., Putnam, R., & Smith, D. (1985). *Action science: Concepts, methods and skills for research and intervention*. San Francisco, CA: Jossey-Bass.

Arizona Department of Education. (2014). Teacher/Principal Evaluation. Retrieved from *www.azed.gov/teacherprincipal-evaluation*.

Baer, D. M., Wolf, M. M., & Risley, T. R. (1968). Some current dimensions of applied behavior analysis. *Journal of Applied Behavior Analysis, 1*(1), 91–97.

Bailey, J., & Burch, M. (2002). *Research methods in applied behavior analysis*. Thousand Oaks, CA: Sage.

Bickman, L., & Rog, D. (Eds.). (2009). *The Sage handbook of applied social research methods* (2nd ed.). Thousand Oaks, CA: Sage.

Blumer, H. (1969). *Symbolic interactionism: Perspective and method*. Englewood Cliffs, NJ: Prentice-Hall.

Bogdan, R. C., & Biklen, S. K. (1982). *Qualitative research for education: An introduction to theory and methods*. Boston: Allyn & Bacon.

Bruyn, S. (1966). *The human perspective in sociology: The methodology of participant observation*. Englewood Cliffs, NJ: Prentice-Hall.

Bryman, A. (2007a). Barriers to integrating quantitative and qualitative research. *Journal of Mixed Methods Research, 1*(1), 8–22.

Bryman, A. (2007b). The research question in social research: What is its role? *International Journal of Social Research Methodology, 10*(1), 5–20.

Burgon, H. L. (2011). 'Queen of the world': Experiences of 'at-risk' young people participating in equine-assisted learning therapy. *Journal of Social Work Practice, 25*(2), 165–183.

Campbell, D. T., & Stanley, J. C. (1963). Experimental and quasi-experimental designs for research on teaching. In N. L. Gage (Ed.), *Handbook of research on teaching* (pp. 171–246). Chicago: Rand McNally.

Carrier, S. (2009). Environmental education in the schoolyard: Learning styles and gender. *Journal of Environmental Education, 40*(3), 2–12.

Carspecken, P. F. (1996). *Critical ethnography in educational research: A theoretical and practical guide*. New York: Routledge.

Cavagnetto, A. R. (2010). Argument to foster scientific literacy: A review of argument interventions in K–12 science contexts. *Review of Educational Research, 80*(3), 336–371.

Centre for Reviews and Dissemination (CRD). (2009). *Systematic reviews: CRD's guidance for undertaking reviews in health care*. York, UK: Author.

Charmaz, K. (2000). Grounded theory: Objectivist and constructivist methods. In N. K. Denzin & Y. S. Lincoln (Eds.), *Handbook of qualitative research* (2nd ed., pp. 509–535). Thousand Oaks, CA: Sage.

Charmaz, K. (2006). *Constructing grounded theory: A practical guide through qualitative analysis*. Thousand Oaks, CA: Sage.

Cheng, E. (2011). The role of self-regulated learning in enhancing learning performance. *International Journal of Research and Review, 6*(1), 1–16.

Chitic, V., Rusu, A. S., & Szamoskozi, S. (2012). The effects of animal assisted therapy on communication and social skills: A meta-analysis. *Transylvanian Journal of Psychology, 13*(1), 1–17.

Chouinard, D. (2011). *Underachieving males in reading: Exploring causes, examining attitudes, changing instruction, and improving literacy*. Unpublished master's action research project, University of Southern Maine.

Clandinin, D. J., & Huber, J. (2010). Narrative inquiry. In B. McGaw, E. Baker, & P. Peterson (Eds.), *International encyclopedia of education: Vol. 6* (3rd ed., pp. 436–441). New York: Elsevier.

Cochran-Smith, M., & Lytle, S. L. (1990). Research on teaching and teacher research: The issues that divide. *Educational Researcher, 19*(2), 2–11.

Cochran-Smith, M., & Lytle, S. L. (1993). *Inside/outside: Teacher research and knowledge*. New York: Teachers College Press.

Cochran-Smith, M., & Lytle, S. L. (2009). *Inquiry as stance: Practitioner research for the next generation*. New York: Teachers College Press.

Cohen, J. (1988). *Statistical power analysis for the behavioral sciences* (2nd ed.). Hillsdale, NJ: Erlbaum.

College Board. (2012). 2012 SAT college bound seniors total group report. Retrieved from *http://media.collegeboard.com/digitalServices/pdf/research/TotalGroup-2012.pdf.*

Connelly, F. M., & Clandinin, D. J. (2006). Narrative inquiry. In J. Green, G. Camilli, & P. Elmore (Eds.), *Handbook of complementary methods in education research* (3rd ed., pp. 375–385). Mahwah, NJ: Erlbaum.

Conners, C. K. (2008). *Conners 3rd Edition (Conners 3)*. Upper Saddle River, NJ: Pearson.

Cook, T. D., & Campbell, D. T. (1979). *Quasi-experimentation: Design and analysis issues for field settings*. Boston: Houghton Mifflin.

Cooper, H., Hedges, L. V., & Valentine, J. C. (Eds.). (2009). *The handbook of research synthesis and meta-analysis* (2nd ed.). New York: Russell Sage Foundation.

Cooper, H., Robinson, J. C., & Patall, E. A. (2006). Does homework improve academic achievement?: A synthesis of research, 1987–2003. *Review of Educational Research, 76*(1), 1–6.

Corey, S. (1953). *Action research to improve school practice*. New York: Teachers College, Columbia University.

Cranham, J., & Carroll, A. (2003). Dynamics within the bully/victim paradigm: A qualitative analysis. *Educational Psychology in Practice, 19*(2), 113–133.

Creswell, J. (2009). *Qualitative, quantitative and mixed methods*. Thousand Oaks, CA: Sage.

Crozier, S., & Tincani, M. J. (2007). Effects of social stories on prosocial behavior of preschool children with autism spectrum disorders. *Journal of Autism and Developmental Disorders, 37*(9), 1803–1814.

Cusick, P. (1983). *The egalitarian ideal and the American high school*. London and New York: Longman.

Darling-Hammond, L. (2013). *Getting teacher evaluation right: What really matters for effectiveness and improvement*. New York: Teachers College Press.

Davies, C. A. (1999). *Reflexive ethnography: A guide to researching selves and others*. New York: Routledge.

Definitions of anthropological terms. (2013). Retrieved from *http://oregonstate.edu/instruct/anth370/gloss.html*.

DeMilk, S. A. (2008). Experiencing attrition of special education teachers through narrative inquiry. *High School Journal, 92*(1), 22–32.

DiBasilio, A. (2008). *Reducing bullying in middle school students through the use of student-leaders*. Retrieved from ERIC database. (ED501251)

Duke, D., & Landahl, M. (2011). "Raising test scores was the easy part": A case study of the third year of school turnaround. *International Studies in Educational Administration, 39*(3), 91–114.

Economic Cooperation Organization (ECO). (2013). *ECO statistical report*. Retrieved from *www.eco-secretariat.org/ftproot/Publications/Annual_Economic_Report/2013/ECO%20Economy%202013.pdf*.

Eisenhart, M. (1991, October). *Conceptual frameworks for research circa 1991: Ideas from a cultural anthropologist. Implications for mathematics education researchers*. Paper presented at the 13th annual meeting of the North American Chapter of the International Group for the Psychology of Mathematics Education, Blacksburg, VA.

Eisenhart, M. (2001, September). *The meaning of culture in the practice of educational research in the U.S. and England*. Paper presented at the VIIIe Congrès International de l'Association pour la Recherche Interculturelle, Geneva, Switzerland.

Ewing, C. A., MacDonald, P. M., Taylor, M., & Bowers, M. J. (2007). Equine-facilitated learning for youths with severe emotional disorders: A quantitative and qualitative study. *Child Youth Care Forum, 36,* 59–72.

Fairclough, N. (1993). Critical discourse analysis and the marketization of public discourse: The universities. *Discourse and Society, 4*(2), 138–168.

Fairclough, N. (1995). *Critical discourse analysis: The critical study of language*. New York: Longman.

Fecho, B. (1993). Reading as a teacher. In M. Cochran-Smith & S. Lytle, *Inside/outside: Teacher research and knowledge* (pp. 265–272). New York: Teachers College Press.

Feldon, D., & Kefai, Y. (2008). Mixed methods for mixed reality: Understanding users' avatar activities in Virtual Worlds. *Educational Technology Research and Development, 56*(5–6), 575–593.

Fernald, J. (2002). *Preliminary findings on the relationship between SAT scores, high school GPA, socioeconomic status, and UCSC freshman GPA*. Santa Cruz: University of California, Santa Cruz.

Fetterman, D. M. (1989). *Ethnography step by step*. London: Sage.

Finfgeld, D. (2003). Metasynthesis: The state of the art—so far. *Qualitative Health Research, 13*(7), 893–904.

Foxx, R., & Meindl, J. (2007). The long-term successful treatment of the aggressive/destructive behaviors of a preadolescent with autism. *Behavioral Interventions, 22*(1), 83–97.

Frechtling, J., & Sharp, L. (Eds.). (1997). *User-friendly handbook for mixed method evaluations*. Washington, DC: National Science Foundation.

Freire, P. (1970). *Pedagogy of the oppressed*. New York: Continuum.

Friday Institute for Educational Innovation. (2009). *Formative evaluation report: North Carolina Virtual Public School*. Raleigh: North Carolina State University.

Gaines, T., & Barry, L. M. (2008). The effect of a self-monitored relaxation breathing exercise on male adolescent aggressive behavior. *Adolescence, 43*(170), 291–302.

Gasiewski, J., Eagan, M., Garcia, G., Hurtado, S., & Chang, M. (2012). From gatekeeping to engagement: A multi-contextual, mixed method study of student academic engagement in introductory STEM courses. *Research in Higher Education, 53*(2), 229–261.

Gaventa, J., & Cornwall, A. (2006). Challenging the boundaries of the possible: Participation, knowledge and power. *IDS Bulletin, 37*(6), 122–128.

Gee, J. (2004). Discourse analysis: What makes it critical? In R. Roberts (Ed.), *An introduction to critical discourse analysis in education* (pp. 19–50). Mahwah, NJ: Erlbaum.

Geertz, C. (1973). *The interpretation of cultures*. New York: Basic Books.

Gencosman, T., & Dogru, M. (2012). Effect of student teams–achievement divisions technique used in science and technology education on self-efficacy, test anxiety and academic achievement. *Journal of Baltic Science Education, 11*(1), 43–54.

Gibbs, G. R., Lewins, A., & Silver, C. (2005). What software does and does not do. Retrieved from *http://onlineqda.hud.ac.uk/Intro_CAQDAS/What_the_sw_can_do.php*.

Glaser, B., & Strauss, A. (1967). *The discovery of grounded theory*. Chicago: Aldine.

Glass, G. V. (1976). Primary, secondary, and meta-analysis of research. *Educational Researcher, 5*(10), 3–8.

Glass, G. V., McGaw, B., & Smith, M. L. (1981). *Meta-analysis in social research*. Beverly Hills, CA: Sage.

Gofin, R., & Avitzour, M. (2012). Traditional versus Internet bullying in junior high school students. *Maternal and Child Health Journal, 16*(8), 1625–1635.

Goldrick-Rab, S. (2010). Challenges and opportunities for improving community college student success. *Review of Educational Research, 80*(3), 437–469.

Guerra, N. G., Williams, K. R., & Sadek, S. (2011). Understanding bullying and victimization during childhood and adolescence: A mixed methods study. *Child Development, 82*(1), 295–310.

Hafeil, M., Stokrocki, M., & Zimmerman, E. (2005). Cross-site analysis of strategies used by three middle school art teachers to foster student learning. *Studies in Art Education, 46*(3), 242–254.

Hancock, D. R. (2002). Influencing graduate students' classroom achievement, homework habits and motivation to learn with verbal praise. *Educational Research, 44*(1), 83–95.

Harry, B., Sturges, K. M., & Klingner, J. K. (2005). Mapping the process: An exemplar of process and challenge in grounded theory analysis. *Educational Researcher, 34*(2), 3–13.

Hattie, J. (2009). *Visible learning: A synthesis of over 800 meta-analyses relating to achievement*. New York: Routledge.

Heron, J. (1996). *Cooperative inquiry: Research into the human condition*. London: Sage.

Holloway, I. (1997). *Basic concepts for qualitative research*. Oxford, UK: Blackwell Science.

Horizon Research. (2000). *Inside the classroom observation and analytic protocol*. Chapel Hill, NC: Author.

Horner, R., Carr, E., Halle, J., McGee, G., Odom, S., & Wolery, M. (2005). The use of single-subject research to identify evidence-based practice in special education. *Exceptional Children, 71*(2), 165–179.

Hull, G. A., & Zacher, J. (2007). Enacting identities: An ethnography of a job training program. *Identity: An International Journal of Theory and Research, 71*(1), 71–102.

International Society for Technology in Education (ISTE). (2008). Standards for teachers. Retrieved from *www.iste.org/standards/ISTE-standards/standards-for-teachers*.

Joe, S. (1993). Rethinking power. In M. Cochran-Smith & S. L. Lytle, *Inside/outside: Teacher research and knowledge* (pp. 290–298). New York: Teachers College Press.

Johnson, B., & Turner, L. (2003). Data collection strategies in mixed methods research. In A. Tashakkori & C. Teddlie (Eds.), *Handbook of mixed methods in social and behavioral research* (pp. 297–300). Thousand Oaks, CA: Sage.

Johnson, R. B., & Onwuegbuzie, A. J. (2004). Mixed methods research: A paradigm whose time has come. *Educational Researcher, 33*(7), 14–26.

Jumpp, D., & Strieb, L. Y. (1993). Journals for collaboration, curriculum, and assessment. In M. Cochran-Smith & S. L. Lytle (Eds.), *Inside/outside: Teacher research and knowledge* (pp. 141–149). New York: Teachers College Press.

Keen, E. (1975). *A primer in phenomenological psychology*. New York: Holt, Rinehart & Winston.

Kemp, K., Signal, T., Botros, B., Taylor, N., & Prentice, K. (2014). Equine facilitated therapy with children and adolescents who have been sexually abused: A program evaluation study. *Journal of Child and Family Studies, 23*, 558–566.

Kerlinger, F. N. (1986). *Foundations of behavioral research* (3rd ed.). New York: Holt, Rinehart & Winston.

Kramer, J. M., Olsen, S., Mermelstein, M., Balcells, A., & Liljenquist, K. (2012). Youth with disabilities' perspectives of the environment and participation: A qualitative meta-synthesis. *Child: Care, Health and Development, 38*(6), 763–777.

Krathwohl, D. (2004). *Methods of educational and social science research: The logic of methods*. Thousand Oaks, CA: Sage.

Krejcie, R. V., & Morgan, D. W. (1970). Determining sample size for research activities. *Educational and Psychological Measurement, 30*, 607–610.

Kuhn, T. S. (1962). *The structure of scientific revolutions.* Chicago: University of Chicago Press.

LaForte, E. M., McGrew, K. S., & Schrank, F. A. (2014). Woodcock Johnson IV Assessment service bulletin number 2: WJIV technical abstract. Retrieved from *http://www.assess.nelson.com/pdf/WJIVASB2.pdf.*

Lewin, K. (1946). Action research and minority problems. *Journal of Social Issues, 2*(4), 34–46.

Li, Q. (2006). Cyberbullying in schools: A research of gender differences. *School Psychology International, 27*(2), 157–170.

Library of Congress. (2011, September 13). Alcove 9: An annotated list of reference websites. Education: General educational resources and directories. Retrieved from *www.loc.gov/rr/main/alcove9/education/general.html.*

Lieblich, A., Tuval-Mashiac, R., & Zilber, T. (1998). *Narrative research.* London: Sage.

Light, R., & Pillemer, D. (1982). Numbers and narrative: Combining their strengths in research reviews. *Harvard Educational Review, 52*(1), 1–26.

Lim, K. Y., Lee, H. W., & Grabowski, B. (2009). Does concept-mapping strategy work for everyone?: The levels of generativity and learners' self-regulated learning skills. *British Journal of Educational Technology, 40*(4), 606–618.

Lincoln, Y., & Guba, E. (1985). *Naturalist inquiry.* London: Sage.

Lynd, R. S., & Lynd, H. M. (1929). *Middletown: A study in modern American culture.* New York: Harcourt, Brace.

Malinowski, B. (1922). *Argonauts of the Western Pacific: An account of native enterprise and adventure in the Archipelagoes of Melanesian New Guinea.* London: Routledge & Kegan Paul.

Marcus, G. E., & Cushman, D. (1982). Ethnographies as texts. *Annual Review of Anthropology, 11,* 25–69.

Marzano, R. J. (2003). *What works in schools.* Alexandria, VA: Association for Supervision and Curriculum Development.

Mathers, M., Canterford, L., Olds, T., Waters, E., & Wake, M. (2010). Pet ownership and adolescent health: Cross-sectional population study. *Journal of Paediatrics and Child Health, 46,* 729–735.

Mathison, S. (2008). What is the difference between evaluation and research—and why do we care? In N. L. Smith & P. R. Brandon (Eds.), *Fundamental issues in evaluation* (pp. 183–196). New York: Guilford Press.

McClelland, J. (1995). Sending children to kindergarten: A phenomenological study of mothers' experiences. *Family Relations, 44*(2), 177–183.

McCormick, S. (1995). What is single subject experimental research? In S. B. Neuman & S. McCormick (Eds.), *Single subject experimental research* (pp. 12–31). Newark, DE: International Reading Association.

McPhail, G. (2009). Teaching the 'bad boy' to write. *Learning Landscapes, 3*(1), 89–102.

McQueen, R. A., & Knussen, C. (2002). *Research methods for social science: A practical introduction.* Upper Saddle River, NJ: Prentice Hall.

Mead, M. (1928). *Coming of age in Samoa.* New York: Morrow.

Mead, M. (1942). An anthropologist looks at the teacher's role. *Educational Method, 21,* 219–223.

Miles, M. B., & Huberman, A. M. (1994). *Qualitative data analysis: An expanded sourcebook* (2nd ed.). Thousand Oaks, CA: Sage.

Minatrea, N. B., & Wesley, M. C. (2008). Reality therapy goes to the dogs. *International Journal of Reality Therapy, 28,* 69–77.

Ming, C. (2007). Families, economies, cultures, and science achievement in 41 countries: Country-, school-, and student-level analyses. *Journal of Family Psychology, 21*(3), 510–519.

Motha, S. (2006). Racializing ESOL teacher identities in U.S. K–12 public schools. *TESOL Quarterly, 40*(3), 495–518.

Narrative Review Literature. (2014, January 6). Retrieved from *http://instr.iastate.libguides.com/content.php?pid=512256&sid=4215505.*

Nesbit, J., & Adesope, O. (2011). Learning from animated concept maps and concurrent audio narration. *Journal of Experimental Education, 79,* 209–230.

Noblit, G. W., & Hare, R. D. (1988). *Meta-ethnography: Synthesising qualitative studies.* London: Sage.

Patton, M. Q. (1990). *Qualitative evaluation methods.* London: Sage.

Pelto-Piri, V., Engström, K., & Engström, I. (2012). The ethical landscape of professional care in everyday practice as perceived by staff: A qualitative content analysis of ethical diaries written by staff in child and adolescent psychiatric in-patient care. *Child and Adolescent Psychiatry and Mental Health, 6*(1), 18.

Penning, S. L., Bhagwanjee, A., & Govender, K. (2010). Bullying boys: The traumatic effects of bullying in male adolescent learners. *Journal of Child and Adolescent Mental Health, 22*(2), 131–143.

Pennington, T., Wilkinson, C., & Vance, J. (2004). Physical educators online: What is on the minds of teachers in the trenches? *Physical Educator, 61*(1), 45–56.

Peters, R. D., Bradshaw, A. J., Petrunka, K., Nelson, G., Herry, Y., Craig, W. M., . . . Rossiter, M. D. (2010). The Better Beginnings, Better Futures Project: Findings from grade 3 to grade 9. *Monographs of the Society for Research in Child Development, 75*(3), 1–174.

Phan, H. P. (2010). Empirical model and analysis of mastery and performance-approach goals: A developmental approach. *Educational Psychology, 30*(5), 547–564.

Pielstick, D. C. (1998). The transforming leader: A meta-ethnographic analysis. *Community College Review, 26*(3), 15–35.

Podeh, E. (2000). History and memory in the Israeli educational system: The portrayal of the Arab–Israeli conflict in history textbooks (1948–2000). *History and Memory, 12*(1), 65–100.

Popham, W. J. (2013). *Evaluating America's teachers: Mission possible?* Thousand Oaks, CA: Corwin.

Powdermaker, H. (1966). *Stranger and friend: The ways of the anthropologist.* New York: Norton.

Prins, E., & Toso, B. W. (2008). Defining and measuring parenting for educational success: A critical discourse analysis of the Parent Education Profile. *American Educational Research Journal, 45*(3), 555–596.

Prothmann, A., Bienert, M., & Ettrich, C. (2006). Dogs in child psychotherapy: Effects on state of mind. *Anthrozoös, 19*, 265–277.

Rademaker, L. L., Grace, E. J., & Curda, S. K. (2012). Using computer-assisted qualitative data analysis software (CAQDAS) to re-examine traditionally analyzed data: Expanding our understanding of the data and of ourselves as scholars. *Qualitative Report, 17*, Article 43.

Rakes, C., Valentine, J. C., McGatha, M. B., & Ronau, R. N. (2010). Methods of instructional improvement in algebra: A systematic review and meta-analysis. *Review of Educational Research, 80*(3), 372–400.

Reisman, C. K. (2002). Analysis of personal narratives. In J. F. Gubrium & J. A. Holstein (Eds.), *Handbook of interview research: Context and method* (pp. 695–710). Thousand Oaks, CA: Sage.

Rhoads, R. A. (1995). Whales tales, dog piles, and beer goggles: An ethnographic case study of fraternity life. *Anthropology and Education Quarterly, 26*(3), 306–323.

Ring, N., Ritchie, K., Mandava, L., & Jepson, R. (2011). Methods of synthesizing qualitative research studies for health technology assessment. *International Journal of Technology Assessment in Health Care, 27*(4), 384–390.

Rist, R. (1970). Student social class and teacher expectations: The self-fulfilling prophecy in ghetto education. *Harvard Educational Review, 40*(3), 411–451.

Rist, R. (2000). Author's introduction: The enduring dilemmas of class and color in American education. *Harvard Educational Review, 70*(3), 131–138.

Rothstein, H. R., & Hopewell, S. (2009). Grey literature. In H. Cooper, L. V. Hedges, & J. C. Valentine (Eds.), *The handbook of research synthesis and meta-analysis* (2nd ed., pp. 103–126). New York: Russell Sage Foundation.

Sacks, G., & Kern, L. (2008). A comparison of quality of life variables for students with emotional and behavioral disorders and students without disabilities. *Journal of Behavioral Education, 17*, 111–127.

Salkind, N. (2004). *Statistics for people who (think they) hate statistics* (4th ed.). Thousand Oaks, CA: Sage.

Savin-Baden, M., McFarland, L., & Savin-Baden, J. (2008). Learning spaces, agency and notions of improvement: What influences thinking and practices about teaching and learning in higher education?: An interpretive meta-ethnography. *London Review of Education, 6*(3), 211–227.

Schreiber, R., Crooks, D., & Stern, P. N. (1997). Qualitative meta-analysis. In J. M. Morse (Ed.), *Completing a qualitative project: Details and dialogue* (pp. 311–326). Thousand Oaks, CA: Sage.

Scriven, M. (1991). Beyond formative and summative evaluation. In M. W. McLaughlin & D. C. Phillips (Eds.), *Evaluation and education: At the quarter century. Ninetieth Yearbook of the National Society for the Study of Education* (Part II, pp. 19–64). Chicago: National Society for the Study of Education.

Scriven, M. (2010). Contemporary thinking about causation in evaluation: A dialogue with Tom Cook and Michael Scriven. *American Journal of Evaluation, 31*(1), 105–117.

Scruggs, T. A., Mastropieri, M. A., & McDuffie, K. A. (2007). Co-teaching in inclusive classrooms: A metasynthesis of qualitative research. *Exceptional Children, 73*(4), 392–416.

Skinner, B. F. (1974). *About behaviorism.* New York: Random House.

Slate, J. R., Jones, C. H., Sloas, S., & Blake, P. C. (1997–1998). Scores on the Stanford Achievement Test–8 as a function of sex: Where have the sex differences gone? *High School Journal, 81*(2), 82–86.

Somervill, J. W., Kruglikova, Y. A., Robertson, R. L., Hanson, L. M., & MacLin, M. H. (2008). Physiological responses by college students to a dog and a cat: Implications for pet therapy. *North American Journal of Psychology, 10,* 519–528.

Spradley, J. P. (1979). *The ethnographic interview.* New York: Holt, Rinehart & Winston.

Spradley, J. P. (1980). *Participant observation.* New York: Holt, Rinehart & Winston.

Stake, R. E. (1994). Case studies. In N. K. Denzin & Y. S. Lincoln (Eds.), *Handbook of qualitative research* (2nd ed., pp. 236–247). Thousand Oaks, CA: Sage.

Starr, P. A. (1993). Finding our way: A deaf writer's journey. In M. Cochran-Smith & S. Lytle, *Inside/outside: Teacher research and knowledge* (pp. 184–194). New York: Teachers College Press.

St John, W., & Johnson, P. (2000). The pros and cons of data analysis software for qualitative research. *Journal of Nursing Scholarship, 32*(4), 393–397.

Strieb, L. Y. (1993). Visiting and revisiting the trees. In M. Cochran-Smith & S. L. Lytle, *Inside/outside: Teacher research and knowledge* (pp. 121–130). New York: Teachers College Press.

Tashakkori, A., & Teddlie, C. (2003a). Issues and dilemmas in teaching research methods courses in social and behavioural sciences: US perspective. *International Journal of Social Research Methodology, 6*(1), 61–77.

Tashakkori, A., & Teddlie, C. (2003b). *Handbook of mixed methods in social and behavioral research.* Thousand Oaks, CA: Sage.

Thomas, J. (1993). *Doing critical ethnography.* Newbury Park, CA: Sage.

Turner, W. G. (2007). Experiences of offenders in a prison canine program. *Federal Probation, 71*(1), 38–43.

Vahey, P., & Crawford, V. (2002). *PALM Education Pioneers Program: Final evaluation report.* Menlo Park, CA: SRI International.

Waller, W. (1932). *The sociology of teaching.* New York: Wiley.

Whyte, W. F. (1955). *Street corner society.* Chicago: University of Chicago Press.

Wilson, A. (1993). Towards an integration of content analysis and discourse analysis: The automatic linkage of key relations in text. Retrieved from *http://ucrel.lancs.ac.uk/papers/techpaper/vol3.pdf.*

Wolcott, H. (1973). *The man in the principal's office: An ethnography.* New York: Holt, Rinehart & Winston.

Wolcott, H. (1987). On ethnographic intent. In G. Spindler & L. Spindler (Eds.), *Interpretive ethnography in education: At home and abroad* (pp. 37–51). Hillsdale, NJ: Erlbaum.

Wunsch-Vincent, S., & Vickery, G. (2006). Participative web: User-created content. Retrieved from *www.oecd.org/sti/38393115.pdf.*

Yarbrough, D. B., Shulha, L. M., Hopson, R. K., & Caruthers, F. A. (2011). *The program evaluation standards: A guide for evaluators and evaluation users* (3rd ed.). Thousand Oaks, CA: Sage.

Ziolkowski, J. (1999). "It's friendship, developing friendship": A teacher action research study on reading buddies. *Networks: An On-line Journal for Teacher Research, 2*(1).

Author Index

Subject Index

Note. *f* or *t* following a page number indicates a figure or a table.

About the Authors

Jeffrey S. Beaudry, PhD, is Associate Professor of Educational Leadership at the University of Southern Maine. His interests include visual learning, assessment literacy, formative assessment, action research, science literacy, educational technology, and program evaluation. The author or coauthor of more than 20 journal articles and book chapters, Dr. Beaudry teaches research methods courses online and in blended media formats.

Lynne Miller, EdD, is Professor Emerita of Educational Leadership at the University of Southern Maine, where she held the Walter E. Russell Chair in Education and Philosophy and directed the Southern Maine Partnership. An experienced teacher and leader in K–12 public schools and higher education, she is committed to linking theory and practice and to promoting research literacy for practitioners. Dr. Miller has authored or coauthored seven books and more than 50 articles. She continues to be engaged as a scholar and activist for equality in education.

CPSIA information can be obtained
at www.ICGtesting.com
Printed in the USA
BVOW05*0606161216
470988BV00004B/8/P